A HUNDRED YEARS OF MEDICINE
WYNDHAM E. B. LLOYD

'How many excellent physicians have written just volumes and elaborate tracts of this subject? No news here: that which I have is stoln from others; *dicitque mihi mea pagina, fur es*. If that severe doom of Synesius be true, *it is a greater offence to steal dead men's labours than their cloathes,* what shall become of most writers? I hold up my hand at the bar, and am guilty of felony in this kind'

Burton's *Anatomy of Melancholy*
(Democritus to the reader).

'Ἱπποκράτης φάος ἦν μερόπων καὶ σώετο λαῶν
ἔθνεα, καὶ νεκύων ἦν σπάνις εἰν ἀΐδῃ
ΝΙΚΟΔΗΜΟΥ, οἱ δὲ ΒΑΣΣΟΥ.

A HUNDRED YEARS
OF MEDICINE

by

WYNDHAM E. B. LLOYD,
M.A.(Cantab), M.R.C.S., L.R.C.P., D.P.H.

London
GERALD DUCKWORTH & CO. LTD.

New York
HUMANITIES PRESS

First Published in 1936
Reprinted in 1938
Second Edition 1968

© 1968 by WYNDHAM E. B. LLOYD

SBN 7156 0401 5

PRINTED IN GREAT BRITAIN BY
COX & WYMAN LTD., LONDON, FAKENHAM AND READING

FOR
JOHN

CONTENTS

7

PREFACE to the FIRST EDITION

IT is hoped that this historical essay may prove to be of value not only to the layman, for whom it is primarily intended, but also to those medical practitioners and students who have not found time for any specialized study of the history of medicine.

The book cannot claim to be comprehensive. In many respects it is necessarily incomplete. The available material is unmanageably abundant. To have included everything in detail would have made the book unwieldy, whereas to have condensed excessively would have made it unreadable. I have therefore presumed to select some of the important and more interesting aspects of the subject while omitting others which may be equally important but which are too technical to be readily described to the non-medical reader. It will be noticed, for example, that there is no description of the immense advances which have been made in the technique of surgery. It would be impossible to do justice to these without inferring a fairly detailed knowledge of anatomy which I cannot assume the reader to possess. It will also be observed that the chapter on State Medicine concerns itself almost exclusively with England. I make no apology for this except to say that the development of modern public health legislation can best be followed through the study of the country where it had its beginnings.

The arrangement of this book has been determined largely by the fact that important medical advances are not made in a single day but are generally the result of a laborious series of steps made by a number of different workers over long periods of years. Consequently the importance of each contribution to medicine can best be understood by tracing it separately from its origins rather than by attempting to survey the whole field of advance in strict chronological order. Furthermore, by treating each subject separately, it is possible to appreciate the train of thought more clearly at a great saving of space and repetition.

I have refrained from using technical terms without explaining their meaning and hope that the ordinary English words which in some places have been substituted for the technical ones will not irritate those with medical knowledge.

Except for those great ones who make it, history is necessarily second-hand. The author is therefore gratefully indebted to many different writers for the material from which this book is made. Many such writers are mentioned in the footnotes, but in a work of this kind it is impossible to give a reference for every statement made. Consequently apologies and thanks are respectfully tendered to those authors both dead and alive from whom facts have been gathered without acknowledgement.

W.E.B.LL.

London 1936

PREFACE to the SECOND EDITION

MORE than thirty years have passed since this book first saw the light: and much has happened since. For that reason the work is now longer than it was. In bringing the history of medicine up to date many difficulties have appeared. The first was the question of the title of the book. Was it to be changed to *A Hundred and Thirty Years of Medicine*? This would have made it a different book and no longer a member of the publisher's 'Hundred Years' series. If the title was to remain unchanged, should the earlier years of the history be dropped? After weighing the pros and cons, it seemed to me best to compromise, at the expense of the absolute accuracy of the title, and so preserve the identity of the book.

In 1943 an American edition was issued in New York with the same title; but the content and the scope of the book were much changed by the co-author, Dr C. D. Haagensen. In particular a long section on the advancement of surgery was added. In the present edition I have used much of this surgical material assembled by Dr Haagensen, with the addition of newer matter.

Today the general public is vastly better informed on scientific and medical matters than it was in 1936, mainly through the press, the radio and television. I have therefore ventured in the new edition to use a number of technical terms without pausing to explain their meaning. In this way it has been possible to record the earlier advances in surgery without circumlocutions, in the firm belief that anatomical and surgical knowledge is more wide-spread than it used to be.

Finally it should be made clear that this work is not intended to give a breath-taking and frenzied account of the 'miracles' of modern medicine ('miracles' which may well be superseded before the ink is dry); but rather to give a sober and balanced account of the changes during the last hundred years, and to explain the arrival of so many of the things that we take for granted today, but which were simply not there in the middle of the nineteenth century. In short, this book is written for those who dislike being shouted at; and I think there are many such.

Devon 1968   W.E.B.LL.

PART I

Introductory

CHAPTER ONE

THE ORIGINS OF MEDICINE

THE importance of studying the history of medicine, or indeed the history of any subject, lies in the fact that a mere summary of concepts and the results obtained therefrom without a knowledge of their evolution cannot give any true picture of the matter. Without being aware of the laborious foundations upon which an edifice is built we can gain but a superficial idea of the great superstructure.

The history of medicine in its entirety would carry us back to the remotest periods of antiquity; but we cannot travel so far in time within the compass of this book. Nevertheless, in order to understand the developments of medical theory and practice during the last century, we must have at least some idea of the state of knowledge which existed a hundred years ago and of the general trend of events which led up to this.

At the dawn of history medicine was by no means a new thing: but the medicine of the ancients, the wisdom of the Egyptians and Babylonians, was in general based upon magic and upon astrology rather than science. However, in the fourth and fifth centuries before Christ, Hippocrates of Cos was the first to insist upon the scientific as well as the ethical aspect of medicine. He founded the profession and from his school came directly or indirectly all the famous physicians, practical observers, of the past. His teaching, essentially scientific, held unchallenged priority for many years, until the time of Galen of Pergamum (A.D. 131–201), who was physician to the Emperor Marcus Aurelius.

The widest and most original discoveries have been accredited to Galen—in anatomy, physiology, pathology and pharmacology. Most of the pathways which Galen had cut through the jungle of ignorance remained as he left them for nearly fourteen centuries, while others were overgrown by the weeds of forgetfulness and dogma which flourished so vigorously in the dark ages. The knowledge of the Greeks virtually disappeared from Europe at the fall of the Western Empire. The ignorance of the barbarians wantonly destroyed that knowledge which the Christians, finding no place for it in their lives, lost through lack of interest rather than through active hostility. Indeed, had not the vigorous peoples of Arabia absorbed the great ideas of the Greeks, it is doubtful how much there would have been left of the early foundations of medicine. Under the Abbassid Caliphs of Baghdad, the Fatimites at Cairo and the Ommiades at Cordova in Spain the civilization of the Arabs was vastly superior to that of the West. 'The age of Arab learning continued about five hundred years, till the great irruption of the Moguls, and was coeval with the darkest and most slothful period of European annals.'[1]

The most famous of ancient text-books of medicine is the *Canon* of the Persian philosopher generally known as Avicenna (A.D. 979–1037). This, his most influential work, follows the ideas of Hippocrates and Galen, intermingled with those of Aristotle, worked up into a great system of medicine. It deals, in five books, with physiology, the study of disease, hygiene, the treatment of sickness and the compounding of physic. This important work contains many fallacies but much good sense and it remained the standard book on medicine for many years.

In the Middle Ages medicine was purely dogmatic. What Hippocrates, Aristotle, Galen and Avicenna had written was right and there was no one to dispute the oracular pronouncements of the past. If we except Roger Bacon, an experimental genius whose discoveries were premature and consequently without any wide influence, until the reawakening of knowledge in the fifteenth, sixteenth and seventeenth centuries, no one dared to question the truth of the old authorities.

The beginning of the modern experimental period may be said to date from Paracelsus, that strange sixteenth-century figure— sorcerer, philosopher, alchemist and physician—who overthrew the absolute sovereignty of Hippocrates, Galen and Avicenna. That men should research into the workings of nature for themselves, that was the keynote of his teaching at the University of

[1] Gibbon, E., *Decline and Fall of the Roman Empire*, Chapter LII.

Basel; and he startled the world by publicly committing the *Canon* to the flames of a students' bonfire.

At the same time Vesalius was laying the foundations of modern anatomy at the University of Padua. Galen's excellent anatomical knowledge had suffered sad mutilation at the hands of Arabian and other medieval scribes. Furthermore a superstitious reverence for the dead had confined both the Greeks and the Arabians to the dissection of apes and quadrupeds. Vesalius, as a result of many personally conducted dissections of human bodies, put anatomical studies on a sure basis of fact. His famous book, *De Humani Corporis Fabrica*, was published at Basel in 1543. At the same university the great Englishman William Harvey, at the beginning of the seventeenth century, acquired that thorough knowledge of anatomy which enabled him to make his far-reaching discovery of the circulation of the blood. Modern physiology, that is to say the study of the functions of the normal healthy organism, had its beginning here. Harvey, like Paracelsus, insisted on the direct experimental approach to nature.

The seventeenth century busied itself mainly with physics and chemistry and it attempted to explain function and disease in terms of these and to apply these principles to the practice of medicine. For example, we find that the vegetable drugs, the 'Galenicals' were beginning to be replaced by the 'chemicals'. But this period also produced a revival of the Hippocratic methods of *observation*, apart from any consideration of theory, in the work of the Englishman, Thomas Sydenham. He believed that all mere theories were valueless and he set out to provide accurate descriptions of the signs and symptoms of diseases. He supposed that each disease was a definite individual species and could be classified like an animal or a plant.

For fuller accounts of the early history of medicine see:

Osler, W., *The Evolution of Modern Medicine*, New Haven, 1921.
Neuburger, M., *History of Medicine*, English translation, London, 1910–25.

CHAPTER TWO

THEORIES OF MEDICINE IN THE EIGHTEENTH CENTURY

IN the eighteenth century theories of medicine abounded. Some of these were quite fantastic, while others, even if fallacious and unworkable, were at least credible. Some, though basically false, led directly to good results, particularly when they indicated the use of mild remedies in place of some of the more drastic and often disastrous measures then in vogue.

There had been many brilliant achievements in other sciences—in chemistry, physics and astronomy. Certain all-embracing theories had had widespread success. Kepler and Newton, for example, had brought the motions of the planets, the tides and the falling apple all under one universal law. Inspired by the results of such wonderful simplicity, physicians began to look for some complete and universal system of medicine. The result of this was a large crop of 'systems', particularly in Germany and in Scotland, which for the most part had a very great effect in hampering positive progress. Some hoped to follow the great mathematicians of the seventeenth and eighteenth centuries and to base their theories on mechanics or arithmetic. A complete mathematical system, for example, was attempted by Richard Mead, the fashionable physician, who had inherited the practice of the successful and insolent[1] John Radcliffe. Incidentally the latter left a huge sum of money which was used for the foundation of a library, an astronomical observatory and an infirmary at Oxford. Mead's teacher, Archibald Pitcairne of Edinburgh, had tried to apply mechanics to physic and to base medicine on geometry. At Halle University Friedrich Hoffmann was teaching that life is based on the presence

---

[1] 'Mead, I love you,' Radcliffe said, 'and I'll tell you a sure secret to make you a fortune— Use all mankind ill.' (Cited by Garrison, F. H. *An Introduction to the History of Medicine*, 4th ed. London and Philadelphia, 1929, p. 390.)

of some universal fluid or ether, while G. E. Stahl postulated a conscious soul whose efforts, often ill-directed, to throw off some adverse influence constituted disease. Stahl's theory was a kind of animism which, rejecting any sort of mechanical explanation, ran contrary to all the scientific ideas then in fashion.

Most famous perhaps among the Scottish physicians was John Brown of Edinburgh, the disreputable boor whose theory had a tremendous impact throughout Europe up to the end of the century. The Brunonian theory, as it was called, held that the phenomena of life depended on stimulus and that diseases were of two kinds, those that were due to lack of stimulus (the asthenic) and those in which there was too much stimulus (the sthenic). Fortunately Brown decided that the great majority of diseases were asthenic and therefore required stimulants. In this respect he made a distinct advance on the drastic weakening measures used by so many practitioners at the time. In practice Brown had two sovereign remedies, the one stimulant and the other depressant. They were alcohol and opium and to these he himself is said to have fallen a victim. The Brunonian system 'destroyed more people than the French Revolution and the Napoleonic wars combined'.[1]

Homoeopathy, which was first put forward as a medical doctrine towards the end of the eighteenth century, was the invention of a German, Samuel Hahnemann of Meissen. Homoeopathy took no account of the causes of disease but studied only the symptoms. It affirmed that symptoms can be cured by those very drugs which would produce these symptoms in a healthy man. Hahnemann added to his theory the extraordinary notion that the physiological effect of drugs is made much stronger by diluting them, pounding them and shaking them. In practice he gave incredibly minute doses such as could generally have had little or no effect either beneficial or the reverse. Here again the theory had considerable success simply because the very mild nature of the treatment gave the *vis medicatrix naturae* the needful opportunity to effect a cure.

In general, the great theories, of which we have given examples, bade their exponents try one or sometimes two kinds of treatment. It was the age of panaceas. We find different practitioners placing

[1] Garrison, op. cit., p. 315.

all their hopes on purges, on clysters, on bleeding, on mineral waters or on whatever remedy their systems demanded.

Among these fanatics we may mention François-J.-V. Broussais. Certainly his theory was better than many others, for he tried to do away with vague notions of mysterious 'disease' and endeavoured to show that any given malady was due to something wrong with some definite organ. Irritation, he declared, was the basis of life— and of disease. Disease occurred when there was some increased irritation in some particular organ. He selected the stomach as the usual seat of such trouble. In practice, however, his system re- sulted in an orgy of blood-letting rivalling the excesses of the great Dr Sangrado in Le Sage's romance *Gil Blas*. As late as 1833 bleeding was still so popular that it was found necessary to import forty-one and a half million leeches into France. Broussais' ideas were widely accepted and blood flowed in cataracts until Laennec and other more advanced clinicians and above all, Louis, with his medical statistics, had made it very obvious that the effects of ill- judged bleeding were not merely worthless, but often fatal.

Good accounts of many of the older medical theories are to be found in:
>Baas, J. H., *History of Medicine* (translated into English by H. E. Handerson, New York, 1889).
>Garrison, F. H., *History of Medicine*, 4th ed. London and Philadelphia, 1929.

CHAPTER THREE

PRACTICAL SCIENTIFIC PROGRESS

THERE were, besides all these theory-mongers, many who devoted themselves wholeheartedly to more scientific medicine. These were trained and highly practical observers and, if they had their theories, they did not allow their work to be hampered by any preconceived notions. It was during the eighteenth and early nineteenth centuries that the foundations of pathology and the principles of hygiene and of sound clinical diagnosis were firmly laid.

The progress that was made during this period in medicine and surgery was the work of several different schools in different countries. Owing to the unsettled state of Europe discoveries and methods did not travel very readily from one country to another. Consequently we find the English and various Continental schools developing along rather different lines.

On the Continent there was Hermann Boerhaave at Leyden whose teaching spread to England through his many English pupils. His was the great centre of medical training and he endeavoured to apply all the available discoveries in every scientific subject to the practical advancement of medicine.

At Padua Giovanni Battista Morgagni laid the very important foundations of morbid anatomy. He examined great numbers of bodies after death and carefully and systematically recorded everything which he found abnormal. The great importance of his work lies in the fact that he also recorded the diseases and signs and symptoms of the diseases in the individuals before they died. In this way he began the scientific study of the changes brought about in the body by disease—a study without which medicine could hardly have made any but purely empirical advance.

Morgagni's great work was followed up by the Scotsman Matthew Baillie, who was a pupil at William Hunter's famous

Windmill Street School, to which we shall have occasion to refer later. Baillie published the results of an enormous amount of work in a systematic treatise *Morbid Anatomy*,[1] excellently illustrated with copperplates.

In England Richard Mead, in spite of his mathematical theories and his conjectures about the power of the sun and moon over the human body,[2] had very definite ideas about epidemic disease. In 1720 he published a *Short Discourse Concerning Pestilential Contagion and the Methods to be used to Prevent it*. This remarkable work contains detailed instructions for quarantine, for the evacuation of towns, for the cleansing or demolition of infected houses, for cleaning the streets, for removing nuisances and for the prohibition of assemblies. He definitely states that lack of cleanliness and overcrowding is the reason 'why the poor are most obnoxious to contagious diseases'. Almost the whole of his recommendations are such as would appeal to any sanitary authority today.

Notable studies of certain infectious fevers had been made in England by John Huxham and John Fothergill. The former made careful reports on typhus and typhoid, scarlatina and diphtheria, though he did not use these names, nor did he always distinguish between the various fevers. He too was a pupil of Boerhaave of Leyden. Fothergill made important contributions towards the study of infectious sore throats.

Another notable Englishman who studied at Leyden was Sir John Pringle. He gained considerable experience as physician to the British forces during the campaigns in Flanders and he wrote a valuable book on the health of the Army. In this he studied the various diseases in connexion with the climate and season of their incidence. He showed that many diseases had removable causes and pointed out the means of removing them. Later he became President of the Royal Society and presented the Copley Medal in 1756 to the representative of Captain Cook who had achieved a

---

[1] London 1793. Plates published separately, 1803.

[2] Of course there is nothing inherently foolish about this conception of disease. That seasonal and climatic variations affect some maladies is obvious enough and it is certain that such influences are primarily controlled by the sun and the moon.

remarkable feat in preserving the health of his crew during a three-year voyage, with only one man dead of sickness. It was Pringle who inaugurated military hygiene by combating damp, filth and bad air in army barracks.

The Royal Navy had its champion in James Lind, who did for the seamen what Pringle had accomplished for the soldiers. His successful essay on the most effectual means of preserving the health of sailors had run into three editions by 1772. His directions against gaol fever (typhus) and scurvy met with well-merited success. To Lind is due the almost complete disappearance of scurvy from the Navy.

In surgery also there had been great advances made in Britain and the most outstanding figure is that of the Scotsman John Hunter. He was the pupil of the celebrated Percival Pott of St Bartholomew's Hospital, whose name is recalled to medical men by Pott's fracture (of the fibula) which he himself sustained through falling from his horse and Pott's disease (tuberculosis of the spine) which he described.

Hunter's activities were multifarious. Besides his medical discoveries on the repair of tendons, on digestion, on teeth, on transplantation, inflammation, wounds, shock and many other subjects, he made important excursions into human anatomy, physiology and the comparative anatomy of beasts, insects and plants. He collected a magnificent private museum of over 13,000 specimens. After Hunter's death in 1793, his executors offered to sell the collection to the Government. But Pitt, then Prime Minister, said, 'What! Buy preparations! Why I have not money enough to purchase gunpowder.' None the less the collection was eventually acquired by the state and placed under the care of the Corporation of Surgeons.

Hunter's importance lies in his methods as well as in his individual discoveries. He began a new era in surgery by the application of the principle of experimental verification. Before his time surgery had been based solely on anatomy and little or no heed had been paid to pathology, that is to say the causes and sequence of changes—the natural history of disease. The work of the great morbid anatomist Morgagni had had no practical application. It was Hunter's great achievement that he showed the importance

25

firstly of applying the available knowledge to surgery, and secondly of making experiments to try the accuracy of his conclusions.

A typical instance of the use to which he put his discoveries was that of his experiment with a deer in Richmond Park. He had tied the artery which supplied blood to one of the antlers of a buck. This antler, deprived of its blood-supply, became cold; but, so far from dying, in a few days the antler had regained its blood-supply, not because the tying had been badly done, but through the enlargement of subsidiary connecting arteries above and below the ligature. Shortly after this he was able to apply the same process in the treatment of those pulsating swellings of arteries known as aneurisms which generally prove fatal if not arrested. Previously surgeons had been forced to cut down on the aneurism and remove its contents after tying the artery above and below. This was often disastrous. The alternative had been amputation. Hunter was able to show that better results could be obtained by tying the artery higher up in a healthy part of the limb without danger of the limb suffering from want of blood.

Personally John Hunter seems to have been a rude and quarrelsome man: in fact, as he himself had prophesied, he met his death from an attack of angina pectoris, to which he was subject, brought on by a fit of rage.

Among Hunter's pupils was one who was destined to have a most profound influence on medical thought and practice. This was Edward Jenner, who starting from the belief popular in Gloucestershire that cow-pox and smallpox were antagonistic to one another, conceived the prodigious idea of vaccination against smallpox. His great discovery, which was published in 1798, was hailed with enthusiasm on the Continent and in America and many thousands of persons had been vaccinated before the close of the year 1800.

Methods of clinical diagnosis received a tremendous impetus from two discoveries of the first importance; namely, the methods of *percussion* and *auscultation*. Both of these methods came from the Continent, the one from Vienna, the other from France.

Percussion is a way of finding out the gross physical conditions inside the body, particularly in the chest, by studying the varying sounds which occur when the body is tapped with the fingers.

Practical Scientific Progress

Leopold Auenbrugger of Vienna made this important contribution to medicine. In 1761 he published his *Inventum Novum* which set forth the principles of the method. The ridicule and sarcasm which this brought upon his head delayed the general application of the invention for nearly fifty years; but in 1808 his book was translated into French and rapidly attained fame throughout Europe. The method itself depends upon the principle that the chest (or abdominal) wall is a kind of drum which, when lightly struck in different places, gives out notes which differ according to whether there is gas, liquid or solid lying inside at the place where the wall is struck.

Auscultation means simply the study of the noises which go on inside the body and is chiefly applied to the heart and lungs. The significance of these sounds was discovered by T.-H. Laennec, a native of Brittany. It was in 1819 that he invented the stethoscope. At first this was simply a tube made from rolled paper. With the stethoscope he made so careful an examination of the sounds that he heard in the heart and lungs of patients both healthy and sick that he put the study of these sounds for the first time upon a really firm foundation. The methods of Auenbrugger and Laennec together are responsible directly for much of the knowledge which has since been gained about the diagnosis of disease in the chest.

It was not until after the close of the Napoleonic wars that these ideas were put into practice in the British Isles. The first English translation of Laennec's work was made by John Forbes in 1821. Three years later he also translated Auenbrugger's book, which had remained almost unknown to English physicians. The famous Dublin school of medicine began to adopt the methods of Laennec at this time. Its leader, William Stokes, brought the stethoscope to the notice of the profession and published much valuable work on heart disease. In the United States these improved methods of physical diagnosis were popularized chiefly by a young group of Boston doctors who took post-graduate training in Paris.

From France too came the first medical statistics. Of course there had been statistics of births and deaths before this time, but it was Pierre-C.A. Louis (1787–1872) who first showed the value of purely medical statistics. By collecting the records of numbers of cases of different diseases and the treatment of each case he was able to show convincing proof of the efficacy, worthlessness or disastrous results of such treatment. Thus he helped to stem the torrent of blood-letting in which Broussais and others indulged, for he brought forward figures to show that in pneumonia, at least, bleeding was worse than useless. To Louis belongs the credit of showing that statistics are an important high-road to the advancement of medicine.

In German medicine at the beginning of the nineteenth century we find numbers of different schools of thought, some of which made great advances while others indulged in such overwhelming masses of verbiage that it is almost impossible to discover any meaning at all in their systems. One group, following the zoologists and botanists, tried to formulate a dogmatic classification which, in the state of medical knowledge existing at the time, could not be very successful. This school was led by Johann Lucas Schönlein, who did valuable work in introducing the use of the microscope and examination of the blood. Schönlein made also one very significant discovery when he showed that the skin disease known as *favus* was due to a parasitic fungus. This was an isolated discovery—the first of the microscopical parasites of which many more were to be found in the course of the next hundred years.

At Vienna a new school of medicine was growing up. Here Josef Skoda made considerable advances in the use of auscultation for the diagnosis of chest diseases. Though he believed that diagnosis could be perfected, when it came to treatment he confessed himself impotent and took a completely defeatist attitude. '*Nichts tun is das beste bei der innern Medizin*', was his philosophy.

The treatment at the disposal of the physicians of these times was necessarily inadequate. Before the discovery of the parasitic nature of many diseases there could be no specific remedies except the few drugs that were known by experience to be effective. Quinine for malarial fevers and mercury for syphilis were used with good effect. Most drugs, however, could only be used to relieve symptoms and could not strike at the cause of the disease, for this was unknown.

CHAPTER FOUR

SURGERY AND ITS LIMITATIONS

IF we look at the surgical writings, the notes and reports of hospitals, the text-books and other publications of the early part of the nineteenth century, we are at once struck by the fact that the diseases commonly treated or most discussed have by no means the same importance today as they seem to have had then. There are three main reasons for this. Firstly the scope for surgery was severely limited by the fact that many of the surgical diseases that we know today were not then understood. The second reason was the lack of means of controlling pain and the third was the lack of any method of controlling infection.

As early as 1799 Humphry Davy had discovered the anaesthetic properties of nitrous oxide, or 'laughing gas'. Although he had pointed out that it might be of great value in surgical operations, the matter had not been pursued. Ether was the substance that first came into general use, but this was some fifty years later. It seems strange that the discovery of Davy should have been allowed to remain for so many years a philosophical curiosity.

It will be readily understood that in the days when operations were done without anaesthetics it was highly desirable that they should be done as quickly as possible. Agony called for speed, which took precedence of everything. The great surgeons of the past justly prided themselves on the dexterity and rapidity with which they could perform operations.

It must be realized that there were only a few surgeons who would undertake big operations and these were found only in the great towns. Operating must have been a ghastly business and he who could perform feats of skill amid the agonizing scenes in the operating theatre must have had nerves of steel. Some surgeons might alleviate the frightful distress by dosing the patients with

29

opium or alcohol, but even this could not have made the pain bearable.

Operation therefore was generally only undertaken with the object of saving life. The patient was not usually cured even if he survived the surgeon's care, because such procedures as amputation, for example, which formed a large part of all the operations performed, could hardly be said to be cures. They were usually undertaken in emergencies where they were the only hope for the patient's life.

Many of the greatest surgeons were fully alive to the opinion that the knife should be the last resort and that wholesale removal of parts of the body was an admission of ignorance and failure. We read, for instance, about the indefatigable Sir Astley Cooper, the most successful and the most popular of all the London practitioners of the early nineteenth century: 'In cases of operation he would show that its performance, although too often considered by the public as the highest point in surgery, was regarded by the profession as an opprobrium to the science, being a want of skill in the knowledge and application of efficient remedies for the *cure* of the disease; a knowledge only to be obtained by constant opportunities for examining the diseases which have hitherto been considered incurable except by their extirpation by the knife.'[1]

The absence of anaesthetics, apart from the patient's point of view, had the further disadvantage that the surgeons were prevented from embarking upon new operations of a more severe or intricate kind such as can now be attempted with success. It was not until the coming of anaesthesia that painstaking attention to detail could take the place of the lightning legerdemain of the older school of operators and that conservative measures could be practised at comparative leisure.

The greatest handicap of all to surgery a hundred years ago was infection. Almost every accidental wound brought to hospital for treatment and every operative wound made in a hospital became infected. This being so, surgery was limited to minor procedures on the surface of the body, such as opening of abscesses or to amputations of limbs which had been irremediably damaged. Because of this risk of sepsis the great cavities of the body, the

[1] B. B. Cooper, *Life of Sir Astley Cooper*, London, 1843, ii, p. 104.

head, the chest and the abdomen were outside any help from surgical interference.

Excellent accounts of surgical practice in the early nineteenth century were published by three young Dutchmen who made a tour of many Continental clinics in 1818.[1] The American surgery of the time is well described in a series of case reports from the New York Hospital taken from a Surgical Register, covering the years 1808 to 1833, published in 1930.[2]

[1] Tilanus, C. B., *Surgery a Hundred Years Ago* . . . edited by H. T. Deelman, London, 1925.

[2] Pool, E. H., and McGowan, F. J., *Surgery at the New York Hospital One Hundred Years Ago*, New York, 1930.

CHAPTER FIVE

THE HOSPITALS: HOSPITALISM AND ITS CAUSES

THE older hospitals in England had their origin in religious foundations and their functions differed essentially from those of today. They were not medical but ecclesiastical. They were for the care rather than the cure of their inmates. Excluding monasteries and friaries there were more than 750 charitable institutions in medieval England.[1] It was from some of these that the oldest of our present-day hospitals grew, but there were others that retained their original characters as homes for the aged and infirm. Of the former type is the hospital of St Bartholomew in the City of London, while a good example of the latter kind is the hospital of St Cross, near Winchester.

In the eighteenth century many of the more famous hospitals of England were built to fill the growing need for purely medical care of the sick. St Thomas's Hospital had previously been founded in 1693, and St Bartholomew's was rebuilt in 1739. The philanthropist Thomas Guy, who spent next to nothing on himself but gave away magnificently, began to build the hospital that bears his name and, when he died in 1724, left the bulk of his fortune, amounting to over £200,000, for its completion and endowment. It was to be further supported by donations which gave the benefactors in question 'free letters' by which they could obtain entry for any sick person whom they might choose. The Westminster, St George's and the London hospitals were all founded between 1719 and 1740, while Edinburgh, Glasgow and other large towns also built for themselves similar institutions.

All these were general hospitals; they took in anyone whatever his complaint might be. There were a few, but very few, hospitals for special diseases. In London, for example, a special smallpox hospital was opened in 1769 and the Children's Hospital in 1769.

[1] Clay, R. H., *The Mediaeval Hospitals of England*, London, 1909.

The Hospitals : Hospitalism and its Causes

The Royal Sea-Bathing Infirmary for scrofula (the King's Evil) was started in 1791, largely through the action of the famous Dr Lettsom. He had in fact been anticipated by Russell who, observing that scrofula seldom or never attacked fishermen, began an institute for sea-bathing at Brighton. The great 'sea-water Russell' himself describes how 'children sent to him for treatment delicate and pale, over-clothed and glandular, had been returned to their parents after sea-bathing bare-necked, their hair shaved, the tumours of the neck cured and the countenances healthy'.[1]

In America also, during the eighteenth century, general hospitals were built in several important cities. The Pennsylvania Hospital in Philadelphia was opened in 1752, the New York in 1776 and Bellevue Hospital in the same city in 1794. The Charity Hospital in New Orleans (originally St. John's Hospital) was established in 1736. All of these played important parts in the development of American medicine.

The new hospitals rapidly lapsed into appalling squalor, largely through overcrowding, lack of cleanliness and inadequate water supplies. A sidelight on the filthiness of the rooms may be gained from the fact that Dr Lettsom, when a student, seemed to think his teacher, the poet Mark Akenside, fussy in not allowing spitting in the wards. Benjamin Rush, an eminent Philadelphia physician of this period, who had worked in the hospitals on both sides of the Atlantic, labelled them 'the sinks of human life'. Overcrowding was the rule. In the Hotel-Dieu in Paris, for example, the sick lay four or even six in a bed—pregnant women along with the diseased.[2]

The surgical wards were veritable forcing-houses for sepsis. They could hardly have been organized in a way that was better calculated to favour the spread of septic diseases. There were four horrible sicknesses which were so much more prevalent in hospitals than outside them that they were called 'hospital diseases'. These were erysipelas, pyaemia, septicaemia and gangrene, mysterious pestilences that came upon the patients and killed them like flies. There seemed to be no rhyme nor reason for these deaths. It

[1] J. J. Abraham. *Lettsom*, London, 1933, p. 281.
[2] Tenon, M., *Mémoires sur les Hôpitaux de Paris*, Paris, 1788, preface.

appeared to be simply a matter of misfortune. The fatalities bore little or no relationship to the care or skill with which the operations had been performed. The scourges came in waves and, once established in a ward, would travel from patient to patient with heart-rending swiftness. Sir James Simpson in his statistical investigation on hospitalism showed that in one hospital five out of every twelve patients who underwent amputation died, for the most part of sepsis; while outside, in private and country practice, only five out of forty-six succumbed. Thus the mortality from amputation was about four times as great in hospitals as in private homes.

In those times wounds were seldom known to heal in the clean and straightforward way in which they mostly do today. Suppuration was the rule, healing 'by first intention' a rarity. Some, indeed, taught that pus formation was one of the essential processes of healing, and they talked of 'laudable pus'. A simple fracture mended very well, but when the fracture was compound, that is to say when the skin was broken, the outlook was black with anxiety. The surgeon waited gloomily, fearing the shivering attack which ushered in the fatal poisoning of the blood.

The methods of treatment varied with different surgeons. There was the 'open' method in which the wound was left uncovered to promote the formation of a scab, for it was noted that when a healthy scab had once formed, then the wound would heal without accident. Other surgeons, believing the air to be the bearer of disease, closed up the wound with airtight dressings such as gold-beater's skin. Where the wound was already infected, this treatment, which shut in the poisons, led to frequent disaster. Perhaps one of the most successful methods was that practised by James Syme, the great Edinburgh surgeon and the teacher of Lister; the drainage of wounds by leaving the long ends of the ligatures hanging out. In this way he sought to drain out the poisons into the dressings; but such drainage must have been at best imperfect.

The last of the pre-antiseptic surgeons were agreed upon one point at least: namely, that sepsis was favoured by dirt and by having other 'dirty' (suppurating) wounds in the same wards and by overcrowding the patients. Little did they realize that in, general, it was they themselves who were unconsciously poisoning their patients every time they used the probe or the knife. The probe was a favourite instrument for the examination of wounds; it was never sterilized and, at the most, was washed between its use on each patient. Who could devise a better means of carrying infection? And these conditions continued until late in the nineteenth century.

The surgeons themselves wore their oldest frock-coats in the operating theatre. These were often heavily encrusted with dried blood and pus. In some instances the surgeons even attached a certain sense of superiority to them. These loathsome coats might be used for six months, a year or more without being changed. When we consider that frequently the pieces of whipcord used for the tying of arteries were kept hanging in the button-hole of such a coat, we can only be astonished that every operation did not end in disaster.

The hospital nurses demand some brief description. They were generally of the charwoman type, unreliable, tipsy and incompetent. 'All drunkards without exception, sisters and all, and there are but two nurses whom the surgeon can trust to give the patients their medicine,' said a London doctor[1]. A nurse went even further in stating that there was also 'immoral conduct practised in the very wards'. Dickens assures us that he considered it 'not the least among the instances of their [the hospitals'] mismanagement that Mrs Betsey Prig is a fair specimen of a Hospital Nurse'.[2]

It is needless to say that there were many vigorous champions of the nurses, who absolutely denied the charges of tippling. Their denials may perhaps be accorded the weight they deserve when we read Lord Granville's ingenuous observation: 'The nurses are very good now, perhaps they do drink a little, but so do the ladies monthly nurses' [Sarah Gamp!] 'and nothing could be better than them: poor people, it must be so tiresome sitting up all night.'[3]

[1] Cook, E. T., *Life of Florence Nightingale*, revised, London, 1925, p. 20.

[2] Preface to *Martin Chuzzlewit*.

[3] Cited by Cook, op, cit., p. 21.

A Hundred Years of Medicine

With this brief description of the hospitals of a hundred years ago, we can hardly be surprised that they were often regarded as death-traps. What is more surprising is the late period at which the reform of the hospitals began. As we shall see later, the person who was pre-eminent in this was Florence Nightingale.

CHAPTER SIX

THE SANITARY CONDITIONS OF THE PEOPLE

IN reading descriptions of the sanitary conditions of the people a hundred years ago it is important to bear in mind that these conditions were in many ways better than they had been for hundreds of years. It must also be remembered that such accounts often described the worst slums that could be found and cannot therefore be accepted as representative of the people as a whole. This is not to say that the hygiene of the people was good; indeed much of what we read appears horrible beyond belief.

Many of the worst features in the lives of the people can be found described in the admirable report on the *Sanitary Conditions of the Labouring Population of Great Britain* prepared by Edwin Chadwick and published in 1842. Here we find conditions that must appear almost inconceivable to us today.

The book deals particularly with the towns. These, largely as a result of recruitments from the country for the new factories, had been growing fast—too fast indeed for any proper scheme of housing to be made. In the big towns it was the speculative builder who supplied the houses for the rapidly increasing additions to the population. In order to obtain the highest yield for their money the builders set about leasing and buying land and cramming as many people as possible on to a given acreage at the least possible cost. The streets were made as narrow as was feasible. The houses were built back to back without drainage or foundations and constructed of the flimsiest and cheapest materials available. There was nothing to stop the builder doing exactly as he pleased, and what he pleased was generally as far removed from any kind of town-planning as it is possible to imagine. There was, in fact, encouragement to build bad houses because, if a house was bad enough, it escaped payment of rates, partly through the inefficiency of the law and partly through the difficulty of enforcing

it. On the other hand there were notable exceptions. Certain enlightened landlords made conditions before granting leases[1] and
insisted on substantial buildings, wide streets and sometimes even
sewers. In general this was not so and the results of such thought-
less building were worse than the most pessimistic landlord could
have supposed.

In the older towns like Edinburgh and Glasgow overcrowding
was as bad as in the newer towns. Large families were living in
rooms that had originally been intended for cellars, without light,
air or drainage. Here might be found twelve or eighteen persons
in as many feet square.[2] The absence of drainage or sewers produced a most lamentable state of affairs. There were low passages
leading into square courts 'occupied entirely as dung receptacles of
the most disgusting kind'. Indeed, part of the rent was paid by the
sale of these heaps for manure.

We read of open drains in Stirling[3] which were flushed only
when there was a hard shower. The filth from the gaol was
washed down the public streets at intervals. Blood flowed from the
slaughter-house down the highways. Often the lower parts of the
houses themselves were used as dung-heaps or pigsties. There
were no 'public necessaries' and the stairs and streets were often
used as such.

In Manchester the streets were barely passable from mud or
tolerable from stench. There were many 'open cesspools, ob-
structed drains, ditches full of stagnant water, dunghills, pigsties,
etc., from which the most abominable odours are emitted'.[4] That
the streets in these and many other towns were not drained would
have been of little consequence had they been properly scavenged;
but attempts at street-cleaning were of the most inadequate and
perfunctory kind.

In many places the sewers that did exist were hopelessly unsuitable and never originally intended for house drainage or indeed
for anything more than rain-water from the streets. They were
often badly constructed, with flat bottoms so that they were rapidly

---

[1] *Health of Towns Commission. Report,* 1844, Appendix.
[2] *Glasgow Medical Journal,* III, 1830, p. 437.
[3] *Sanitary Condition of the Labouring Population, London, 1842,* p. 34.
[4] ibid. p. 38.

silted up, or through carelessness or ignorance they were built without regard to geographical levels so that frequently, especially during floods, the contents of the sewers were regurgitated into the houses. This was particularly likely to happen when the drains opened into a tidal river. Nauseous gases too often found their way from untrapped sewers into dwelling-houses. Where efficient main sewers existed there was more likely to be a considerable charge for connecting a house to the main rather than a penalty for omitting to do so.

In places where house-drainage was connected up with sewers these generally ran directly into the local river, canal or stream with the natural result that such water became a stinking open drain. The Thames had become horribly polluted. 'What was the use of praying to be delivered from plagues and pestilences so long as the common sewers ran into the Thames?' wrote Florence Nightingale. 'The Serpentine itself, intended . . . as an ornamental water, became an open sewer which drained Kilburn, Paddington and Bayswater.'[1]

The absence in many places of an adequate supply of water had a large effect in increasing or perpetuating intense squalor. In certain districts the shortage was pitiful. In Hampstead and Hendon water was bought by the pailful, while in Edinburgh many persons had to carry it for long distances and then perhaps to the top of a five- or six-story house. In many places the supply was intermittent and turned on for very inadequate periods. Generally the only supply of running water that was available for private houses was to be had at considerable expense from private water companies. A notable exception to this was Bath, where there was a plentiful supply which, owing to the geography of the town, needed no mechanism to arrive at any part.

Often the little water that was available was of the most disgusting kind, filthy, unwholesome, malodorous and discoloured. A water supply was not an unmixed blessing where it enabled people to have their own cesspools. London, for example, was riddled with these contrivances which were often liable to leak or overflow and as a result any neighbouring water supply might be contaminated.

[1] Hammond, J. L. L. and B., *The Age of the Chartists*, London, 1930.

Lack of light and ventilation was by no means confined to the cellar dwellings which we have described. The notorious window tax, though reduced in amount, still set a price on these necessities. It is true that the duties were levied only on houses which had more than eight windows; but in many places there were large houses inhabited by several poor families, and these were taxed on the total number of windows.

If such abominations were to be found in the larger towns, what sort of sanitation was there in the villages? Little or none. It must be remembered, though, that conditions that create squalor in towns can be comparatively harmless in the country. If one were to apply the standards of many small villages in England today to a town of considerable size, the results would be horrible. The villagers had no piped water supply and no need for sewers; but if they had overcrowding in their cottages, they had also the fresh air of the countryside and lived for the most part out of doors. The country folk were liable to the same diseases which attacked the townsmen; but it is significant that the death-rate of the country was lower. This circumstance may be partially accounted for by the fact that many who were born in the country went to die in the towns.

There has been an unfortunate tendency to idyllize the village life of 'those days', but the legend of the healthy villages of the eighteenth century is probably no truer than that of the 'healthy savage' of today. Goldsmith's 'Sweet Auburn' must have been an insanitary place even before it became deserted. In George Crabbe's *The Village* we find a graphic account of the sorrow and squalor in the parish poor-house and of the 'consequential apothecary who gives an impatient attendance in these abodes of misery . . .'

'A potent quack long versed in human ills
Who first insults the victim whom he kills;
Whose murd'rous hand a drowsy Bench protect
And whose most tender mercy is neglect.'

It has been customary to blame the Industrial Revolution for the unhealthy state of the towns and to some extent this is justified: but the industrialists were not wholly to blame. That there was sweated labour under vile conditions there can be no doubt. The descriptions of the badly ventilated overheated and candle-lit workrooms of the London journeymen tailors, for example, make sad reading. The depressing effect of long hours in foul air, laden with moisture and sweat, drove them surely to the habit of break-fasting off gin. Small wonder that numbers of them were 'taken with a decline'. The master tailors attributed this ill-health to drink, whereas it seems fairly clear that heavy drinking was but one of the appalling results of the conditions under which the journey-men lived.

Industry drew countless men, women and children into towns too small to hold them. Overcrowding was the inevitable result. If the new houses of the speculative builder were 'unfit for human habitation' (in the language of the modern sanitary inspector) they were probably no worse and sometimes better than the normal artisan's house of the day. Drainage and water supply there had been none before and they were not missed.

It is necessary to view the advantages of industrialism as well as its drawbacks. Commerce, improved agriculture and new facilities for transport had made the food of the people more plentiful, more varied and, above all, more certain. Manufacturers had given them cheap cotton—a circumstance which, next to water, did more towards keeping them clean than any other single factor. The truth of the matter is that the great evils which had been present for many hundreds of years were simply accentuated by the Indus-trial Revolution. There was nothing new about them. They were a legacy from the Middle Ages. It has been pointed out that the reason we hear so much of these distressing circumstances is that the masses were becoming articulate. Previously they had suffered in silence, but with leadership they could make themselves heard. The Victorian novelists, too, were to do much to draw attention to the abuses that were current: but to convince ourselves that these things were not new, we have only to read some of the novelists of the eighteenth century—for example, Tobias Smollett, himself a doctor of medicine, who gives us so graphic a description of the methods of sewage disposal in Edinburgh, of the food supply of London and of the waters of Bath.

From the foregoing paragraphs it must not be assumed that

Great Britain alone was affected in this way. In America the Industrial Revolution also brought bad sanitation, but to a lesser degree than in England, mainly because the new factories were usually built on water-power sites in the country and not right in the middle of the old towns. Moreover the factory system had developed in England a generation earlier, so that its evils were already apparent and so could to some extent be forestalled. When Dickens toured America in 1842 he visited tenement districts, hospitals and prisons wherever he could find them. His descriptions were full of praise. In Lowell the conditions under which the factory workers lived, their pianos, circulating libraries and literary magazines delighted him.

Of course there were black spots and the New York slums were the worst. The best description of these slums, where the very poor, together with hordes of immigrants, lived under horrible conditions, was written by John H. Griscom in his book *The Sanitary Condition of the Laboring Population of New York*, published in 1845. Here he described misery and disease comparable to that related by Chadwick in England. Dickens saw some of these conditions and wrote: 'There is one quarter, commonly called the Five Points which in respect to filth and wretchedness, may be safely backed against Seven Dials, or any other part of the famed St Giles.' The scavenger pigs on Broadway added a touch of local colour that did not escape his eye.

CHAPTER SEVEN

THE HEALTH OF THE PEOPLE

W HEN we come to study the health of the people in the early nineteenth century we find ourselves seriously handicapped by lack of material. There is plenty of information about individual institutions, doctors and diseases, but about the health of the public in general the data are meagre. In order to make a reliable estimate of the prevailing health conditions it is essential to know the population at any given time, the number of births in each succeeding period, the number and the causes of the deaths and the age of each person at death. None of these can we find accurately.

The London Bills of Mortality, from 1605, were compiled by the parish clerks, who also entered the cause of death which was discovered by official searchers, generally persons ignorant of the elements of medicine. There are also the parish registers, but these contain many defects. Firstly there are many omissions, for it is baptisms and burials, not births and deaths that are entered here. Dissenters might not be entered, while Jews and Roman Catholics often had separate cemeteries. In many places, too, the registers were kept with the utmost carelessness. In making up the Bills of Mortality the information was taken from the parish registers, so that the same mistakes occur in both.

The first census in England was taken in 1801, but through lack of efficient control it was unreliable. Consequently it is only from information obtained later in the century that we can obtain by retrospective computation the best, but by no means accurate estimate of the population of this country. The United States Constitutions provided for a decennial census and thus America became one of the first countries to make a regular enumeration of its inhabitants. However, the systematic registration of vital statistics, upon which so much of our modern information about

43

public health depends, was started far earlier in the Scandinavian countries. Sweden has an unbroken series of such statistics, dating back to 1749, a unique contribution to public health.

Meagre and uncertain as our information is, we can see certain tendencies which stand out quite clearly; there are movements which occurred on so large a scale that they show obviously through all possible sources of error. First and foremost is the undoubted fact that, whereas previously the population had not increased very quickly, an enormous increase occurred in the latter half of the eighteenth century throughout Europe. If we discount immigration and emigration (which were not on so large a scale as to affect the general conclusion), this can have arisen only from an increased birth-rate or a decreased death-rate, or both.

It has often been assumed that the birth-rate rose rapidly, but there is really very little good evidence for this. If on the other hand we can point to many good reasons for a drop in the death-rate. We can show the disappearance of a number of factors which had combined to kill off the people in previous times and we can point to the active measures which had been carried out to achieve this.

In the Middle Ages famine had been a destructive agent of enormous scope. Agriculture was primitive and a failure of crops in one area led to a scarcity of food through lack of efficient transport from other districts. The same factors led furthermore to a lack of variety of foods, especially of fresh food during the winter months. By 1830 improved methods of farming and better transport had to a large extent banished the fear of famine from the land.

The other great enemy was pestilence. If we inquire into the diseases which took a heavy toll of life in previous times we shall find that many of these were decreasing, some of them to vanishing point. Some diseases may have disappeared of themselves for no obvious cause, but with others we can point to some excellent reasons.

Leprosy was virtually extinguished and this has been claimed as a triumph for the method of segregating the sick; but the disappearance of leprosy may well have been due to some quite different cause; for the exact method of infection is as yet unknown.

Plague, too, had disappeared from London and, except for occasional epidemics, from Europe. The reason for this is by no means clear. Strict quarantine against the dreaded pestilence may have had much to do with it, but other reasons have been advanced. For example it has been suggested that it might have been due to the fact that the black rat, chief carrier of the disease, was largely displaced by the brown rat of Norway, whose habits are not so domestic as those of his black cousin.

Smallpox was always present in Europe and America in the eighteenth century, attacking principally the very young, killing enormous numbers, particularly of infants, disfiguring and often blinding those it did not kill. No class was exempt: indeed in the previous century it had carried off the Queen of England herself. Smallpox hospitals were founded for the reception of the sick. Purposed inoculation of mild smallpox to guard against a more virulent attack was freely practised. This certainly achieved its effect in making many people immune, but it was highly dangerous and must have helped to keep the disease alive after the coming of vaccination. Jenner's discovery that inoculation with cow-pox was effective and safe was announced in 1798 and gave new hope against the scourge. In the years that followed, vaccination began to be practised on an increasing scale. The results must have helped materially to swell the population by saving the lives of thousands of infants every year.

The chief diseases of London had been 'intermittent and remittent fevers and dysentery',[1] in fact such diseases as would be diminished by proper drainage and a good water supply, for hidden in this list, but unrecognized, were the diseases now known as malaria and typhus (gaol fever). The latter was not clearly distinguished by the physicians of the period from typhoid fever (enteric) and relapsing fever. It was an American, W. W. Gerhard who first clearly differentiated typhoid from typhus, in Philadelphia in 1837.

Some of the observers of the day fully recognized that both typhus and relapsing fever were diseases of dirt and starvation. As we have seen, Pringle and Lind had shown the way to rid the Army and Navy of typhus fever. John Howard, the great prison reformer,

[1] Bateman, T., *Reports on the Diseases of London,* London, 1819.

at great personal risk and with immense energy, made a tour of the gaols in England and Wales. The shocking squalor of these pestilential dens is recorded in his famous book. *The State of the Prisons of England and Wales*, first published in 1777. Howard, however, was not merely an observer, for he added to his description many sound hygienic suggestions for remedying this deplorable state of affairs. His recommendations have a modern flavour: baths, soap and water, smooth floors, ovens for baking the louse-ridden clothes of the prisoners, segregation of the sick and the provision of the services of doctors. Later these methods, with fumigation, ventilation and lime-washing, were taken up by others and applied, for example, in hospitals. Later still separate wards were reserved for those with infectious fevers. The energetic campaign included eventually the provision of separate fever hospitals in some of the larger towns. Typhus began slowly but surely to decline. Howard's lesson, though successfully adopted in other spheres, was rapidly forgotten in the prisons themselves. In 1812 James Neild visited the prisons as Howard had done and found them 'relapsing into their former horrid state of privation, filthiness, severity and neglect', so that he had to fight Howard's battle anew.

Agues, many of which were undoubtedly malaria, were also rapidly diminishing in many parts of England, though they were not finally extinguished until much later. The disappearance of these fevers almost always followed the efficient drainage of marshlands. Such drainage was not made with this object primarily in view, but rather for the reclaiming of land or the prevention of floods. Whether the dying out of malaria in England can be attributed entirely to this cause is more than doubtful, for mosquitoes capable of conveying malaria are not uncommon in this country today; but, historically speaking, we may say that the sequence of events looks temptingly like cause and effect.

In America malaria was prevalent as far north as the Canadian border during Colonial times. During the first half of the nineteenth century the disease gradually retreated from the northern states, for reasons that are not entirely clear. It continues to be endemic in the southern states, mainly along the coast and in marshy regions.

The Health of the People

In viewing such statistics as there are for the early nineteenth century, we find that a large decrease in death-rate seems to have occurred among infants and young children apart from all considerations of infectious fevers. This has been attributed, with great probability, to better standards of living, healthier dwellings and better medical advice. Unquestionably there had been a relative improvement in the conditions of living. Many English medical writers of the period, Bateman[1] and Farr,[2] for example, are almost lyrical about the improvements that had taken place in the health of the metropolis and in the whole of England and Wales in their lifetime. These advances were observed on all sides and were attributed to more hygienic habits, to cleaning and scavenging, to drainage, to greater temperance, to better agriculture and to better medicine.

[1] Bateman, op. cit.
[2] Farr, W. Section on Vital Statistics in J. R. McCullough's *A Statistical Account of the British Empire, 1837.*

CHAPTER EIGHT

SOME COMMON INFECTIOUS DISEASES

Now that we have outlined the abject conditions under which the people struggled for life, it will not be surprising to find that the towns were very hotbeds of infectious disease. 'Low' or 'putrid' fevers were hardly ever absent from the worst of these Augean stables. We hear much more of epidemic infectious disease than of other kinds for an obvious reason. A sudden attack of a pestilence produces a profounder stir among the people than does the toll levied continuously by more insidious diseases. An unexpected outbreak obtrudes itself where the more ordinary of the killing maladies are accepted as part of the scheme of things. We tolerate the occurrence of a hundred or more deaths every week on the roads of this country, whereas a similar number in railway accidents would leave us profoundly shocked.

We hear much of typhus fever throughout England and Ireland, but rather less of the other diseases which carried off so many lives. The reason for this is not far to seek. Typhus attacked the adolescent and adult breadwinner, while smallpox wrought havoc among infants and young children and was taken more as a matter of course. These contagions must have been readily spread by all the circumstances of squalor and overcrowding which we have mentioned, as well as by the wholesale pawning of bedding and clothing and the migrations in search of work that took place in times of scarcity. Other diseases were carried, above all, by contaminated water supplies.

There was, in fact, one terrible disease for which a magnificent welcome had been prepared and which, though it may never have invaded this country before, was expected with alarm. In the year 1831 the Asiatic cholera, which had been laying waste the continent of Asia for the past dozen years, made its dreaded appearance in

48

Europe, where the evils of war helped to propagate the contagion. It reached Germany by three separate routes, via Poland, Danzig and Austria. In Hungary the havoc was fearful. More than a quarter of a million persons took the infection and of these some hundred thousand died.

In England a rigorous quarantine was instituted and the people waited with anxiety. The pestilence reached Hamburg in October and it was not long before some vessels from Europe evaded the quarantine and the cholera disembarked at Sunderland. The disease quickly killed some two hundred persons and then spread with undiminished violence to other towns.

Early in January of 1832 the cholera was at Newcastle and on its way to Edinburgh. Scotland began to suffer and the disease, as is its wont, took its chief toll in regions where dirt and depression most prevailed. Glasgow acted promptly by providing a cholera hospital, by closing the theatres and places of public entertainment and by discouraging shipping, but neglect of sanitation brought its own reward. The disease appeared with explosive violence in the pauper infirmary and, before the epidemic waned, Glasgow had lost more than three thousand souls.

London was attacked in February and Parliament hurriedly conferred large powers on the Privy Council to make arrangements against the danger. The *Annual Register* stated that 'the alarm was infinitely greater than the danger' and, indeed, it is true that England suffered less, proportionately, than France or Hungary; but nevertheless the total deaths amounted to 21,882 in England and Wales, 20,070 in Ireland and 9,592 in Scotland.

The importance of this epidemic, which was the first of a series of visitations, lies not in the actual mortality which it caused but in the psychological effect which it produced on the rulers and the people, to say nothing of the medical profession. There does not seem to be much doubt that it was the fear of the cholera which was largely responsible for the acceleration of the movement towards the improvement of the towns. The actual mode of propagation was not discovered until much later, but it was generally agreed that, whatever the primary cause of the disease, squalor was its meat and drink.

It is well to bear in mind this agreement among the doctors.

The disease had been excellently described, the pathology studied, a variety of remedies had been tested and hospitals had been provided. True, the origin, the cure and the mode of spread were yet unknown, but the cholera did not leave medical men as it found them. The attention of thinking people was concentrated on the state of the towns, for here was an obvious and *removable* cause of disease.

Influenza is a disease which is regrettably prevalent today. It has been epidemic for as long as we can trace it back. When we follow it into the eighteenth century it becomes inextricably mixed up with the various agues and other fevers which were not then sufficiently well distinguished from one another. In Europe there was an undoubted epidemic of influenza in 1803 and between 1830 and 1833 it became general in both the Eastern and Western Hemispheres. The influenza of 1833 in England seems to have claimed many deaths among the rich and, in this respect, it differed from the cholera of the preceding year.[1] One observer stated that he had heard of 'no less than nine lords or ladies who had been carried off by it or through its indirect agency in the course of the last week.'[2] The monthly bills of mortality rose suddenly to double their previous total, but they sank again fairly soon.

This epidemic seems to have been very widespread indeed and there was no place or class exempt. A doctor is reported to have made the following observations: 'I have not a moment to spare. In the very thick of my best harvest. Best thing I ever had: quite a Godsend: everybody ill, nobody dies—so the recoveries are all cures you know.'

The doctors did not at first realize the seriousness of influenza. When they did so we find them eagerly discussing the pathology and treatment, but without coming to much agreement even about the advisability of blood-letting. The consensus of opinion was against the belief that influenza was contagious. They declared it to be no more so than the last year's cholera. The rapidity of the spread and the way in which it jumped from one part of the

[1] Creighton. C., op. cit. II, p. 380.
[2] *Lancet* 1832–3, II, p. 145.
[3] ibid., p. 125.

country to another were against the contagion theory. Evidently at this time contagion was very much out of vogue.

That this disease was not at first considered serious may have been due to an effect on statistics which is now known to be highly characteristic of influenza. This illness kills directly only a proportion of its true victims. Attacks occur frequently among sufferers from consumption, asthma or other respiratory disease, or among the aged who have little resistance to infection. The result is that many deaths are recorded as being due to some other cause than influenza, although they might not have occurred without the super-added influenza. The consequence of this is that an epidemic of influenza sends up the figures of the 'deaths from all causes' out of proportion to the deaths from the disease itself.

Measles has been widespread ever since it was properly distinguished from other eruptive fevers. Deaths from measles were comparatively rare in the eighteenth century, but for some reason the mortality had been steadily increasing at the close of the century and continued to do so throughout the nineteenth. Both measles and whooping-cough were gradually becoming more and more important causes of death. Smallpox was declining. This is to be accounted for, partially at least, by the increasing number of children who were being inoculated with cow-pox according to the teaching of Jenner. Measles generally attacks later in life than smallpox. Weakly children may die of it, but if they are prevented from dying of smallpox, then they may well die of measles or of something else later on. The mortality of diseases other than smallpox therefore rises.

Scarlet fever came also in epidemics during the eighteenth and nineteenth centuries, though it is difficult always to be sure whether an account of a 'throat distemper' refers to this or to some other disease.

Diphtheria became common quite suddenly in England as late as 1858, though it had been prevalent on the Continent of Europe and in America in the eighteenth century. It remained a very serious menace until well into the present century.

These are the very brief histories of a number of common infectious diseases which attacked our forefathers. Some of these diseases are still with us. Our list has been far from complete, but those who would study further the history of infectious diseases in this country are recommended to Charles Creighton's *History of Epidemics in Britain*,[1] to which the writer is indebted for much of the information contained in the preceding paragraphs.

[1] Cambridge, 1891 and 1894.

CHAPTER NINE

THE MEDICAL PROFESSION: ITS ORGANIZATION
AND EDUCATION

AT the beginning of the nineteenth century the medical profession was not organized as it is today. A man could be a
physician or he might be a mere quack. For the general
public there was no means of distinguishing one from another.

In Tudor times attempts had been made to prevent unautho-
rized persons from practising. In 1511 it was enacted that no one
should practise medicine or surgery in London unless he was first
examined and approved by appropriate authorities. But this
arrangement did not work, because the poor became neglected by
the surgeons, so that a further Act was passed to allow persons with
botanical knowledge to attend the sick poor.

From the time of the Renaissance onwards we find a sharp distinction drawn between the physicians and the surgeons. The
physicians were considered to constitute a superior profession. In
1518 they were formed into a college which was to become in 1851
the Royal College of Physicians. Surgery, on the other hand, was a
less distinguished calling and was practised by the barber-surgeons,
for in the time of Henry VIII the Barber's Company was united
with the Guild of Surgeons to become the Barber-Surgeons
Company. This union lasted until 1745 when the surgeons were
separated and eventually, in 1800, obtained the charter which in-
corporated them as the Royal College of Surgeons. To them was
entrusted the care of John Hunter's great medical collection.

The two colleges could issue degrees and diplomas, the fees for
which paid for the upkeep of the colleges. These were not the only
bodies which issued permits to practise. Each university, as well as
the Apothecaries' Hall, could issue similar qualifications without
interference or supervision from any higher authority. In this way
there came to be many ports of entry to the medical profession and

this strange multiplicity still obtains in England today. It was not until the Medical Act of 1858 that the State began to exercise any real control over the profession.

By contrast this distinction between physicians and surgeons did not gain a foothold in the American colonies, in spite of the fact that most of the doctors in the early days had been trained in Britain. Eventually, after the Revolution, the various individual states of America passed laws establishing the requirements for medical practitioners. Thus it has come about that each state has its own licensing board. The standards required by the different boards vary considerably, even today. There is no national regulation of medical practice.

In 1832 the British Medical Association was founded by Charles Hastings at Worcester. This was a private organization of doctors, intended to represent the highest standards of the profession in this country. Its aims included the advancement both of learning and of the social status of medical men. The Association has done much good work in pressing for reforms in matters of public health and can well claim to represent the opinion of the majority of general practitioners in the country.

The American Medical Association, a similar private body of doctors in the United States, was founded in 1847. It likewise has been a powerful agent in bringing about public health reforms such as the Pure Food and Drug Act, in suppressing medical quackery and in raising the standards of medicine.

We have seen that in the seventeenth century there were medical schools in different parts of Europe and that these were generally formed round some eminent teacher. In the eighteenth century these centres of teaching began to expand and to become more numerous. Anatomy was taught in Paris, Berlin, Strasbourg and in Edinburgh, Cambridge and Glasgow. Clinical instruction was more of a novelty. Professorships of clinical medicine were founded in Edinburgh in 1741.

It was largely at the voluntary hospitals that students in this country gained experience and knowledge while they worked under the great physicians and surgeons of the time. From these beginnings, at Guy's, St Thomas's and St Bartholomew's, for example, have grown up the great medical schools of today. A number of private medical schools which were run for profit by individual teachers constituted another important source of medical education. Among the most famous of these in London were William Smellie's school for obstetrics, William Cullen's for internal medicine, Joseph Black's for chemistry and William Hunter's school in Windmill Street, where some of the greatest surgeons of their day received instruction in anatomy, surgery and obstetrics. These extra-academic schools were of immense importance elsewhere besides in London. It was largely due to these that Edinburgh attained its great reputation as a medical centre.

In America, on the other hand, the early medical schools developed within the academic organizations. The first of these began in 1765 as part of the College of Philadelphia. The second was the Medical School of King's College in New York (later to become the College of Physicians and Surgeons of Columbia University), set up in 1768. The Harvard Medical School, the third of its kind in the American colonies, was opened in 1783.

There was little specialization in teaching. The leading surgeons were also teachers of anatomy, which they studied sedulously in such spare time as they could find. We read of Sir Astley Cooper rising at six o'clock to put in an hour or more in his private dissecting-room before starting the day's work. The private teachers who kept their own schools may have been more specialized.

The chief obstacle in the way of teaching anatomy lay in the difficulty of obtaining corpses, or 'subjects', as they were called, for dissection. The law on the matter was not helpful. Under Henry VIII it was granted that the Company of Barbers and Surgeons should have the bodies of malefactors and in 1752 it was ordered that the bodies of murderers executed in London and Middlesex 'should be conveyed to the hall of the Surgeon's Company to be dissected and anatomized'. Since this was the only legal supply in the early nineteenth century, there was consequently a shortage of subjects, for the general public was naturally reluctant to hand over the bodies of its dead to suffer a murderer's fate.

A knowledge of anatomy was obviously essential, and indeed was insisted on by the Corporation of Surgeons for practitioners who otherwise must have experimented blindly on their patients. The result of the inadequacy of the law was that there grew up an illicit traffic in dead bodies, conducted by the notorious body-snatchers or 'resurrection-men'. This gruesome occupation was in the hands of a few 'regular men', although outsiders also plied the same trade. The rivalry between different factions of the resurrectionists was so keen that there was no kind of ingenuity or artifice to which they did not resort to obtain their prey or injure their rivals. Ordinarily they merely robbed newly filled graves, bribing the custodian if necessary. Sometimes, however, they would pose as relatives of the deceased and lay claim to the body from a hospital or workhouse. They would even seize a body already on the dissecting-table and convey it elsewhere to be sold anew. Brawls in the very graveyards between rival gangs were far from rare.

The price paid for a subject rose at one time from two guineas up to fourteen or even sixteen, and besides this the teachers had to pay the men 'opening money' at the beginning of each course to secure a monopoly of their services and a regular supply of bodies, as well as a retaining fee during the vacation and compensation for any man who was unfortunate enough to get a spell of imprisonment. Some of the buyers formed an 'Anatomy Club' in an attempt to regulate the prices and limit the extortion: but this was never very successful. Some teachers refused to pay the extra fees and of these men the resurrectionists made an example. A Mr Joshua Brookes of Great Marlborough Street was rewarded by having decomposed bodies left on his doorstep and on one occasion was sold a live confederate of the resurrectionists done up in a sack.

As may be well imagined, popular feeling grew to a white-hot pitch of fury. Guards were instituted over recent graves and frequently came into conflict with the body-snatchers, whom they sometimes severely manhandled. The Government was reluctant to act. The need for subjects was imperative, but the popular outcry made it probable that any attempt at legislation might be fatal to the intended object.

Both the private teachers and the surgeons were hand in glove with the resurrection-men. Sometimes a surgeon would specially commission one of these miscreants to obtain for him the body of one of his patients who had been subjected to some interesting operation, or who had suffered from some disease which made a post-mortem examination desirable. When giving evidence before the Select Committee on Anatomy (at which some of the snatchers themselves were anonymous witnesses), Sir Astley Cooper said: 'The law does not prevent our obtaining the body of an individual if we think proper: for there is no person, let his situation in life be what it may, whom, if I were disposed to dissect, I could not obtain. . . . The law only enhances the price and does not prevent the exhumation.'

Some enlightened people saw the necessity for dissection and saw too how unwise it was to drive all the would-be doctors to Continental universities to learn anatomy. Jeremy Bentham went so far as to set the example of leaving his own body to be dissected. When he died in 1832 this was done by a friend in accordance with his instructions and his skeleton is still preserved in University College, London.

It was not until this same year, four years after the Select Committee had presented its report, that the Anatomy Act was passed. This was undoubtedly expedited by the still greater public feeling which was aroused when it came to light that certain malefactors, Bishop and Williams in London, and Burke and Hare in Edinburgh, had resorted to cold-blooded murder with the object of selling bodies for anatomy.

The Act abolished the dissection of the bodies of murderers, thereby removing the stigma attaching to being dissected. It provided that properly qualified practitioners, teachers and students should be given licences to practise dissection. It insisted upon proper death certificates and a decent burial afterwards. It allowed executors or any persons having lawful possession of a body to give it up provided no relative objected. The Act was successful, for it secured a reasonable number of bodies and it also put the ressurection-men out of business.

PART II

*Medical Scientific Discovery
in the last Century and a half*

CHAPTER ONE

THE NEW PATHOLOGY

T HE nineteenth century brought a fundamental change of outlook, which has coloured the whole of medical thought ever since. The decisive factor was the discovery of the animal cell, which led to the conception of the living body as a vast organization consisting of millions of tiny individual cells. It is difficult to give any adequate idea of the tremendously far-reaching results of this or of the immensely fertile field which it was to lay open to medical science. Suffice it for the moment, before we go on to describe the development of the Cell Theory, that every doctor of today thinks of health and disease ultimately in terms of these cells.

In 1665 the initial discovery had been made by Robert Hooke, who found that if he cut a sufficiently thin slice of cork, then he could see under the microscope that the whole substance of the cork was made up of little bladders of air with little wooden walls separating them from one another. The same was found to be true of green plants except that, as the great botanist Robert Brown showed more than a hundred and fifty years later, each little cell contained an essential structure called the 'nucleus'. Incidentally Brown was also the discoverer of the important fact that the pollen of the plant played the part of the male element in the process of fertilization.

Germany, however, was to have the distinction of elaborating the new biological theory. Mattias Jacob Schleiden of Hamburg in 1838 conclusively showed that every part of a plant was made of groups of cells and that the nucleus was the controlling influence inside each cell.

Stimulated by these discoveries in the vegetable kingdom, Theodor Schwann began to look for cells in animal tissues; and he found them everywhere. He had received a sound biological training in the laboratories of Johannes Müller at Bonn and Berlin and was already an experienced scientist when he began his study of the microscopical appearances of animal matter. Among other achievements he had disproved the theory of spontaneous generation which held that life might arise *de novo* from dead materials under suitable circumstances.

The stronghold of the supporters of that idea was the proved appearance of small organisms in material which was undergoing fermentation or putrefaction. Schwann was able to show that these processes were in fact the *effect* of the growth of the organisms and not by any means the *cause*. This will be seen to be of great significance when we come to discuss the work of Pasteur.

Schwann proved that all vegetable and animal tissues are composed of and developed from cells. The cells of each individual tissue are all alike. Different tissues have different kinds of cells, but any cell of a given tissue is like all the rest in the same tissue. He showed too that the ovum, the 'seed' from which all plant and animal life developed, was itself a cell. He noticed also that the cells had some kind of internal substance besides the nucleus and pointed out the movements occurring in this stuff which today we call protoplasm. It is noteworthy that Schwann's religious convictions made him secure the approval of the Archbishop of Malines before he gave to the world his remarkable work.[1]

It was Rudolf Virchow, the most influential of all Germany's medical thinkers, who applied the discoveries of Hooke, Schleiden and Schwann to the intimate study of disease. Virchow was above all a man of science and he believed that practical medicine must be based only upon the firm structure of applied theoretical medicine, which must in turn rest upon pure scientific physiology and pathology.

In 1839 Virchow arrived on the scene in Berlin just when the tremendous discovery of animal cells had been published from Müller's laboratory. To this he added the important truth that no cell ever arises except by direct formation from another cell. Life is continuous: *omnis cellula e cellula*. Before this it had been assumed that in certain circumstances cells could develop from the

[1] *Mikroskopische Untersuchungen über die Uberreinstimmung in der Struktur und dem Wachsthum der Tiere und Pflanzen,* Berlin, 1839.

'organization' of some more homogeneous animal substance, much as foam is formed from soap. This supposition had been found necessary to explain, for instance, how a homogeneous clot in a wound could be converted into a living scar composed of cells. Virchow showed quite definitely that these cells were not formed from the clot, but grew out into the clot from the living cells of the surrounding tissues.

Virchow's academic career very nearly came to an untimely end owing to his left-wing political views. In 1848 there was an outbreak of relapsing fever in Upper Silesia and he was sent by the Prussian Government as a member of a commission to investigate the cause. He quickly saw that famine and unwholesome conditions were the precipitating if not the ultimate cause of the pestilence. Accordingly his report, detailing the villainous conditions which he found, showed a political rather than a medical bias and, in the storm of indignation which it aroused, he was suspended from his post at Berlin.

Happily he was invited to take up a position at Würzburg where, as professor of pathology, he turned his attention to more scientific matters. He worked for years at the study of the animal cells in disease. He returned later to Berlin and two years later, in 1858, he gave to the world his great work on cellular pathology.[1] In this he enunciated the doctrine that every diseased tissue consists of cells which arise only as the offspring of pre-existing cells. This may seem to us today suspiciously like a truism, but it was not so regarded at the time. Indeed the very fact that this truth seems so obvious goes to show how deeply the fundamental idea enters into our mental make-up.

In the eighteenth century Marie François Xavier Bichat, the great French anatomist, began to observe animal tissues under the microscope in an attempt to make some sort of systematic classification. He found, as was to be expected, that certain tissues recurred in different parts of the body. He counted as many as twenty-one distinct types of tissues or 'membranes'. He observed only the grosser features of each and that is why he supposed there were so many.

[1] *Die Cellularpathologie in ihrer Begründung auf physiologische und pathologische Geweblehre.*

Disease, he decided, must ultimately be some change in one or more kinds of tissue. Any tissue in any organ might be affected while the other kinds of tissue in the same organ might undergo no change. Indeed this is what so often happens. This conception would account for multiple changes all over the body in some generalized disease. Rickets, for example, affects the same kind of tissue wherever it occurs. The fact that the disease attacks the tissue of the growing parts of the bones accounts for the bony deformities which occur in every region of the body.

Bichat had carried pathology one step further than Morgagni. The latter considered an *organ* to be the seat of the disease, whereas the former showed that it was a particular *tissue* that was at fault. Virchow thought, as we all do now, in terms of *cells*. Disease is simply the life of the cell under abnormal conditions which naturally cause abnormal life. In other words, sickness is the reaction of the cell to altered conditions. If the conditions become altogether too anomalous then the cell dies. Speaking prematurely in terms of the germ theory, we might add that the disease is not the germ but the behaviour of the body-cells towards the germ.

Virchow made many individual discoveries extending over a wide field, not only in pathology, but also in anthropology and archaeology; but it is by his cellular pathology that his name will live. Upon this rests the whole edifice of the modern study of disease and its influence extends to every branch of medical thought. Virchow's doctrine has been extremely fertile. Because of it the microscope has become a necessary part of the equipment of every doctor. In the diagnosis of cancer, of blood diseases and of kidney disease, to name but three examples, the present-day pathologist is looking daily and hourly through the lenses of his microscope to observe the minutest variation from the normal appearances of the cells. Here lies the key not only to diagnosis but to the discovery of the fundamental nature of disease.

Virchow became the Grand Old Man of German Medicine. He was to medicine what Liebig was to chemistry, an acute thinker, an oracular figurehead and an influence which is still felt in every corner of the civilized world.

In 1862 he returned to the political stage as a member of the

Prussian lower house and later in 1880 of the Reichstag, where he was among the most formidable of the opponents of Bismarck. Municipal affairs also claimed some of the attention of the indefatigable professor and it is largely to him that Berlin owes its excellent water supply and drainage system. He died in 1902 at the age of eighty-one, but his work is being carried on in every pathological laboratory in the world—a supreme tribute to this great man—while his name survives in the periodical which he founded and which is known to every doctor as Virchow's Archives.

CHAPTER TWO

NEW AIDS TO DIAGNOSIS

ONE of the most striking changes in medical practice is the addition, during the last century, of various scientific weapons, physical and chemical, to the armament of the diagnostician. The important principle underlying most of these new inventions is that of accurate measurement, replacing the mere qualitative observation of the signs and symptoms of disease.

Before the invention of the modern thermometer attempts had been made to estimate the temperature of the human body. In the seventeenth century Santorio had used a bulb filled with air and opening into a tube. The other end of the tube opened under the surface of some water in a vessel. He placed the bulb inside a person's mouth and the air inside expanded as it became warm and issued in bubbles through the water. By counting these bubbles he could gain some idea of the 'hotness' of the person in question. This was an extremely rough-and-ready method, but it was not until nearly two hundred years later that the researches of the physicists, notably Helmholtz and Sir William Thomson (Lord Kelvin), improved the thermometer and placed thermometry on a sound basis.

Although Boerhaave and others had certainly made some use of the thermometer, it remained for Karl August Wunderlich to show its real value to medicine. He collected careful records of the variations in temperature of the human body in health and disease. Working at Leipzig, he showed that in 'fevers' the variations of temperature were an essential feature and indeed a guide to the precise nature and course of the disease. He published numbers of papers on this subject and followed them up in 1868 with his comprehensive work *Das Verhalten der Eigenwärme in Krankheiten* (Body Temperature in Disease).

It is certainly due to Wunderlich that the thermometer has

become an instrument for the everyday use of the bedside physician. The first instruments began to be used in hospitals in England about 1866 and their use rapidly became universal. These
early thermometers were unwieldy, being generally some ten
inches long and the quantity of mercury that they contained so
large that five or more minutes were necessary if a reliable reading
was to be obtained. Sir Clifford Allbutt saw these grave disadvantages and it is to him that we owe the use of the accurate little
pocket thermometers which everyone knows so well today.

Physics again came to the help of medicine with a whole series of
optical instruments for the examination of various parts of the
body. The first of these was the ophthalmoscope, the invention of
the German physicist and physiologist Hermann Ludwig von
Helmholtz. He argued that since the eyes of an animal shone by
reflected light when the surroundings were dark then, if a suitable
optical system were devised, it should be possible to see into the
interior of the living human eye. The problem was to obtain a
source of light which would shine directly into the eye without
being interrupted by the head of the observer—to find a source of
light which was virtually proceeding from the observer's eye. This
he solved in 1851 by placing a lamp at the side of the patient's head
and reflecting the light into the eye by means of a concave mirror.
This mirror was pierced in the centre by a small hole through which
Helmholtz looked. He was thus able to see for the first time the
living human retina.

With the ophthalmoscope the retina, that is the light-sensitive
part of the eye can be studied in health and disease. Much useful
information can be gained in this way, not only about diseases of
the eye itself, but also in more general ailments. For example, the
changes in the retina in diabetes, kidney disease and arteriosclerosis
are all quite characteristic. Besides this invention Helmholtz made
other valuable contributions to the study of eyesight. For example,
he worked out in considerable detail the mechanism of binocular
vision.

Following the ophthalmoscope came a number of scopes of all
kinds. In 1855 a Spanish singing teacher living in London,
Manuel Garcia, made the first laryngoscope. In the capable
hands of the physiologist Nepomuk Czermak, of the university of

Pest, this invention became an important instrument for the examination of the larynx. Later still came instruments for looking into the urethra, the bladder, the gullet, the stomach and the rectum. These, however, had to await the invention of the electric light by Edison in 1879 before they could be really workable, because the natural cavities of the body are, of course, dark inside. It was not until it was possible to obtain tiny electric lamps which were small enough and cool enough to be introduced harmlessly into the various organs that the new instruments could be used with advantage. All these devices, particularly the cystoscope, the invention of the Viennese Max Nitze, with which the interior of the bladder can be examined have proved of immense value in diseases of the urinary system.

Machines were also devised from 1881 onwards, for measuring the blood-pressure in the arteries and veins and for recording the pulse-waves in graphic form. These have been very useful in examining the condition of the heart and blood-vessels. Sir James Mackenzie (1853–1925) was the greatest exponent of the value of these instruments in the study of heart disease, and he has been regarded as the founder of modern cardiology.

Another machine which shows in even more detail the working of the heart is the electrocardiograph, invented, in 1903 by Willem Einthoven of Leyden. It was known that the heart-beat was accompanied by electrical changes, but these, being of a very small order, were not easy to measure with the ordinary galvanometers or electrometers. Einthoven therefore set out to make a highly sensitive machine especially for the purpose. He stretched a very fine thread of quartz, coated with silver, between the poles of a powerful electro-magnet, at right-angles to the magnetic field. He connected up the two ends of the thread with two pads, soaked in salt solution, which were applied one to each arm or leg of the patient. The magnetic field was turned on and at each heart-beat the fine thread pulsated. Einthoven was able to photograph these pulsations by throwing the shadow of the thread on to a moving photographic dry-plate. In this way he obtained graphic representations of the electrical changes accompanying the heart-beat. These electrocardiograms, as he called them, have been carefully analysed and used to study the different kinds of heart disease. Today an electrocardiogram has become an essential step in the investigation of every case of suspected heart disease.

During the nineteenth century the science of chemistry also contributed much to medical diagnosis. The first important discovery was that of Apollinaire Bouchardat and E. M. Peligot who proved that the sweet substance in diabetic urine was identical with grape-sugar (glucose). Ten years later, in 1848, Hermann von Fehling devised his famous method of testing for and estimating the quantity of sugar in the urine by means of the alkaline copper solution that bears his name today. A more reliable test was developed much later by S. R. Benedict.

During the present century advances in our knowledge of the chemical processes within the body have been so enormous that they now constitute a separate branch of learning called biochemistry, which has an important place in the medical curriculum. The new science has given us a whole series of quantitative tests for substances present in blood and urine which are among the most valuable aids to diagnosis. Many of these resulted from the ingenuity of Otto Folin of Harvard. Among other inventions he devised methods of measuring constituents of body-fluids by means of colour reactions and he introduced the colorimeter—a simple, but accurate instrument for measuring the intensity of colours.

These chemical methods quickly proved their value to clinical medicine. They have been so refined that they can be carried out with minute amounts of blood. These micro-chemical methods are now an indispensable part of medical practice, and their usefulness increases as our knowledge of biochemistry grows.

CHAPTER THREE

THE COMING OF ANAESTHETICS

WE have already given a short account of the horrors of surgery in pre-anaesthetic days. It seems quite extraordinary that this problem of pain should not have been solved decades before it actually was. Before Davy's discovery, in 1799, of the anaesthetic properties of laughing gas, attempts had been made to lighten the burden of pain by means of drugs. Of these hashish, opium and mandragora, 'the drowsy syrups of the east', had been used with some success, but with no little danger. Alcohol too was freely used by some surgeons. Others had even resorted to the highly dangerous practice of compressing the carotid arteries until unconsciousness supervened.

A successful method of conducting painless surgery was the use of hypnotism. This process was known hundreds of years ago by the Indian Yogis and others, and there is no doubt that many surgical procedures were carried out under hypnotism. In the Western schools the subject seems to have fallen into the hands of mountebanks, who invented a whole jargon of pseudo-science with which they surrounded the mysteries of 'mesmerism' so that even the very existence of such phenomena became discredited. John Elliotson, who made a serious attempt to introduce hypnotism into surgery, was forced to resign his appointments. James Esdaile[1] succeeded in conducting many painless surgical operations in Hindus, but unfortunately found that Europeans were not so susceptible to his hypnotic influence. His results were received by the medical journals with incredulity and a black stream of abuse which stigmatized mesmerism as an odious fraud. Here was a typical example in medical history of the way in which the strength

---

[1] J. Esdaile, *Mesmerism in India 1846 and The Introduction of Mesmerism (with the Sanction of the Government) into the Public Hospitals of India,* 2nd edn. London, 1856.

of the reputation of the pundits was able to discredit not only opinions but very facts.

Thirty years after Davy's discovery, Michael Faraday showed that ether could produce much the same effect as Davy's gas. Again the seed fell on barren soil and the idea failed to take root. The miraculous properties of ether were relegated to the use of pleasure parties who inhaled the vapour for its exhilarating effect.

It was in America that gas and ether were first used to achieve painless surgery. There has been considerable dispute about who was the first to use anaesthetics in this way, but probably the earliest instance was the removal of a tumour under ether by C. W. Long of Georgia in 1842; but his friends ridiculed his discovery to such an extent that he waited until 1849 before publishing his account of the use of ether. The Georgia Medical and Surgical Association certainly hailed him as the discoverer of anaesthesia, but nevertheless Long seems to have received little or no credit during his lifetime. It was a dentist Horace Wells, who called public attention to the use of gas in 1844. While watching a demonstration of the effects of laughing gas at a popular lecture, he noticed that one of the subjects of the experiment injured his leg while under the gas and felt no pain. The following day Wells had a tooth drawn from his own head under gas and thus inaugurated 'a new era in tooth pulling'. Unfortunately, at a public demonstration which he staged, the operation was bungled and brought the unfortunate Wells nothing but ridicule.

After this failure, W. T. G. Morton, a Boston dentist, who was a pupil of Wells, began to look for something stronger than gas and, with considerable courage, to experiment on himself. In this way on September 30th, 1846, after inhaling ether from a handkerchief, he 'speedily lost consciousness and in seven or eight minutes awoke in possession of the greatest discovery that had ever been revealed to suffering humanity'.

Almost at once he began to use ether for the extraction of teeth. Shortly afterwards Morton arranged for a demonstration of his discovery, but luckily met with a better reception than Wells had had. At the Massachusetts General Hospital both the surgeon and his audience were more than sceptical, but with Morton as the anaesthetist, a tumour was removed with the knife without any vestige of pain. 'Gentleman, this is no humbug' was the verdict of Dr Warren, the operating surgeon.

It must be confessed at this point that Morton had carefully concealed the fact that ether was the drug he had been using. He intended to patent his discovery and make a fortune. He did in fact file his papers before revealing that the drug was ether, but through some legal difficulties, he did not make the fortune on which he had counted. He became involved in arguments and recriminations about the originality of his discovery and finally lost both his dental practice and his mental balance and died in 1868, penniless and dishonoured.

In Britain, James Young Simpson took up the subject of ether anaesthesia. In January 1847, though not yet thirty-six, he had been for nearly seven years Professor of Midwifery at Edinburgh. He started his investigations without delay and by March 1847 he was already able to publish a series of successful births conducted under ether.

Simpson, however, was by no means satisfied that ether was the best substance for his purpose, so he set about to look for something better. Night after night, when his busy professional day was finished, at great personal risk, he would inhale the vapours, one after another of all the likely drugs which he could obtain. Having failed with the likely he had recourse to the rarer and less likely, but for some time without success, until, on November 4th, 1847, the great discovery was made. Chloroform had been invented by von Liebig in 1831, but had remained a chemical curiosity. Professor Miller, Simpson's colleague, tells of the historic evening when Dr Simpson 'with Drs Keith and Duncan sat down to their hazardous work in Dr Simpson's dining-room. It occurred to Dr Simpson to try a ponderous material which he had formerly set aside on a lumber-table and which, on account of its great weight, he had hitherto regarded as of no likelihood whatever: that happened to be a small bottle of chloroform. . . . And with each tumbler newly charged, the inhalers resumed their vocation. Immediately an unwonted hilarity seized the party—they became bright-eyed, very happy and very loquacious—expatiating on the delicious aroma of the new fluid. . . . But suddenly there was talk of sounds being heard like those of cotton mills louder and louder;

a moment more then all was quiet—and then crash! On awakening Dr Simpson's first perception was mental—'This is far stronger and better than ether', he said to himself. His second was to note that he was prostrate on the floor and that among the friends about him there was both confusion and alarm.'[1]

Six days later Simpson had already used the new substance in several cases of labour and had convinced himself of the superiority and harmlessness of chloroform. But, alas, chloroform is not entirely innocuous and a little later, when it was found that deaths could occur from chloroform, Simpson's adversaries armed themselves with this additional weapon. It must be understood that, important as was the discovery of chloroform as an anaesthetic, Simpson's real claim to the gratitude of posterity lies in the brave fight which he made against the opposition which arose on all sides.

Almost every important medical discovery has been received with ridicule and prejudice, amounting sometimes to a denial of the basic facts. In Simpson's case, however, no one seems to have attempted to deny that chloroform abolished pain. The opposition was on medical, moral and religious grounds. Firstly his critics said that the use of chloroform in childbirth certainly resulted in an increased maternal and infantile death-rate and they prophesied haemorrhages, convulsions, pneumonia and palsies. Such positive criticism could be refuted by an appeal to the facts and Simpson's statistics showed that, so far from an increase, the new anaesthetic produced a decrease in the mortality of the mothers and the children. The critics then put forward the astonishing argument that pain itself is beneficial. Here again Simpson was able to show that pain is a potent contributing cause of shock and that shock often leads to death. He mocked his opponents for the originality of their discovery that the agony of the operating theatre was so salutary for its victims.

Simpson went on to point out the perversity of those who had rejected other great inventions such as Jenner's vaccination. But this is a dangerous line of reasoning which makes use of a false syllogism. Every great discovery is repudiated. My discovery is

[1] Cited by H. Laing Gordon, *Sir James Young Simpson and Chloroform*, London, 1897, pp. 106, 107.

repudiated. Therefore my discovery is a great one. Furthermore it is unhappily the truth that twenty years later Sir James Simpson was himself to be in the forefront of the bitter and discreditable attack on Lister and his antiseptic system.

The religious objections to the new painless delivery were based on selected Biblical quotations and on the general belief that Divine Providence knew its own business and could be relied upon to have chosen the best possible way of managing it without any presumptuous interference from Simpson. The latter showed that he could secure better results than unaided 'Nature', but of course statistics cannot be the answer to religious convictions. He found counter-quotations from the Bible. He pointed out that 'In *sorrow* thou shalt bring forth children' does not mean 'In *pain* thou shalt bring forth children', and reminded his opponents that, in the creation of Eve, before removing a rib, 'the Lord God caused a deep sleep to fall upon Adam'. Simpson won his battle and almost single-handed he forced the adoption of chloroform anaesthesia in the British Isles, not only in obstetrics, but in all forms of surgery.

It was perhaps unfortunate that Simpson insisted on chloroform, because it began to be realized that this was a dangerous toxic substance. It was true that deaths occurred with ether as well as from chloroform, but evidence began to accumulate that, while chloroform induced anaesthesia more quickly and easily than ether, it was more dangerous. The use of chloroform was abandoned very soon in the United States, but in England, and indeed throughout most of Europe it continued in use, mainly as a result of Simpson's prestige.

Various methods of dulling pain locally, such as applying pressure or freezing the skin with a fine spray of liquid ethyl chloride, had been used without much success. Cocaine was the first substance known to have a powerful inhibiting effect on pain. It is the active principle of the leaves of the plant *Erythroxylon coca* which, mixed with clay or ashes, are chewed extensively by the natives of Peru and other South American countries. The drug was isolated chemically as early as 1855 and its power of numbing the tongue noted in 1862. It was not until twenty years later that cocaine was suggested as a local anaesthetic. The man responsible was none other than Sigmund Freud, who will be known to readers from his studies of the psychology of sex. One of his colleagues Karl Koller was the first to use cocaine as a local anaesthetic for operations on the human eye and the drug quickly came into use among oculists all over the world.

The use of local anaesthetics was extended very much by W. S. Halsted, then a young surgeon at the Roosevelt Hospital in New York. He established the method of injecting the anaesthetic into the main trunks of the nerves which supplied the part to be operated on. Halsted and his colleagues conducted many experiments on themselves and in some cases with disastrous results. At that time it was not known that cocaine was a habit-forming drug, and before they knew what was happening Halsted and his co-workers found themselves addicts. Several of them became utter wrecks and died in pathetic circumstances. Fortunately for surgery, Halsted himself overcame the addiction, though it cost him a full year to do so.

More daring still, another New York doctor, J. L. Corning introduced spinal anaesthesia by injecting cocaine into the cerebro-spinal fluid. Corning used this method to relieve pain in medical cases. It was first used in surgery in 1889 by August Bier in Berlin.

The use of cocaine has certain drawbacks apart from its habit-forming nature. For one thing it is a powerful poison and it is not easy to prognosticate how dangerous it may be in any given case. it was not until its chemical structure had been worked out that chemists could set about making less toxic substances from it. In 1905 A. Einhorn at Munich produced the synthetic drug novocaine or procaine which has the anaesthetic properties of cocaine without its disadvantages.

Yet another form of anaesthesia has now been perfected, namely intravenous anaesthesia. As long ago as 1872 L. L. G. Oré of Lyon used chloral hydrate for this purpose, but this was not found satisfactory. Numerous other substances were tried from time to time, but fifty years elapsed before really effective and safe drugs became available. The first of these was *evipal*, a derivative of barbituric acid, prepared by H. Weese in the pharmacological laboratory of the *I. G. Farben-industrie* at Elberfeld in Germany.

The original sedative drug of this class was *veronal* which had been made by Emil Fischer, the great German chemist, in 1903 and he called it veronal after the city of Verona, the most restful place he had ever known.

Other more potent intravenous anaesthetics have since been introduced and they are now used almost everywhere to supplement the older methods and, where only short duration of anaesthesia is required, they are used alone. There is no doubt that the induction of anaesthesia by the intravenous route is the one preferred by the patients.

CHAPTER FOUR

FOOD: ITS CHEMISTRY AND DIGESTION

I. THE CHEMISTS

THE scientific study of foodstuffs and of nutrition may be said to have begun in the eighteenth century when the chemist Lavoisier, who perished in the French Revolution, first recognized the true nature of combustion. He had proved that 'organic' foods contain carbon and hydrogen and that in the process of burning these elements became combined with oxygen to form carbon dioxide and water. He also showed that respiration was a precisely similar phenomenon, and again carbon dioxide and water were the end products. It is true that he wrongly supposed that the process of burning went on in the lungs, but this was shown to be a mistake by Lagrange, who demonstrated that the lungs were simply a mechanism whereby oxygen was taken up by the blood from the air and the products of combustion given up to the air. The actual combustion went on all over the body and the blood acted as a transport service in bringing up supplies of oxygen and removing waste products.

It was not possible to make much further progress until the chemists had worked out in detail the essential nature of foodstuffs. The greatest of all the nineteenth-century chemists was Justus von Liebig. His most important contributions to chemistry were three in number.[1] Firstly, he devised and perfected a way of analysing organic matter. The essential groundwork of this method still forms the basis on which all our analyses are made today. Secondly, he invented a number of entirely new substances of which chloral and chloroform are not the least important. Thirdly Liebig introduced the far-reaching idea of 'compound radicals'. These he showed, were special groups of atoms which might undergo many

[1] Tilden, W. A., *Famous Chemists*, London, 1921.

77

different chemical combinations with other atoms or groups of atoms, but which all through these changes maintained their existence as identical groups. This conception has had an immense influence on chemical thought ever since.

Liebig paid particular attention to organic compounds, that is to say those obtained from plant or animal products. All these contain carbon. These substances are of very great importance in that they alone can be utilized as food for animals. Having made his great discoveries in pure chemistry, Liebig spent the last thirty years of his life investigating the processes of life. He recognized the new idea that the heat of the animal body comes from the carefully regulated burning up of food, and accordingly he divided foodstuffs into two classes, those that went to supply energy—the respiratory foods, as he called them, consisting of sugars and fats—and those that went towards building up new tissues and repair of wear and tear—the plastic foods, which are the nitrogen-containing foods or proteins. He saw that all food comes eventually from plants which obtain their carbon from the carbon dioxide of the air and not, as had been previously supposed, from the soil.

All these discoveries Liebig made by clinging to the idea that the processes of life are purely chemical and physical. He would not believe that the processes of fermentation or putrefaction were in any way due to special living organisms and he treated bacteria with derision. Yet, undoubtedly, he really believed in some sort of vital force. Lord Kelvin relates that once he 'asked Liebig if he believed that a leaf or a flower could be formed or could grow by chemical forces. He answered, "I would more readily believe that a book on chemistry or on botany could grow out of dead matter by chemical processes".'[1]

Liebig's tremendous importance lies not only in his own discoveries, but in the fact that he pointed out the best methods of studying and of teaching chemistry. In this way his influence flourished long after his death and is still a fruitful inspiration to science. He virtually invented the chemical laboratory as we know it today. His pupils and their successors have made immense

[1] Kelvin, *Popular Lectures and Addresses*, London, 1894, p. 464. (Cited by Garrison, op. cit.)

strides in every branch of chemistry and in his *Annalen* he founded one of the first and most important of chemical journals.

It had always been considered that there was some essential difference between mineral or non-living chemical compounds and those which were found in animal or vegetable products. These latter were held to be formed by 'vital' forces. Hence the former were called inorganic and the latter organic compounds. In 1828 Friedrich Wöhler, a personal friend of Liebig, shattered for ever the distinction between the organic and the inorganic. He was able to prepare artificially the substance known as urea, which had previously been found only in animal excreta. For the first time an organic material had been made out of inorganic materials without any 'vital' interference. The two names still remain, but organic chemistry now means simply the chemistry of the carbon compounds, whatever their origin.

This discovery started a whole train of work on the artificial synthesis of substances, which has thrown a flood of light on the essential structure of foodstuffs. Wöhler made one other very significant discovery when he showed that benzoic acid is converted in the animal body into a more complex substance, hippuric acid. This does not sound a particularly startling announcement: but when we recall that before this it had been held that the animal body was incapable of manufacturing the complicated substances it needs and had to receive all such requirements in the shape of food, then we can more readily appreciate the striking nature of Wöhler's discovery. The animal body is able to build up at least some more complex compounds from relatively simple ingredients. The chemical processes of the body can be constructive as well as destructive.

II. THE PHYSIOLOGISTS

The next phase in the elucidation of the problems of digestion came not from the chemists but from the physiologists, and of these the most important from this point of view was Claude Bernard.[1] He was the son of a Burgundian wine-grower and early in life he worked in a pharmacist's shop at Lyons. Here he was

[1] Michael Foster, *Claude Bernard*, London, 1899.

speedily disillusioned about the value of the mixtures prepared for the cure of customers. There was a famous syrup for which he was always being asked. Bernard was astonished to discover that the syrup varied very much in composition; in fact it was compounded from all the odds and ends and spoiled drugs of the shop.

Claude Bernard turned his attention to writing plays and his vaudeville comedy '*La Rose du Rhône*' met with some fair provincial success: but a critic who read his next work, a tragedy, advised him to take up medicine. Thus instead of a playwright he became one of the most famous physiologists of his day.

Before his time physiology in France was much handicapped by the teaching of the 'vitalists' who held that the phenomena of living bodies could never be the subject of exact experimental inquiry. Whether this is true or not, it is certain that anyone who adopts this attitude in a laboratory will not be likely to progress very far. It is a defeatist and stultifying doctrine to presuppose that the business of the physiologist is merely to describe and to make no attempt to explain.

Bernard's teacher, François Magendie, made many important discoveries through experimenting: but it has been said that he gave too little attention to the interpretation of his results—that he substituted experimentation for thinking. Bernard's method was far sounder. He would think out a matter thoroughly and then test the conclusion of his rational speculation by experimental appeal to nature.

Bernard's researches into nutrition began with his discovery that, if he injected a solution of cane-sugar into the veins of a dog, the sugar reappeared in the urine: but if the sugar had previously been treated with gastric juice (the secretion of the stomach) of the dog, then this did not happen. The inference he drew was that unaltered cane-sugar was useless for nutrition and so was discarded in the urine: but that the stomach juices altered the sugar in some way so that it became acceptable. This was the first clue to the now well-known fact that all the more complicated sugary and starchy substances must be broken up by 'ferments' in the bowel until they are reduced to the simplest kinds of sugar, and that until this is done sugar cannot be used by the body tissues.

Claude Bernard's next line of inquiry was to discover what

happened to fats in the animal bowel. He noted that fat in the stomach was not changed by the action of the gastric juice, but that as soon as ever the fat reached the point where the pancreas (sweetbread) poured its juices into the intestine, then the fat began to be digested. This was a big step forward, for up till then it had been assumed that digestion took place almost entirely in the stomach itself.

As early as 1833 an American army surgeon, William Beaumont, had made many valuable observations on the digestive processes of the stomach. This he was enabled to do by a curious accident whereby a gunshot wound had made a permanent hole leading from the abdominal wall into the interior of the stomach of a Canadian half-breed named Alexis St Martin. Beaumont carefully described the movements of the stomach during digestion and showed that the gastric juice is not manufactured continuously but is poured out only when there is food present. He also showed that the juice contained hydrochloric acid and a highly active milk-clotting ferment. These discoveries are of fundamental importance, as every doctor who has a patient with indigestion well knows. For example it is known that gastric indigestion is often associated with an excess or deficiency of this hydrochloric acid. The doctor is accordingly able to remedy this by giving alkalis or acids as the case may demand.

Bernard followed up this work by showing that the digestion in the stomach is simply a preliminary phase and that both fat and protein are not fully digested until they encounter the pancreatic secretion. Next he turned his attention to sugars because he was aware that in the chemistry of the sugars lay the key to the cause of diabetes. What happened to the glucose that he injected into the veins of the dog? It must be stored or destroyed somewhere in the body: and surely if this 'somewhere' were put out of action the glucose would accumulate in the blood—a condition of diabetes would be established. He discovered that the liver was able to produce glucose and, later, that it could do so because it had a store of some substance which it could turn into glucose. This substance, now called glycogen, is a kind of 'animal starch' and it is made in the liver from the glucose in the blood. It can be turned back again into glucose when occasion demands.

This discovery was a blow to the well-established theory that each organ had one function. The consequence of this belief had been that once the function of an organ had been discovered there was a tendency to assume that there was nothing more to be found out about it. It had long been known that the function of the liver was to secrete bile: and now Bernard had shown that it had also this glycogenic function.

These were by no means the only contributions that Claude Bernard made to physiological knowledge. For example, he discovered that the flow of blood in the arteries is controlled by an elaborately balanced system of nerves of two kinds, the one set constricting and the other dilating the blood-vessels. This has a very important bearing on our present-day physiological outlook. These systems are called into action every moment of our lives. They ensure supplies of blood to our digestive organs after meals, they control the temperature of our skin and through this they regulate that of our whole body and, furthermore, they make sure that our brain is properly supplied with blood at the right pressure whatever posture we assume.

The next steps in the elucidation of the mechanism of digestion were taken by Karl von Voit, who developed a method of measuring the total amount of food eaten by an animal, while at the same time he also measured the amounts of carbon dioxide and nitrogen given out in the breath and excreta. In this way he was able to calculate how much of each kind of foodstuff (sugar, fat and protein) was actually being burned up to supply the needs of the body.

Max Rubner, a pupil of von Voit, began to investigate these problems from the point of view of the heat-value of the foods (that is to say, how much heat they give out when completely burnt) and of the amount of heat given out by the animal body. A whole host of workers have given their attention to this, and many elaborate machines have been invented for measuring the heat given off by animals. Some of them have been large enough to contain a man. Rubner was able to show that the food burnt up by a resting animal was proportional to the area of body-surface.

By these heat-measuring experiments the energy-values of the various kinds of foods were found. These values are measured in

Calories, or units of heat. A Calory is the amount of heat required to raise a kilogramme[1] of water through one degree centigrade. It was shown that starches, sugars and other members of the carbohydrate family each provided 4·1 Calories for each gramme of their weight. The nitrogen-containing substances, that is to say the proteins (lean meat and white-of-egg, for example), have about the same heat-value as the carbohydrates. Fats, on the other hand, give as much as 9·3 Calories per gramme.

From all these findings have gradually emerged the true principles of diet. It began to be realized that the total energy put out by the body must be exactly equal to the energy obtained by the combustion of foodstuffs and tissues in the body *at the same time.* It immediately follows from this that, given the knowledge of how many Calories are necessary for people following various modes of life, we can calculate the exact food requirement for any individual following any definite occupation. It is now pretty generally agreed that the average requirement for an adult is about 3,000 Calories per day, but heavy manual workers need more. In calculating suitable diets it is important to bear in mind that there is always some wastage. Everything is not digested, especially with vegetables. A purchase of food furnishing 3,400 Calories makes allowance for this and for loss in the preparation of the meals.

It must be understood that quantity is not the only requirement: for, if this were so, two pounds of sugar would more than supply energy for anyone but the hardest manual worker. It is obvious that no one could live on such a diet. There must be a proper balance of foodstuffs, with a proper proportion of each of the three main kinds of food. An easily remembered formula for a daily diet giving 3,390 Calories consists of 100 grammes of fat, 100 grammes of protein and 500 grammes of carbohydrate. Today it is held that not all the proteins have the same biological value and that most of the animal products are superior to the vegetable. Consequently an assured minimum of first-class animal protein is desirable.

The animal body always contains fat and it might be thought that it was necessary to provide all this in the food. It appears, however, from the classical experiment of Lawes and Gilbert, that

---

[1] To avoid confusion it should be explained that 1 physiological Calory (with a capital C) equals 1,000 calories of physics.

fat can be manufactured inside the animal. They took two pigs from the same litter, ten weeks old and of almost equal weights. The first they killed at once and measured the total fat and nitrogen in its body. The second pig was fed on barley (which contains very little fat.) The amount eaten was carefully measured and analysed, as were also the excreta of the pig. After four months the second pig was killed and its fat and nitrogen estimated. The experimenters then drew up a balance sheet showing the amount of fat eaten and that present in the pig at the end of the four months. They conclusively proved that at least five kilogrammes of fat must have been manufactured by the pig out of the carbohydrate in the food.

Fat forms a reserve of nourishment which can be drawn upon when necessary. It can be manufactured from carbohydrates or can, of course, be obtained directly from fat in the food. In this connexion the experiment of Lebedev is very interesting. He took two dogs and, after slimming them, he fed one on a diet containing much mutton fat, while the other was given food containing linseed oil. Later he killed the two dogs and found that while the fat of the first was solid even when heated to 50 degrees centigrade, that of the other was still liquid at the freezing-point of water. It seems from this result that fat is stored in the body without much alteration. Cows fed on an excess of oilcake produce too soft a butter.

Sugar or carbohydrate is used primarily for the immediate energy requirements of the body. There is a nicely balanced adjustment whereby the blood is kept supplied with the right amount of sugar. If there is too much the surplus is stored as glycogen or converted into fat. In diabetes the arrangements for dealing with excess of sugar are upset and consequently glucose accumulates in the blood and is eventually passed out in the urine. If there is too little sugar in the blood then the normal processes are reversed, glycogen or fat being reconverted into sugar ready for use as fuel. A feeling of faintness after exertion may be due to there being too little sugar in the blood, and a timely administration of cane-sugar, or better still glucose, will quickly relieve the symptoms.

Sugar is eaten mainly in the form of starch (in potatoes, bread, peas, beans, etc.), cane-sugar and also in fruits, vegetables and milk. Sugar in one form or another comprises about three-quarters of the weight and half the energy value of all our food. It appears that sugar is necessary to us for reasons other than its energy value. No man can live long without some sugar. Deprived of it he develops a condition of *acidosis* (too little alkali in the blood), which is a characteristic of diabetes. It seems that the presence of sugar is in some way essential for the proper combustion of fats. In its absence the fats are only partially burnt and give rise to poisonous substances. The sugar has been compared to the draught without which the fats burn with a smoky flame. In this lies the crux of diabetes. We cannot say that there is not enough sugar in the diabetic's blood; indeed there is too much. As will be seen later, the trouble is that the mechanism for dealing with it has gone wrong.

As Liebig had taught, the proteins are required for two purposes; firstly the building up of the body tissues, that is to say for growth; and secondly, to replace the loss of body-substance from wear and tear. The case of gelatin puzzled him because, though obviously very like other proteins, it had no value as a body-building food. He explained this by saying that gelatin was converted into the gelatinous material of bones and tendons. This unconvincing explanation was widely accepted until about 1912.

The German chemist Emil Fischer and his co-workers probed much deeper into the essential structure of proteins during the first decade of the present century. All proteins, they found, were built up by combinations of large number of smaller units, called amino-acids. Some twenty-three of these amino-acids were discovered. Some or all of them combine in different ways and different proportions to form all the known animal and vegetable proteins. In the process of digestion all the food proteins are broken down into their constituent building-stones, the amino-acids, which are absorbed into the blood-stream and later on are built up into the complicated proteins of the living animal tissue. These animal proteins consist of combinations of the individual amino-acids arranged together in a way which may be quite different from those occurring in the foodstuffs. The whole process of digestion, absorption and reconstruction may be compared to the pulling down of a building into its original bricks and then using these to construct another building which may be of quite another architectural style and may subserve an entirely different purpose. The amino-acids may also be compared with the letters of the alphabet which are used to form long words which can be rearranged into various anagrams. This is perhaps a better analogy because the number of different amino-acids is roughly the same as that of the letters of the alphabet.

It further appears that the body can synthesize some of these amino-acids, but that certain individual amino-acids cannot be so made and consequently are absolutely essential constituents of food. Hopkins and Wilcock,[1] for example, fed animals on a diet in which the only available protein was zein, which is derived from maize. This contains no tryptophane, which is one of the essential amino-acids. The animals soon sickened. This showed that the body was incapable of manufacturing tryptophane. In 1912 Osborn and Mendel fed a rat for 178 days on a protein called gliadin, together with milk from which all the proteins had been removed and to which some carbohydrate and fat was added. It appeared that all the necessary factors for growth were present. Four young rats were then born and were fed for thirty days on their mother's milk. Then three of the young were put on a normal diet while the fourth was fed on the same food as the mother had received. The three grew up normally while the fourth ailed. From this it appeared that a diet which could keep an adult in good health could be quite inadequate to support a growing infant.

In the case of gelatin, which had so perplexed Liebig, chemical analysis showed that it was totally lacking in no less than three of the essential amino-acids and for that reason was useless for tissue-building purposes. From these examples it became obvious that not all proteins had equal biological value. The best proteins are found in the more readily digested meats and in milk. The worst is gelatin, with no growth value at all. In between come the proteins of vegetables and cereals, with something like half the growth-value of meat. In other words it would take about twice the amount of protein in the form of bread to promote the same rate of growth in a child as would be needed if milk or meat were

[1] *Journal of Physiology*, 1906, 35. pp. 88–102.

given. For this reason meats and milk are said to provide 'first class proteins'.

Besides the three main kinds of food there are other essential requirements. The need for water is obvious enough. Water is being lost continuously through the skin and from the lungs and, furthermore, a supply must be available at all times for washing out of the blood all the waste products of the chemical processes of life. Salts, too, are absolutely necessary to replace those lost in the urine and sweat. Certain particular salts must be present to fulfil special functions. Iron, for example, is needed for the oxygen-carrying part of the blood, while lime-salts are required for the bones and the teeth as well as being necessary for the proper clotting of the blood in a wound. These salts should be present in any reasonably well-balanced diet provided it is properly cooked.

For the elimination of waste products from the bowel it is desirable that these should have a large bulk so that the action of the bowel should be stimulated. The food should therefore contain a considerable amount of indigestible material to make up this bulk. Such 'roughage' is generally composed of cellulose which is abundantly present in all fruit and vegetables. Without these the bowels will act badly. Pure concentrated food will not do.

Armed with all these and many other facts, the physician faced with a patient suffering from digestive or other troubles is in a strong position to give his advice on the subject of diet. In fever, for example, the patient burns up far more than the normal energy requirements. So far then from 'starving a fever' it is important to supply as much food as can be used; but we must compromise about this, because a sick man has a weakened digestion and an increased diet would not be absorbed. We start off with a lowered diet and then feed up the patient as soon as ever we think his digestion will stand it.

Another way in which the physician takes advantage of the new knowledge follows directly from Claude Bernard's discovery that some substances are not digested until they reached the pancreatic juice. When it is desired to administer a drug which would irritate the stomach-wall, or a drug which would be destroyed by the acid stomach-juices, or again one that the doctor does not wish to act on the stomach but on the intestine, then all that it is necessary to do is to enclose the drug in a little capsule made of some substance which is not dissolved until it reaches the juices of the pancreas.

In the case of a drug which is irritant to the stomach it is sometimes possible to combine it chemically with another substance and so form a non-irritant compound which is split up into its original parts only when it reaches the small intestine. Such a drug is salicylic acid which is irritant to the stomach but when combined to form acetyl-salicylic acid (more commonly known as aspirin) acts in the way described above.

Yet another important application of the basic principles of diet is found in the management of diabetes. Here the problem is that there is already too much sugar in the blood, but that sugar is vitally important for the proper utilization of fats. Noxious acids are formed from incomplete combustion of the fats. It is necessary for the doctor to prescribe a diet so balanced that it will produce in the patient the very least possible quantity of these noxious acids. Such diets have been worked out very carefully, but the problem has been much simplified, as we shall see later, by the discovery of insulin.

By the turn of the century it was generally thought that our knowledge about foodstuffs was almost complete. In 1900 Seebohm Rowntree published a terrible account of life in the slums of the city of York.[1] He laid particular stress on bad housing and sanitation, but he also pointed out the hopelessly inadequate food the poor were compelled to eat. Most of the poorer families lived almost exclusively on bread (and it was white bread, be it noted) and many were suffering from near-starvation. These exposures carried little weight at the time and the Government took no notice, or at any rate no action.

A year later the complacency in high places received a rude shock when Sir William Taylor, Director General of the Army Medical Service, reported that the Inspector of Recruiting could not find enough men of satisfactory physique for service in the Boer War.[2] The rejections, mainly for bad teeth, defective sight or hearing and gross deformities, were as high as 60 per cent in some areas. These defects were almost certainly the result of dietary deficiencies, but

[1] Seebohm Rowntree, *Poverty. A Study in Town Life*, 1900.

[2] Watt Smyth, A., *Physical Deterioration, its Causes and Cure*, 1907.

this was not known at the time. Investigators paid much more attention to housing and sanitation. It was an era when domestic hygiene was making rapid progress. Much had been discovered about the value of pure water and adequate sanitation, but the influence of malnutrition (apart from obvious starvation) was not appreciated. Indeed doctors were so obsessed with the quantitative viewpoint on diet that every problem was regarded in terms of calories, sugars, proteins and fats.

Reluctant to admit that the findings of the Inspector of Recruiting were anything new, the Royal College of Physicians and the Royal College of Surgeons both advised the Government that there was no case for an inquiry. None the less an Inter-Departmental Committee was set up and in due course presented its report.[1] It is understandable that they stressed such factors as overcrowding, bad sanitation, gin-drinking, working conditions and ignorance, but did not recognize the devastating effects of dietary deficiencies. At that time defective nutrition seemed a much less likely cause than the environmental factors. As will be seen later, the discovery of vitamins during the following twenty years revolutionized the whole science of nutrition.

[1] Report of the Inter-Departmental Committee on Physical Deterioration, London 1904.

CHAPTER FIVE

THE GERM THEORY

I. INFECTIVE ORGANISMS

(a) Early Conceptions

FROM the remotest periods of history we find mention of plagues and pestilences and it is scarcely surprising that mankind should have invented many different hypotheses to account for the undoubted fact that many diseases are epidemic. From antiquity to the Middle Ages these ideas about the cause of disease varied from cosmic influences (hence 'lunacy' and 'influenza') to witchcraft and from the will or vengeance of the gods to the poisoning of wells by the Jews.

The doctrine of contagion is not a new one. The writer of Leviticus, in Chapters XIII–XV, clearly recognizes this as the method of spread of leprosy and gonorrhoea when he lays down the law that persons who are suffering from these diseases must be prevented from mixing with their fellows. Thucydides, too, in his description of the plague at Athens, recognized that the disease was conveyed directly from one person to another. More recently, in the eighteenth century, the practice of inoculating smallpox from person to person was brought[1] into this country from the East and clearly showed that contagion was accepted as the means of spread of this disease at least.

Another theory of epidemics that received wide recognition appears under a variey of names. In general it assumes that there is an 'atmospheric influence' or 'epidemic miasma' which may pass over a country and that its progress may be shown by outbreaks in different places where there is some determining factor, such a condition being found where there are present all the well-known

[1] By Timoni and Pilarini's communications to the Royal Society 1713–16, and later by Lady Mary Wortley Montagu.

circumstances that make a place unwholesome. In other words the air is to blame: there is a bad air, a *mal aria*, and from this comes the name of a disease which, whereas it was once common in England under the name of ague, is now found chiefly in tropical and sub-tropical lands. This hypothesis of epidemic miasmata is by no means worthless; for, while it shows us no means (other than flight) of avoiding the miasma, at least it teaches that filth is a predisposing cause of disease. It was believed pretty generally until the actual living germs of certain diseases were discovered. The theory of contagion was forced on medical opinion by outbreaks which were quite obviously contagious, epidemics which swept over Europe—notably the Black Death (probably the bubonic plague) which killed more than sixty million people and entered Europe about 1348 after having ravaged Asia and Africa. There were also the waves of syphilis in the fifteenth, smallpox in the eighteenth and cholera in the nineteenth century.

Before the discovery of disease germs, attempts to prevent such epidemics were for the most part unsuccessful. Isolation of the diseased and quarantine for those who had been in contact were the only available methods. The greatest triumph claimed for the isolation method was the disappearance of leprosy from Western Europe. This disease, which was possibly introduced and probably spread by the crusaders, had been so far eradicated in France, Italy, Spain, England, Denmark and Switzerland by the middle of the sixteenth century that we hear little after this of the lazar houses, of which there had existed in this country more than two hundred in the previous century. However, since the exact mode of transmission is yet uncertain, we must not assume that the segregation of the infected was the sole cause of the disappearance of leprosy from England.

More recently by strict quarantine for dogs and by muzzling all dogs when there is any source of rabies about, this disease has been completely eliminated in this island: but of course this result depends on the fact that we live on an island. The same result cannot be obtained easily on the Continent. On the other hand the quarantine method had conspicuously failed to keep the plague from Venice in the fourteenth century and, in the light of our present knowledge, this is not surprising.

There is no doubt that in some instances the method of propagation of the contagion and the means of prevention had been well understood many years before the actual microbes were known. A conspicuous example is found in the death-dealing spectre of the lying-in chamber, puerperal fever. As early as 1795, Dr Gordon of Aberdeen had shown that this disease 'seized such women only as were visited or delivered by a practitioner, or taken care of by nurses who had previously attended patients affected with the disease'.[1] He gave tables to show that this was not an assertion, but a fact admitting of demonstration and he added that it was a disagreeable declaration for him to make that he himself was the means of carrying the infection to a great number of women.

The same subject was taken up in 1843 by Oliver Wendell Holmes of Boston; but the opposition he aroused from his American colleagues was heated indeed. They argued that the transmission of the disease by themselves was very improbable, that a doctor who had a series of cases consecutively of puerperal fever was merely 'unlucky'. In answer to this Holmes, taking into account the total incidence of the disease compared with the total number of births 'had the chances calculated that a given practitioner A. shall have sixteen fatal cases in a month' and declared that 'there was not one chance in a million million millions that such a series should be noted . . . chance, therefore, is out of the question as an explanation of the admitted coincidence'. The fact was that medical men naturally found it extremely inconvenient to admit that so many women had died from the poison conveyed to them by the doctors themselves. Holmes added 'the facts shall reach the public ear: the pestilence carrier of the lying-in chamber must look to God for pardon, for man will never forgive him'. He went on to point out the remedy. No doctor, he advised, should attend a woman in childbirth if he had recently a case of puerperal fever, or if he had attended post-mortem examinations. He extended these recommendations to include the nurses and advised repeated washing of hands and changes of outer clothes.

Elsewhere the discovery was made again, but Ignaz Semmelweiss saw more deeply than the others. In the Allgemeines Krankenhaus in Vienna he noticed that the deaths from puerperal

[1] O. W. Holmes, *Medical Essays 1842–82*, London, 1891, p. 134.

fever in the first ward greatly exceeded those in the second. The first ward was used for teaching students who came unwashed from the dissecting-room, whereas the second ward was used by the midwives. In 1847, as he watched the post-mortem on the body of one of his colleagues who had died from blood-poisoning contracted from a dissecting-wound, the light suddenly dawned. The appearances in the body were just like those in the dead mothers from the first ward. Puerperal fever was a form of blood-poisoning and the cause was the dead infective material brought in by the students. Here was the greatest piece of good fortune; for, where all had been doubt ('only the great number of the dead was an undoubted reality') he had shown the plain truth. By insisting on cleanliness and rinsing the hands in a solution of chloride of lime, he quickly reduced the mortality to 1 per cent. Again the truth was unwelcome, but he put up a vigorous fight for his discovery. He was ridiculed and his opinions derided: but his memorable book[1] remains to show the lasting debt which every mother owes to Semmelweiss, who died in 1875 embittered and insane. Though the case was proved, it was not until Lister's teaching had spread, that the principles of cleanliness and asepsis were widely applied to save the lives of women in childbirth.

(b) The Discovery of Bacteria

The discoveries of Gordon, Holmes and Semmelweiss had been made years before the casual streptococcus had been found. Many micro-organisms had long been known, but it was left to a chemist, Louis Pasteur, to point to some of these as the true and only causes of certain diseases. Pasteur did not 'discover' germs in the sense that he was the first to see any microbes through his microscope. In the latter half of the seventeenth century the Dutch microscope-maker, van Leeuwenhoek, had described a variety of such minute organisms. Bacteria in fact are found almost everywhere on earth in enormous numbers and countless species. Fortunately only a very few species can produce disease in human beings. Pasteur's researches led him to the discovery that putrefaction is a kind of

[1] Semmelweiss, I., *Die Aetiologie, der Begriff und die Prophylaxis des Kindbettfiebers*, Budapest, Vienna and Leipzig, 1861.

fermentation, that both these processes are due to micro-organisms and that putrescible material (such as blood, for example) can be kept indefinitely if care is taken to exclude all living micro-organisms. These are, in fact, absolutely necessary to, and the cause of putrefaction.

He began by trying to find out what turns milk sour. He pointed to the little globules seen down the microscope, living globules that budded and multiplied, so that just a trace of these globules could sour milk. Alcoholic fermentation he showed to be due also to self-producing globules; but these were different from the others: they could produce alcohol from sugar, but they could not turn the milk sour. Each fermentation had its own kind of organism and vice versa. This is the important principle of *specificity*.

Pasteur showed that these ferments came from the atmosphere and multiplied in the fermenting liquids: they were present in very different numbers in different places: they swarmed in towns and rooms, but were scarce in the high mountain air. He showed that by heat, or by filtering the air through plugs of cotton wool, the germs could be prevented from reaching any vessel, although the air itself flowed freely in and out.

In the agent which produces the butyric acid, that causes the smell of rancid butter, he found something quite unforeseen. Here was an organism which would grow only in the absence of air, or rather of oxygen. This was the first of the *anaërobic* bacteria, as he called them.

All these fermentative changes he showed were due to these *living* microscopic beings and to them alone. The opposition which this idea aroused was so enormous as to seem almost incredible to us now, but Pasteur had against him the full crushing weight of the terrific Baron von Liebig, the leading chemist of his day. Liebig's dicta were looked up to by an enormous following, but since while denying Pasteur's ideas he absolutely refused to look through a microscope, the matter could not very well be argued to a conclusion. This kind of attempt to stultify his activities occurred to Pasteur more than once. He spent much time in proving his point about micro-organisms against Liebig's assertion that fermentation and putrefaction were processes akin to slow chemical combustion and that the dead portion of the yeast was alone responsible for the production of alcohol: but he spent even longer over his celebrated controversy with Pouchet over the 'spontaneous generation' of life. Were the germs the cause or the effect of the fermentation? After a bitter fight in which his experimental proofs were met with flowers of oratory and his arguments with rhetoric, in 1862 he succeeded in convincing the Academy of Sciences at Paris that 'spontaneous generation is a chimaera' and that all life comes from life alone. Pasteur had a negative point to prove and that is not easy; but he convinced them all.

The wine industry in France was losing huge quantities of wine every year from a wine-disease of unknown origin when Pasteur turned his mind to the matter. As he expected, the wine-disease was due to an organized ferment and he showed that by heating the wine for a short time to a temperature of between 50 and 60 degrees Centigrade, this ferment could be destroyed, and the wine remained unaltered and would keep indefinitely. The wine, as we say, had been 'pasteurized'.

Pasteur's researches extended into diseases of silkworms and into the brewing of beer and from these he turned to diseases of man. As early as 1863 he said to the Emperor, to whom he had been presented by the great French chemist Dumas, that his 'ambition was to arrive at the knowledge of putrid and contagious disease'.

Before Pasteur there had been isolated discoveries of microscopic beings associated with disease. The little rod-like organisms in the blood of animals dead of anthrax had been seen as early as 1838, but it was not until Davaine heard of Pasteur's work on fermentation that he began to inoculate rabbits with these organisms and to reproduce the disease. In 1839 Schönlein had discovered the fungus which causes the skin disease called *favus*; but it was Pasteur and his pupils who put the germ theory upon a sound footing and the whole structure of the science of bacteriology is built directly on his work.

To a German, Robert Koch, we owe the beginnings of modern bacteriological technique. He it was who first laid bare the natural history or life story of the anthrax bacillus and showed how to grow the bacillus and how to obtain it unmixed with other organisms in 'pure culture'. From these first discoveries an enormously complicated technique has grown up, which enables the bacteriologist to separate and identify the different disease-producing agents. But even today the subject is far from being a complete and orderly one and this is largely due to the fact that bacteriology has been an *applied* science and 'investigators have been more interested in what bacteria do than in what they are and much more interested in the ways in which they interfere with man's health or pursuits than in the ways in which they function as autonomous living beings' as Topley and Wilson have said.[1] The general natural history of germs has been neglected for the study of the particular habits of a few species.

Pasteur had previously shown how to cultivate the germs in his liquid media which he prepared synthetically in his laboratory. He had realized that different bacteria needed media which differed not only in the varying quality of the nutrient material, but also in the amount of oxygen or the degree of acidity. He had grown an organism in a tube and then sown one drop of the liquid into another tube, waited, then sown one drop from this into a third tube and so on through a long sequence of tubes, so that any extraneous, non-living substances which might have been present in the first tube were inconceivably dilute in the last tube, but the organisms were alive, reproduced themselves and were as numerous and had the same disease-producing properties in the last as in the first tube. It was the organisms and they alone which produced the disease.

Koch had shown how to separate different kinds of bacteria by growing them on solid media. He also showed how organisms could be distinguished from one another by the way they took up different dyes from solutions. Thus began the important technique of 'staining' bacteria to make them more easily seen under the microscope, as well as to help in identifying the various species.

Following the work of these two leaders came the discovery of a large number of the bacteria responsible for many different diseases. Some were discovered by the masters and more by their pupils. Before the close of the nineteenth century there had been discovered the causative organisms of leprosy, gonorrhoea, suppuration, typhoid fever, malaria, tuberculosis, cholera, diphtheria, pneumonia, cerebro-spinal meningitis, Malta fever, tetanus (lock-

[1] *The Principles of Bacteriology and Immunity*, London, 1929.

jaw), plague, botulism and dysentery; while more recently, in the present century, observers have found the organisms of sleeping-sickness, syphilis, whooping-cough, infective jaundice and scarlet fever. This list is far from complete and there are numbers of organisms which are almost certainly the cause of different diseases, but the absolute proof is sometimes lacking. Until it can be shown that the organism is always present in every case of the disease, that it can be cultivated through several generations and that the last generation can reproduce the disease with certainty, it cannot be claimed that this organism is the cause of the disease beyond any shadow of doubt.

The bacteriologists have worked out a complicated technique for studying germs and for distinguishing one kind from another. Firstly the appearance of the micro-organisms is important. They are of different sizes and shapes, they may have granules in them, or they may be surrounded with a kind of capsule. They may have one or more thread-like appendages called flagellae, or they may be grouped together in definite formations such as clumps or long chains. Furthermore a large group or 'colony' of bacteria, which is big enough to be seen with the naked eye, has characteristics which often vary according to the species. The colonies are of different sizes and shapes and have different surface textures. Certain bacteria, when stained with aniline dyes and then washed in a solution of iodine, are easily decolourized by subsequent washing in alcohol; other kinds retain their colour under this process. There are some which remain coloured when acted upon by strong mineral acids. By these and other micro-chemical means many bacteria can be distinguished from one another.

Other methods depend upon the behaviour of growing cultures of the bacteria. Some will liquefy gelatin, others not. Some can set free the red blood-pigment of mammals from the containing corpuscles, while others are unable to do this. Some can ferment different kinds of sugar with the production of carbon dioxide, while others cannot alter the sugars at all. There are some bacteria that need oxygen for their growth, some can do without it, while others still cannot grow at all except in the complete absence of free oxygen. There are many other delicate biological tests too, but we have not space to describe them here.

It began to be assumed, then, that every infectious disease had its own particular organism which caused this disease alone; but today we know that the matter is not quite so simple as this. For example, the pneumococcus, though a common and important cause of pneumonia, is not the only germ that can cause it. As an antithesis to this, we know that certain species of bacteria can cause more than one disease. There seems little doubt that scarlet fever, puerperal fever, infectious sore throat and erysipelas, besides some forms of wound infection, are all due to streptococci. These can be seen under the microscope as tiny rounded bodies arranged in chains. Controversy has raged between those who believe that these streptococci are all of one kind and those who think that there is a separate kind for each of the diseases in question. One fact remains undisputed, that there has been a very great decline in epidemics of these streptococcal diseases. Since puerperal fever, when it does occur, still has an undiminished violence (if untreated), this decline seems to be more the result of hygiene than any decrease in the virulence of the germs.

(c) The Viruses

Bacteriologists had met with one big difficulty in their search for the microbes of disease. There were a number of diseases which were undoubtedly infectious since they could be produced by inoculation, but no one, search as he might, had been able to see the organisms, or at least nothing resembling the known germs of other diseases. Later it was shown that these infections were due to very minute bodies, called *viruses*, each virus being specific for a given disease, in the same way that most pathogenic bacteria are specific. The viruses differed in many ways from bacteria. Besides being invisible, they could not be grown on artificial culture media. They grew and multiplied only inside living material, a whole living animal, a developing egg or a living tissue-culture.

The earliest virus to be discovered was that of a plant disease, the mosaic disease of the tobacco plant, so called because of the typical patterns it produces on the leaves of infected plants. In 1892 a Russian botanist, Ivanovsky, showed how the disease could be transferred by infecting a healthy plant with the sap of a diseased one. Furthermore the sap was infectious even after being passed through a Pasteur-Chamberland filter, which effectively removed all forms of bacteria. The invisible agents so demonstrated became known as the *filterable viruses*. Ivanovsky himself does not seem to have grasped the full significance of what we now see to have been a discovery of immense importance.

Little progress in this direction was made until 1935 when an American, W. M. Stanley, showed how a virus could be isolated by purely chemical means from filtered solutions. This is done by adding weak acid drop by drop until the virus particles become without either positive or negative electric charge (the so-called isoelectric point) when they are thrown out of solution as a fine precipitate which is the very virus itself. Some viruses can be crystallized out, like chemical salts, and so be obtained in very pure form.

It turned out later that a virus is a protein with a very big molecule, that is to say with a molecular weight of many millions. This raises the question of whether these viruses are in fact living beings or dead chemical agents. They appear to be living in that, under suitable conditions, they can reproduce themselves indefinitely, generation after generation. Equally they seem to be dead in that they can be produced in pure crystalline form and can be kept dormant for indefinite periods. Another method of separating viruses depends upon the very fact that they are large molecules, that is the use of a very high-speed centrifuge. This, the ultra-centrifuge, works at some 30,000 revolutions per minute—in a vacuum, to avoid the heat which air friction would otherwise engender at such enormous speeds.

Why was it that these viruses, demonstrably present, could not be seen? The melancholy fact is that there is a limit to the power of the usual compound microscope. When an object is much smaller in diameter than the wave-length of the light used to view it, the light, because of its wave nature, bends round the object, so that the effect is as though the light came uninterruptedly through; in other words the object is invisible; and this is true however 'powerful' the microscope may be.

If we throw a very bright beam of light on to a small body and view the body sideways—that is at right-angles to the beam—we may be able to see the body by virtue of the light which is scattered. In theory the smallest bodies might be seen by this method which is an extension of the principle whereby the little motes, otherwise invisible, can be seen dancing in a sunbeam. In practice there are a number of difficulties which severely limit the resolving power of such a microscope. We can, of course, use light of shorter wave length. In 1925, J. E. Barnard succeeded by means of ultra-violet light in photographing (for we cannot *see* such 'light') objects as small as 75 mμ.[1] The difficulties are enormous; for example, the microscope lenses must be made of quartz, since glass is opaque to this kind of light.

About 1925 the first electronic lenses were developed. The principle is simple, though the technical difficulties are immense. Instead of light we use a beam of cathode-rays. These are streams of rapidly moving electrons which, since each bears a negative electrical charge, can be deflected by a magnet. In practice these beams, after striking a microscopic object, can be 'focused' by a suitable arrangement of powerful electromagnets. Thus, in 1931, was born the electron microscope which can photograph objects as small as 2 mμ in diameter. With this powerful new weapon even the smallest viruses can be made visible.

Among the important diseases for which viruses are responsible are smallpox, cow-pox, infantile paralysis, rabies, foot and mouth disease, yellow fever, encephalitis lethargica—the so-called sleepy sickness, a comparatively new disease which was first reported in Vienna in 1917 and of which an outbreak caused 4,000 deaths in Japan in 1924—and distemper, which attacks dogs and other carnivorous animals. There is also an important virus-produced group of diseases which attack mainly the breathing mechanism of the body. This includes measles, influenza, the common cold and psittacosis (the parrot disease). Unfortunately it has been shown that influenza and colds can be produced by many different strains of virus. Indeed the Common Cold Research Unit at Salisbury, Wiltshire, has recently shown that there are at least 90 different strains of virus which cause the common cold, so that attempts to

[1] One μ (mu) = a thousandth of a millimetre.
One mμ (milli-mu) — one millionth of a millimetre.

produce immunity to this scourge are likely to encounter serious difficulties.

The viruses, as photographed by the electron microscope, vary very much in size and shape. The largest are the *Rickettsiae*, the causes of typhus (gaol fever) and trench fever. They are named after H. T. Ricketts who discovered them. These bodies are big enough to fall just within the range of visibility of the compound microscope. The virus of vaccinia (cow-pox) is as large as 275 mμ in diameter, whereas that of infantile paralysis[1] is as small as 15 mμ. The electron miscroscope gives excellent pictures of all these viruses and with modern 'scanning' technique the pictures give an impression of three-dimensional photography.

In reviewing the expedients to which experimenters have resorted in the war against disease-producing bacteria and viruses —pathogens is a useful word to include them all—it will be convenient to abandon direct chronology and trace separately the two phases of the battle. Firstly we shall describe the attack on the germ outside the body and then go on to consider the means both natural and artificial whereby the germ can be checked or killed within the body.

II. THE ATTACK ON THE GERM OUTSIDE THE BODY

(a) Listerism

The distressing condition of the surgical wards in hospitals before the days of antiseptics has already been described. The frightful mortality, not only among those who came into hospital with open wounds, but worse still those who became victims of sepsis through the direct intervention of the operator, was a mysterious Nemesis which came swiftly and suddenly to wreck the handiwork of even the most skilful surgeon. Of course no one could have failed to notice that these hospital diseases attacked only those patients who had broken skins. A simple fracture with the skin intact mended quite readily, whereas a compound fracture with its open wound often ended in tragedy.

Joseph Lister, born in 1827 of Quaker parents, was teaching surgery at the Royal Infirmary in Glasgow in 1865 when he began

[1] *Acute anterior poliomyelitis* (a name often abbreviated into 'polio').

his researches on wound infection, but even before this he was pointing out to his class that anyone who should explain this difference and enable an open wound to behave like a closed one would be among the greatest benefactors of his age.

Now that Pasteur had shown that decomposition was due not to the air but to the living organisms carried by particles of dust, Lister saw that here in the work of the French chemist lay the beautifully simple key to the situation. His patients were suffering 'from the evils alluded to in a way that was sickening and often heart-rending, so as to make me feel it a questionable privilege to be connected with the institution';[1] and all because, as he rightly surmised, there were living organisms which found their way on to the open surfaces of wounds. His object, then, must be to destroy the germs in the wound and, by insisting on the absolute cleanliness of the instruments, the dressings and anything that might come in contact with the wound, so prevent the infection. Pasteur had shown how to destroy organisms by heat or how to remove them by filtration and there was the third method of antiseptic chemical solutions. This was the one that Lister thought would be best. As all the world knows, carbolic acid (phenol) was the substance he chose and this, in a way, was unfortunate because it was falsely asserted that Lister had claimed to be the first to use this compound. This led to endless bitterness, although he repeatedly stated in public that he set no store by any specific virtue in carbolic, but that the principles of the Antiseptic Method were strict attention to technique in preventing the access of organisms to a wound, and that without this there was no magic in any chemical whatsoever.

His carbolic spray (depicted on the Lister Centenary stamps) he abandoned later when he found that it could never do what he had supposed it to be doing—namely destroying the organisms in the air. Attention to the hands of the surgeon, the skin of the patient and the dressings and instruments were what really mattered. Unfortunately his giving up the spray was misinterpreted into his having given up his faith in antisepsis.

Of enormous importance was his discovery of the sterile catgut

[1] Lister, J., *Collected Papers*, Oxford, 1909, Vol. II, p. 123.

ligature, which became absorbed by the tissues of the patient and so did not form a source of irritation and sepsis like the usual unabsorbable silk ligature. From his Christmas holiday in 1868 throughout the whole of his active life he was constantly experimenting and improving his ligatures at a cost in sheer labour that cannot be easily appreciated. His first discovery of the absorbable ligature was made by tying the carotid artery of a living calf which was killed a month later. The result exceeded all expectations. He found the catgut gone and its site occupied by a living ring of fibrous tissue. It is well to note this circumstance, because animal-lovers have constantly belittled the humane results which have flowed directly from animal experiments. Lister, himself, in spite of a personal appeal from the Queen that he should condemn such practices, asserted before the Royal Commission on Vivisection,[1] that without animal experiments his results could not have been achieved.

It is not possible here to trace in detail the early experiments of Lister, with various mixtures containing carbolic acid or metallic antiseptics—his carbolized oil, his cyanide gauze—which have led gradually, but directly, to the elaborate aseptic ritual which can be seen daily in the operating theatre of any hospital. It may here be mentioned that the use of rubber gloves by surgeons and nurses was introduced by William S. Halsted at Johns Hopkins Hospital, Baltimore, in 1889. His primary purpose was to protect the operators' hands from the antiseptics, but it soon became evident that the gloves protected the patient too. The gauze face-masks were first advocated by Johann von Miculicz at Breslau (now Wroclaw) in 1896, following the discovery by his bacteriologist colleague Karl Flügge that even during quiet speech droplets containing bacteria are sprayed into the air.

The importance of Lister's work lay not in the discovery of antiseptic chemicals (indeed, as Sir R. J. Godlee pointed out in his Life of *Lord Lister*, antiseptics have been used empirically from time immemorial; for example, the Good Samaritan poured into the wounds oil and wine), but in his practical application of Pasteur's discoveries, his tireless work in perfecting details of technique and not least in the vigorous fight in which he was

[1] London, 1876, *Royal Commission. Minutes of Evidence.*

forced to engage before his work was accepted by all. The astonishing results achieved by the Antiseptic Method will be further considered when we come to discuss the reform of the hospitals.

(b) *Infection from Water and Food*

The channels of infection are by no means confined to cases of surgical wounds. There are a number of diseases which are acquired by actually swallowing the germs in food or water. Two striking instances of this mode of infection are seen in typhoid fever and cholera. From the fact that the infection is through the alimentary tract, the expectation is that an epidemic will follow the distribution of food or water; and such indeed was the case, which we may take as an example, of the great cholera epidemics which occurred in the British Isles between 1831 and 1866.

It was John Snow[1] who put forward a mass of evidence to show that cholera was in general a water-borne disease. It had long been noticed that the pestilence came out of the East along the great trade routes, from port to port, 'never going faster than people travel'. Snow clearly stated that some material passes from the sick to the healthy, 'which has the property of increasing and multiplying in the systems of the persons it attacks. . . . As cholera commences with an affection of the alimentary canal . . . it follows that morbid material producing cholera must be introduced into the alimentary canal . . . must, in fact, be swallowed accidentally'. He went on to point out how by uncleanliness the swallowing of 'minute quantities of ejections and dejections' is favoured; how cholera spreads most easily and rapidly among the dirt of the very poor; and how the mining population suffered so much because they worked eight hours at a stretch and consequently took down their food which they ate with unwashed hands in the pits which were little better than 'one huge privy'.

In some districts of London the water supplies were nothing more or less than diluted sewage, the water being polluted by leaking sewers and overflowing cesspools. A fearful outbreak of cholera occurred in Broad Street, Soho, and caused 500 deaths in

[1] Snow, J. *On the Mode of Communication of Cholera*, 2nd ed., London, 1855.

ten days—and the mortality would have been worse had not the populace taken refuge in flight. Snow traced nearly all these deaths to the pump which stood in Broad Street and he tried to stop the outbreak by the simple manœuvre of removing the pump handle.

More convincing than this was the information he collected in London, south of the river. This area was supplied with water by different companies which overlapped in some areas. 'It is extremely worthy of remark,' wrote Snow, 'that whilst only 563 deaths occurred in the whole metropolis in the four weeks ending August 5th (1853), more than one-half of them took place amongst the customers of the Southwark and Vauxhall company and a great proportion of the remaining deaths were those of mariners and persons employed in the shipping in the Thames, who almost invariably drew their drinking water directly from the river.'

Of course the matter was hotly contested. Many adhered to the old theories of miasmata and epidemic influences. It was only reasonable to blame the air, and besides there was no vested interest in the atmosphere and so, unlike the water, which had sturdy champions in the directors of the various water companies, the air went undefended.

Snow gave excellent advice, including cleanliness about the sick and the sterilization of infected bed-linen, the importance of obtaining clean, or failing this, boiled water for drinking. He added that it was unwise to hide from the people that cholera was communicable with the object of preventing panic. A true knowledge of the cause was likely to be far more helpful.

Cholera in epidemic form has not visited this island since 1866, and there is no doubt that this is due not only to quarantine measures, but more than anything to the excellent sewerage systems and pure water supply which we now enjoy; in fact to the application of the knowledge that cholera is a water-borne disease. It was not until 1884 that Koch was able to announce that the Berlin Conference that he had isolated the causative organism, called the comma bacillus, which he had found in Egypt and in India.

Water is not the only article of diet that can spread disease. Tuberculosis germs were found often enough in cow's milk. The diphtheria bacillus too can grow in milk without giving rise to any change in the appearance or taste. Malta fever is spread through drinking raw goat's milk. There is also an important group of diseases which are spread by food. One used to hear much of 'ptomaine' poisoning, but when it is realized that ptomaines are chemical products of putrefaction and that any food containing enough to do anyone a serious mischief would be likely to be extremely offensive both to the nose and the palate, we cannot suppose that more than a small fraction of all cases of food-poisoning can be simply due to the presence of ptomaines. The truth is that in most cases living germs are swallowed. These produce various forms of gastro-enteritis. One of the most destructive of such organisms is the dysentery bacillus, discovered by Kigoshi Shiga in 1898. Dysentery was rife among the troops engaged in the Crimean War and again in the ill-fated Gallipoli campaign in 1915, during the First World War. Indeed, in the course of history, this one species of bacillus has destroyed whole armies.

Botulism is another form of food-poisoning which, though less common, has a very high mortality. In August 1922 eight people died within a few days of eating sandwiches of wild-duck paste at Loch Maree in Ross-shire, and the lethal *bacillus botulinus* was isolated from the paste. Apart from three deaths in London in 1935 from botulism after eating nut-meat brawn, this is the only recorded outbreak in these islands. Such poisoning, however, occurs from time to time in Europe and America, so that we may expect that sooner or later further outbreaks may happen here. Fortunately meat containing this poison almost always looks and smells peculiar. At Loch Maree no doubt the strong flavour of the wild-duck paste masked the peculiarity. The toxin of botulism is one of the most powerful poisons known.

(c) Carriers of Infection

It has been shown that an unsuspected source of infection lies in certain individuals who, though in perfect health themselves, carry about and distribute pathogenic bacteria among those who come into contact with them. These 'carriers', as they are called, have sometimes suffered shortly before from the disease in question. This is usually so with typhoid carriers. With diphtheria on the other hand the carriers have often not had the disease themselves, while with the meningococcus, the organism of cerebro-spinal meningitis, we find the extraordinary fact that the number of carriers enormously exceeds that of the persons who actually take or have taken the disease. The importance of carriers in keeping diseases endemic among populations is at once obvious, though, as we shall see later, we now have means of protecting the community so effectively that diphtheria and typhoid can be abolished altogether if the community will take proper precautions. The danger from carriers has been enormously increased by the speed of modern travel. An infective person may be distributing cholera or typhoid for days or months and in that time have travelled round the world scattering infection broadcast. Quarantine methods therefore cannot be totally effective and we must rely upon active immunization, as will be apparent in the next sections of this book.

Animals other than man can act as carriers. The fatal disease hydrophobia may follow the bite of a mad dog, but, it has been possible to eradicate this disease in Great Britain by strict quarantine for dogs and muzzling orders when necessary. On the Continent the matter is much more difficult owing to the impossibility of effective quarantine. Another difficulty is that dogs are not the only animals which can spread rabies (as the disease is called when it affects animals). Cats, jackals, wolves, ruminants and even human beings have been the rabid biters. In Trinidad certain bats have been found to carry the infection. One further example of illness caused by animal bites is the rat-bite fever of Japan, in which rats can inoculate man with the organism called *Spirochaeta morsus-muris*.

Insects are responsible in a far greater degree for some disastrous afflictions, from which enormous numbers of persons have perished in the past and are likely to do in the future. The first discovery of insect-borne disease was made in 1879 by Patrick Manson,[1] who showed how the embryos of a worm which causes a

[1] Manson, P., *Journal of the Linnaean Society*, London, 1879, XIV, pp. 304–311.

common tropical disease are taken from the blood of an infected man by a female mosquito; how these embryos develop inside the mosquito and are then injected into another man when he is bitten by the same insect. This was a discovery of tremendous importance, though it was not so regarded at the time. None the less it was directly due to this theory of insect-borne disease that Ronald Ross, in 1898, was able to prove that the parasite of malaria (which had been discovered eighteen years earlier by Alphonse Laveran[1] in Algeria) is conveyed from man to man in just the same way. He demonstrated that the parasite has a double life-cycle; One set of changes occurs in the body of man *at regular intervals*, which accounts for the well-known regularity of the recurring fever of malaria (men spoke of quotidien, tertian or quartan agues, according to the interval between the feverish bouts). The other cycle of change goes on inside a definite species of mosquito, until the spit-glands are heavily charged with malarial spores, ready to infect the next victim of the hungry mosquito.

The cause found, the remedy becomes evident. Malaria is no longer a bad air, an exhalation from the marshes, but a phase in the life-cycle of a known organism. To abolish the spread of malaria it is necessary to break the life-cycle at some point. The first and most obvious method is to avoid being bitten by the mosquito and, since its habits are nocturnal, the provision of fine-mesh nets in windows and mosquito-proof nets over beds can protect those who stay indoors after dark.

The next method is to try to destroy the mosquitoes themselves. The anti-mosquito campaign began in 1901 and has met with considerable success, though constant vigilance and perseverance are needed, because in the absence of preventive measures the mosquitoes breed at an alarming rate. The eggs are laid on the surface of stagnant water. Little wriggling larvae are hatched and the full-grown insect emerges from the water in from seven to ten days.

There are four main methods at our disposal for destroying the insects. We can dry up their breeding-grounds or convert the stagnant pools into running streams, we can poison the larvae, we can asphyxiate them or we can employ predatory animals to eat

[1] Laveran, A., *Comptes Rendues de l'Academie des Sciences*, Paris, XCIII, p. 627.

them. The poisoning has been done with 'paris green' (aceto-arsenite of copper). The asphyxiation is brought about by pouring oil on the surface of the stagnant water—diesel oil, kerosene or waste oil is commonly used—so that the larvae cannot come up to breathe. Small predatory fish will feed with avidity on the 'wrigglers' and have proved of great value. In spite of all these ways of killing off mosquitoes (supplemented more recently by the newer insecticide sprays for indoor use) there are often many difficulties in practice; for example, it is almost impossible to deal with every collection of stagnant water, and any small quantity, such as might occur in the fork of a tree or a puddle is quite sufficient for the breeding of mosquitoes provided it remains in existence for the few days required for the eggs to develop completely.

Furthermore there is more than one species of mosquito which can carry malaria and the species often have different habits. One kind may breed in small pools, puddles, quarries or wheel-ruts, whereas another may prefer large fresh-water swamps or a third brackish swamps. 'Only about one species of anopheles in ten carries malaria and care must be taken to do nothing that would increase the number of the dangerous species. Indeed the unwary medical officer may easily stir up a virulent outburst of malaria by the adoption of a method that would be 100 per cent successful in another type of land perhaps only a few miles away.'[1]

Yellow fever—or the yellow jack—the appalling pestilence which has played such havoc in the tropics, had its chief seats in Central America and the West Coast of Africa. At the beginning of the present century it had already been suggested that a mosquito was the vector of the infection, when the American Army Board, under the leadership of Walter Reed, was sent to Havana to investigate the matter. The story of the fight against yellow fever is one of heroism and tragedy, but the struggle ended in a magnificent triumph.

The main difficulty was that it had not been possible to transmit the disease to any animal and consequently, if experiments were to be done, there must be human volunteers willing to run the risk of taking this loathsome disease. One of the Board, James Carroll, was

[1] Sir Malcolm Watson, *The Times*, July 1st, 1932, p. 15.

the first volunteer to be bitten by an infected mosquito and he was fortunate to survive the attack of yellow fever which resulted. Carroll found that the disease could be produced by the injection of blood or serum, even if it were filtered, as effectively as by mosquito-bite. This was proof that yellow fever was caused by a virus. On the other hand the seven men who volunteered to sleep in bedding of yellow fever patients failed to take the disease, provided they were protected from mosquitoes. This proved that the fever was not communicable except by inoculation.

Other investigators were not so fortunate as Carroll. J. W. Lazear, also a member of the Board, died of yellow fever through being accidentally bitten. In 1928 the brilliant Japanese bacteriologist Hideyo Noguchi met a similar fate in Africa, where he had gone to search out the true cause, because the spirochaete which he had claimed as the causative organism had been exonerated. So also died Adrian Stokes, whose great contribution was his discovery that certain Asiatic rhesus monkeys could be successfully inoculated.[1] This discovery did away with the necessity for human volunteers.

The results of this brilliant piece of research have shown that these men did not die in any useless cause. War was declared on the swarms of death-dealing insects. In 1901 William C. Gorgas, the chief Sanitary Officer of Havana, began by screening all the yellow fever patients from mosquitoes, thus preventing the infection of the insects. Then, by an unbelievably energetic campaign against the vector mosquito, *Stegomyia fasciata*, also known as *Aëdes aegypti*, he succeeded in three short months in clearing Havana of a plague that had hardly been absent in recent history. In 1900 there had been 1,400 cases in Havana; in 1902 there were none. Through the efforts of the same man Panama, which had long been a veritable pest-hole, became one of the healthiest of places. Without this work the canal could never have been completed. It had been started by de Lesseps as long ago as 1882, but the work had been abandoned because of the yellow jack. The project was resumed once the Americans had the disease under control and they were able to complete the canal in 1914 (though it was not formally opened by President Wilson until 1920).

[1] Stokes, Bauer and Hudson, *Amer. Jour. Trop. Med.*, 1928, 8, p. 103.

The Germ Theory

In spite of the successful campaigns against yellow fever, the danger of its spread is very real. The distribution of *Aëdes aegypti* has been widely studied and it has been found to extend over immense tracts of the earth, in every continent, not excluding Europe, so that presumably it is only necessary for some one with yellow fever to travel to such areas to provoke an explosive outbreak. Furthermore it has been shown that the disease occurs naturally in certain monkeys who may therefore keep the disease going as an enzootic one. In addition there is good evidence that *Aëdes aegypti* is not the only vector, for in South America, in the emerald-mining village of Muzo, for example, epidemics have occurred in *spite of the absence of Aëdes aegypti*.[1] Apart from mosquito control, which is always difficult, active immunization of people against yellow fever is the best method of protection.

In parts of Africa there is a disease with which the inhabitants are only too familiar, which kills slowly with long fever, protracted wasting and increasing lethargy. This is the African sleeping-sickness (not to be confused with the European encephalitis lethargica, called sleepy sickness).

An organism of the kind known as trypanosome had been found, in New Zealand, by David Bruce, in the blood of cattle suffering from nagama, which causes fever, oedema, anaemia, emaciation and death. In 1894 Bruce showed that these trypanosomes were conveyed from big game to domestic animals by the tsetse fly, *Glossina morsitans*. Undoubtedly the wild animals were the sole source, because where there was no game there was no nagama.

Aldo Castellani, a graduate of the University of Florence, and later trained at the London School of Tropical Medicine, was one of three members of the Royal Society Commission sent to Africa to investigate sleeping sickness in Uganda. In 1902 Castellani found trypanosomes in the cerebro-spinal fluid in patients suffering from the disease. He suspected that tsetse flies were the vector of the parasites. By carefully mapping the geographical distribution of the various species of fly and that of sleeping-sickness cases, he was able to show that *Glossina palpalis* was the species involved.

The means of prevention were firstly the destruction of the flies

[1] League of Nations, *Epidemiological Report on Yellow Fever*, Geneva, 1935, p. 120.

and secondly the temporary clearing of the population from the fly-areas, so that the infected flies would die out. This last method proved ineffective, either because there was a reservoir of illicit population living in or near the fly-area, or because animals also carried the trypanosomes. If the animal hypothesis was true, it was suggested that the big game should be wiped out; but such a course would be difficult, expensive and repugnant. There is little doubt that the destruction of the flies can be made effective by the proper reclamation of land, because tsetse flies cannot live in intensively cultivated areas. A capital example of a really successful campaign in a limited area was that carried out in the three years from 1911 to 1913 in the Portuguese island of Principe off the west coast of Africa. Here, in addition to clearing the thickets draining the land and segregating those infected from the flies, an ingenious method was used for trapping the insects. Ten men, in white clothes with protective headgear, each carried on his back a square of dark-coloured cloth spread with bird-lime. They were set to walk in pairs through the infested clearings. In this way 470,000 flies were caught. Principe was cleared completely of a scourge which had previously accounted for one third of the total deaths on the island. *Glossina palpalis* became extinct.[1]

A further interesting proof that the tsetse flies are the sole vector can be seen in retrospect. Many negro slaves imported into the New World died of African Sleeping-Sickness; but the tsetse flies remained in Africa and the disease did not spread.

The bubonic plague in epidemic form is now a matter of history in this country, but history which is gruesome enough when we recall that the Black Death in 1348–9 accounted for one half of the inhabitants of this island and probably one quarter of the population of the known earth. But the plague is not dead and may yet come again out of the East, where it dwells widely but patchily endemic. Indeed in the last years of the nineteenth century the old scourge threatened the whole world. From Hong Kong in 1894 it spread to India, Japan, Turkey and Russia. In 1897 it was at Madagascar and the Mauritius; by 1899 it was in Europe again and in the same year it reached Hawaii. In India alone, between 1898

[1] League of Nations Health Organization, *Further Report on Tuberculosis and Sleeping Sickness*, Geneva, 1925, p. 62.

and 1918 there have been recorded more than ten million deaths from plague.

It was in 1893–4 at the beginning of this pandemic, that the plague bacillus was identified independently by Shibasaburo Kitasato and Alexandre Yersin at Hong Kong. Later it was found that the disease spread in a way quite unlike anything then known. The plague is, in the first place, a disease of rodents and in particular of rats and is conveyed from rat to rat by the bites of fleas. These same fleas may bite human beings. When the rat dies of the plague, the fleas leave the body as it cools and seek fresh victims and so the plague is spread.

This discovery throws some light on various pestilences recorded in history. When the Philistines had carried the ark of God to Gath, the Lord 'smote the men of the city both small and great, and they had emerods in their secret parts'. In order to appease the Lord the priests and diviners advised offerings of golden 'images of your emerod and images of your *mice* that mar the land.'[1] Surely it is significant that the rodent and the bubo (or emerod) should be connected in this way.

The prevention of plague therefore consists in keeping down the number of rats, avoiding human contact with them and protecting people from flea-bites with the newer insecticides. There are certain foci where there is always some plague among the rodents; for example a district in the South-West Himalayas. Besides rats, other rodents which carry the plague are the ground-squirrels of California and the gerbilles in Africa. It is important to prevent the rats from migrating from one country to another in ships and to stop them landing large metal discs are placed on the mooring-ropes of ships in port. If any ship arrives with the plague on board, the essential work is to destroy the rats by chemical fumigation.

The louse is yet another parasite that can carry serious disease. The three fevers, relapsing fever, trench fever and typhus are all conveyed by lice. In these instances it seems that it is not the bite that conveys the infection, but that irritation causes scratching and thus the victim inoculates himself with the virus present in the excreta of the lice.

Relapsing fever, or famine fever is a malady of which we hear

[1] Samuel, V and VI.

little in this country today, though it still flourishes in eastern Europe, Asia and Central and South America; but during the last century this disease, together with typhus (gaol fever) and dysentery caused frightful distress in Ireland. These three furies came savagely on the unfortunate people in the middle of the appalling potato famine in 1847. A correspondent, writing from Dingle, says; 'The state of the people of this locality is horrifying. Fever, famine and dysentery are daily increasing, deaths from hunger daily occurring, average weekly twenty—men, women and children thrown into the graves without a coffin—dead bodies in all parts of the country, being several days dead before discovered—no inquests to inquire how they came by their death, as hunger has hardened the hearts of the people.'[1]

The causative organism of relapsing fever is a spirochaete, discovered by Otto Obermeier during the Berlin epidemic of 1867–8 and it has been found to be transferred by blood-sucking parasites. In the Congo and in Central and South America it is carried by a tick and accordingly is known as 'tick fever', whereas in Europe, Asia and North Africa it is lice which are responsible.

Gaol fever, or typhus, is uncommon where sanitation and hygiene have left their mark, but it was with us in Britain well into the nineteenth century. It is still endemic in some parts of the globe and, indeed, it follows closely the geography and the history of dilapidation and dirt, wretchedness and war. Typhus used to occur regularly, not only in goals, but also in the armed forces. It has been suggested that the fever of the Royal Navy was constantly recruited from the prisons by the press-gangs who impressed the newly discharged convicts.

The causative organism was named by da Roche Lima, in 1916 *Rikettsia prowazekii*, to commemorate Howard Ricketts and Staislaus von Prowazek who had both fallen martyrs to the study of this disease. The Rickettsiae are minute organisms which form a class by themselves. They are not only much smaller than ordinary bacteria, being near the optical limits of the compound microscope, but are difficult to stain. They were first described, in 1909, by Ricketts in the blood of patients ill with Rocky Mountain spotted

[1] O'Rourke, J., *History of the Great Irish Famine of 1847*, 2nd edn., Dublin, 1879(?), p. 409.

fever, a disease akin to typhus. In 1910 he found similar organisms in the blood of typhus patients and in the excreta of lice. Von Prowazek confirmed these observations in Serbia in 1916.

The prevention of these louse-borne diseases is simple in principle and consists essentially in preventing the louse from changing its host, by stopping overcrowding and thoroughly 'delousing' the inhabitants. This process has been greatly simplified by the introduction of D.D.T.

The story of D.D.T. is of great historical interest. Chemically it is one of the chlorinated hydrocarbons, the initials standing for the substance dichlor-diphenyl-trichlor-ethane. It was first made in a laboratory in 1874, but more than sixty years elapsed before its extraordinary value as an insecticide was discovered. In the First World War the three louse-borne diseases, typhus, relapsing fever and trench fever had caused terrible havoc among the troops engaged in trench warfare, where any form of personal hygiene was impossible. In 1939 the authorities in this country were well aware that the new war would see a repetition of the disaster if nothing was done.

Fortunately D.D.T. was found to be an almost perfect insecticide, for it killed lice in dilutions at which it was quite harmless to man. It was only necessary to impregnate underwear with a solution of D.D.T. to secure immunity from lice for a matter of weeks at a time. As a result of this discovery louse-borne infections were completely controlled among the British troops during the Second World War. It was a secret weapon, unknown to the enemy and it certainly went a long way towards securing final victory for the Allies.

(d) Air-borne Diseases

There is another important channel by which disease germs may enter the human body, namely the respiratory tract. Pasteur had shown that the air in inhabited places was swarming with micro-organisms; but most of these are harmless. None the less harmful germs certainly do get loose about the air. A person coughs or sneezes and throws into the air a fine spray of innumerable droplets. A patient may be suffering from some respiratory disease or he may be a 'carrier'. He may be coughing diphtheria or scarlet fever into the air. When a person with consumption spits into the street, the sputum dries to form a fine powder which may be carried to others on the wind. There has been much dispute about whether pulmonary tuberculosis (consumption) gains entry by the air or by the mouth, but it is now fairly generally agreed that most cases arise from inhaling the bacilli.

The air, as we have seen from the miasma theory, from time immemorial has been suspect. The great prison reformer, John Howard, believed that the poisonous effluvia of the noisome dungeons he inspected were the cause of gaol fever. Florence Nightingale too declared her belief that fever arose *de novo* from bad air and filth. Diseases were seen to spread rapidly and mysteriously and it is therefore not surprising that the air was blamed. In 1750 the prisoners at the Old Bailey conveyed their typhus fever (surely through the air, it was thought) even to the Bar and Bench, so that many died, including the Lord Mayor and other notables.[1]

More than a hundred years ago Maidstone gaol was rid of typhus by the energetic use of soap, water, quicklime, clean clothes, sulphur and nourishing food.[2] The same methods are used today with fuller knowledge of the rationale. Thus we see that gradually the number of diseases for which the air can be blamed is declining, but it seems certain that some of the respiratory diseases at least will remain in this category.

In some cases the remarkable rapidity with which a disease will spread almost forces us to the conclusion that it is conveyed through the air. For example, it is stated that in the island of Wharekauri, 480 miles east of New Zealand, the visit of a ship to the island was followed by a four-day illness, called 'murri-murri', of both whites and coloured, 'The mere appearance of murri-murri is proof to the inhabitants even at distant parts of the island, which is thirty miles long, that a ship is in port.[3]

[1] Creighton, op. cit., II, p. 93.

[2] Sweating, *The Sanitation of Public Institutions*, Howard Prize Essay, London, 1884.

[3] Creighton, op. cit., II, p. 432. See also Boswell, J., *Journal of a Tour to the Hebrides with Samuel Johnson, LL.D.*, where the latter 'disputed the truth of what is said, as to the people of St Kilda catching cold whenever strangers come'.

In many of these influenza-like illnesses it is certain that the air is the channel of infection, but can germs travel long distances in the air and appear spontaneously at some distant site? Considering the fact that disease can almost always be kept out by strict quarantine this seems unlikely. On the other hand it was shown by the United States Bureau of Plant Industry that the spores of black stem rust, a serious menace to American wheat, could be collected on glass microscope slides, by means of an aeroplane, at the astonishing height of ten thousand feet. These spores fall so slowly that it has been calculated that regions a thousand miles and more to the leeward of the original source *might* become infected. We must therefore not be too sure about how far germs may travel in air; but it is important to remember that viruses are essentially parasitic and are always found in association with living matter, so that it does not seem likely that they are borne passively for long distances on the wind. We have also to consider that common pests like the house-fly can, and often do, act in the rôle of disease-carriers, infecting our food with their germ-laden feet as they fly from dunghill where they breed to the dinner-table where they feed.

III. THE ATTACK ON THE GERM INSIDE THE BODY

(a) The Conception of Immunity

It must have been noticed at a very early stage in the history of man that certain infectious diseases rarely, if ever, attacked the same person twice. Thucydides plainly states that no one was ever attacked a second time, or not with a fatal result, by the plague at Athens in 430 B.C., and this belief was so strong in those who had recovered that they even entertained the innocent fancy that they could not die of anything else.

The practice of inoculation of smallpox with the idea of 'getting it over' and in the hope of inducing a mild attack came to us first from eastern Europe. It is supposed that this practice originally contained no idea of engendering in the body antidotes to the contagion, but was intended either by magical symbolism or scientifically to rid the patient of the disease by passing it on to another

[1] *Nature*, 1932, cxxlx, p. 754.

person or animal. It is said that this idea is shown in the scapegoat of the Israelites and in the miracle of the swine of Gadara. This kind of belief, which still exists, regards a disease as an entity, a sort of possessive devil, as it were, which goes from one person to another. Our modern concept, in contrast, is that contagious disease is due to infecting organisms and that any immunity that develops is due to the building up by the body of specific substances which either kill the germs in the body or neutralize the poisons given out by them.

Inoculation of smallpox matter from a mild case was almost always successful, if it produced an artificial attack, in preventing a subsequent natural one. The method was widely used in the latter part of the eighteenth century, but unfortunately it was not always possible to gauge the virulence of the inoculated matter, so that the results were sometimes fatal and often disfiguring. Nevertheless numbers of people were successfully protected from smallpox by this means and without disfigurement, if we may judge from the remark of Mrs Hardcastle in Goldsmith's *She Stoops to Conquer*: 'I vow, since inoculation began, there is no such thing to be seen as a plain woman.' The story of Jenner's substitution of vaccination (the inoculation of cow-pox) for the more dangerous practice has already been told. This was the beginning of the science of immunology.

No further progress was made until the time of Pasteur. Following his brilliant demonstration of the microbic nature of disease, he went on to discover preventive inoculation. It began almost accidentally. He had been studying the disease of fowls known as 'chicken cholera', of which the causative organism had already been found. One evening he inoculated a bird with a stale culture of chicken cholera germs, some six weeks old. The bird sickened slightly and then recovered. Using the same bird and a fresh tube of virulent germs, he was interested to find that the bird was now resistant to the infection, although the germs were fully virulent to any normal chicken. He was quick to see the prime importance of his discovery. The oxygen of the air was responsible for the attenuation of the germs. He could now cultivate germs to any lessened virulence that he desired and with these produce an immunity to future infection.

These studies led him to try to provide a preventive inoculation for sheep and cattle against anthrax (splenic fever). With the discovery that the virulence of germs could be attenuated or reinforced by passing the germs through different animals—that is by inoculating the animals and recovering the germs later in a fresh culture from the animal—he brought this line of research to a triumphant conclusion. In 1882 he completely annihilated the opposition of those who had contradicted his opinions and impugned his scientific honesty by the world-famous and classical experiment on the farm of Pouilly-le-Fort near Melun. Here he had three groups of sheep. The first group, consisting of ten sheep, were the control animals. Of the remaining fifty, twenty-five had previously been inoculated with an attenuated culture of living anthrax germs and twenty-five had not. In the presence of an interested audience of friends and sceptics, Pasteur publicly injected all but his control group with a virulent culture of anthrax germs. To the confusion of his enemies and jubilation of his friends all of the unprotected sheep died, just as he had predicted, while the inoculated ones remained alive and well.

Hydrophobia was the first human disease which he tried to prevent by inoculation. He started with the assumption that the rabid virus was in the spittle of the mad dog. He was unable at first to transmit the disease to animals by inoculating them with human saliva from a patient with hydrophobia. It then occurred to him that, from the nature of the symptoms, it was likely that the virus attacked the central nervous system. He found that he could convey the disease to animals by trephining them. Thus he came to use the central nervous system of rabbits as a culture medium for growing the virus, which of course he could not see with the microscope since it belongs to the class of 'filterable viruses'. By drying the infected spinal cord from rabbits for varying lengths of time, he could produce samples which might have their virulence attenuated to any degree he required.

It was clear from the outset that it would be impossible to inoculate all the dogs in France, because there were some hundred thousand in Paris alone and two and a half million in the provinces; and each dog would have had to have several injections. Pasteur therefore decided that the method must be one which could be applied to human beings *after* they had been bitten by mad dogs. Courageously, but with some mistrust of a treatment which up to then he had used only on dogs, he began by inoculating with increasing strengths of virus a little Alsatian boy of nine years old, Josef Meister, who had been bitten in fourteen places by a mad dog. There was no doubt at all that the dog had rabies and Pasteur adopted the method as the only hope of saving the boy from a certain and very painful death. The result was successful and, as all the world soon knew, the boy remained well. This was in 1885 and it marked the beginning of the justly celebrated Pasteur treatment for the prevention of hydrophobia. It was followed by the inauguration of the Pasteur Institute in Paris in 1888. At present there are Pasteur Institutes scattered throughout the world and in these persons bitten by rabid animals are given one or another modification of Pasteur's original treatment.

Pasteur looked on these inoculations as preventive and not curative. His high hope was that every infectious disease could be combated in the same way, but unfortunately success with attenuated living viruses was limited until more recent times.

(b) Immune Sera

A further phase in the fight against infectious disease can best be traced by studying the history of diphtheria. This was a mysterious sickness. Before the middle of the nineteenth century it was little known and the older epidemics of 'throat-distemper' cannot be definitely assigned to diphtheria or to scarlet fever. Quite suddenly between 1856 and 1859 diphtheria, as we know it, became common. In 1884 Friedrich A. J. Loeffler isolated the bacillus (which had first been observed by Theodor Klebs) from the throats of diphtheria patients and was able to reproduce the disease in animals. Later it was found that this bacillus does not spread throughout the body like anthrax, but remains localized in the throat or wherever it first takes root. In 1885 it was shown by Pierre Roux and Alexandre Yersin that the serious and often fatal complications of diphtheria were caused by a powerful toxin which is produced by the bacillus and which circulates in the blood.

At the Pasteur Institute it was shown that by inoculating a horse with gradually increasing doses of this toxin, it was possible to make the horse immune to further large doses. (We are reminded of the method used on himself by Mithridates IV, king of Pontus, to protect himself from death by poison.) The horse is bled, the blood allowed to clot and the serum filtered off. The antitoxic strength of this serum is standardized by measuring its protective action on guinea-pigs against a standard dose of toxin. This antitoxic serum proved of enormous value in treating diphtheria, but it had to be used promptly and in large amounts. As a result there were often complications, some of them serious. More recently purification and concentration of the antitoxin by purely chemical means enabled much smaller doses of serum to be thoroughly effective without the risk of untoward side effects.

It must be noticed that the principles involved in vaccines and sera are quite different. A vaccine consists either of living or dead germs which provoke the formation of resistance in the body. An antitoxic serum, on the other hand is an animal blood-serum containing substances that can neutralize bacterial poisons.

Diphtheria antitoxin can be used not only in the treatment of the disease, but also during epidemics to immunize those at risk. The antitoxin brings about rapid immunity, but unhappily it is not a lasting one and it disappears in a few days or weeks. Such a 'passive' immunity is therefore of limited use. The next step was to try to procure some lasting immunity. If the horse can produce antitoxin when injected with toxin, cannot the same process be applied to man? Unfortunately the toxin as such is far too dangerous, but it was found that it could be modified by treatment with formalin in such a way that the virulence was lowered, but the power to confer immunity was retained. A similar effect could be produced by using a judicious mixture of toxin and antitoxin. By this method von Behring, in 1907, started the practice of 'active immunization,' which was shown to confer a lasting immunity to diphtheria.

Statistics have shown that diphtheria is more prevalent in certain social classes and in certain age-groups. This is because some people have antitoxin circulating in their blood, giving them a natural immunity. In 1913 Bela Schick invented the intradermal test for susceptibility to diphtheria. A minute and measured dose of standardized toxin is injected into the thickness of the skin of the forearm. A positive reaction is a red flush, appearing at the site of the injection a day or two later and this means that there is little or no resistance to diphtheria. Those who show no reaction are immune. In this way it was possible to decide which individuals needed active immunization.

In the decade between 1914 and 1924 the new methods of immunization had produced very striking results in New York where the incidence of diphtheria fell dramatically. In England the use of the Schick test, followed by active immunization of all those negative to the test, was started as a public health service in 1921 in the borough of Holborn. By this time it was clear that immunization gave almost certain protection against the disease. The modified toxin, now called toxoid, was much safer than the toxinantitoxin mixture and had the advantage that only one injection was needed. Later it was decided to dispense with the Schick test for general purposes and offer active immunization to all children. In England and Wales, before the National Immunization Campaign began in 1940, more than 50,000 cases were notified annually, with some 3,000 deaths. With the provision of free immunization, especially for infants, the position so far improved that in 1959 there were no deaths from diphtheria. The complete disappearance of the disease could not last, but today diphtheria is an uncommon occurrence and the annual deaths can normally be reckoned on the fingers of one hand.

In tetanus (lock-jaw) the causal organism gains entry through a wound. The germs produce a powerful toxin, without themselves being disseminated throughout the body, in this respect behaving like the diphtheria bacillus. It was found that antitetanic serum, prepared in a similar way to the anti-diphtheritic serum, was very effective in lowering the incidence of tetanus. Here the circumstances are ideal for the use of passive immunity, because the risk is only for the short time during which the wound remains infected. This technique is now used as a routine measure in all cases where there are dirty wounds, especially those contaminated with mud or manure.

During the First World War the use of anitetanic serum was introduced in October 1914. In September 15·9 per thousand of the wounded in the British forces developed tetanus and by October the figure had risen to 31·8; but the following month saw a dramatic drop to 1·7. In the Second World War a still more important measure was introduced, namely active immunization against tetanus by the use of toxoid. Again it was found that treatment of the toxin with formalin deprived it of its toxicity while preserving its power to confer immunity. Active immunization was introduced into the British Army in 1938 and was always supplemented by an injection of antitoxin to any man wounded. In the United States all personnel were immunized with three doses of toxoid, with a 'booster' dose after a year had elapsed. The result of these wholesale immunizations was that tetanus, which was formerly one of the most destructive elements in warfare, was reduced to an insignificant factor. In the Peninsular War, by contrast, the incidence of tetanus among the wounded had been as high as 12·5 per thousand.

Passive immunity had also proved of value in other diseases, in the form of sera prepared from the blood of human beings convalescing from some infectious condition. In 1901 Francesco Cenci began to use convalescent serum in the treatment of measles, and in 1910 it was also shown that convalescent sera from cases of poliomyelitis could protect monkeys from paralysis if given early enough after they had been infected. It is clear that such convalescent sera are only likely to contain protective factors in diseases where one attack gives lasting immunity. Measles is a notable example of this. It was also found that by timing the injection judiciously, that is by giving it between the fifth and ninth days after contact with the infecting case, it was possible to ensure a very mild attack of measles which conferred the same lasting immunity that a full-scale attack invariably brings about.

Many other specific sera have been tried, but with varying success. Many of them, especially in respiratory diseases, have now been superseded by the newer chemotherapeutic and antibiotic agents.

A Hundred Years of Medicine

(c) Vaccines

Pasteur believed that immunity could be acquired only by infection with living pathogens. It is to Sir Almroth Wright that we owe the introduction of vaccines made from *dead* organisms. This has the big advantage that it rules out any possibility of producing the disease itself. The classic example is the anti-typhoid inoculation. Typhoid was a disease deadly enough at home in England and Wales, where it was still causing over 5,000 deaths annually as late as the last decade of the nineteenth century. In the Crimean War it had caused greater mortality among British troops than the war itself. Wright began by trials of vaccines, made from killed typhoid bacilli, on himself and the surgeons of the Royal Victoria Hospital at Netley, and was able to show that their blood-serum developed bactericidal powers.

A beginning of wholesale inoculation of British troops was attempted in the Boer War, but owing to bitter opposition from influential persons less than 4 per cent of the soldiers had the vaccine. As a result of this blunder the Army had some 58,000 cases of typhoid (enteric) fever and about 9,000 deaths. Today all troops proceeding abroad are given vaccines made from killed typhoid bacilli, supplemented with the related para-typhoid A and B strains. There is no doubt that it is to this that we can attribute the remarkably low level of typhoid fever among the armed forces of two world wars. In the First World War, it is true, there were as many as 20,000 cases of typhoid, with over 1,000 deaths in the British Army in France; but it has been calculated that without the use of the triple vaccine (T.A.B.) one could have expected a million cases and 125,000 deaths.

It is impossible here to analyse the enormous mass of information which has been discovered about the way in which immunity is produced. Briefly it may be said that a number of substances having a hostile action on the invading germs have been demonstrated. In general they have not been isolated, but their presence is surmised from the properties of immune sera. These agents have been named, rather unhappily 'antibodies'. There are also the white blood corpuscles which can ingest and digest the germs of disease. These white cells are the 'phagocytes' of which we read in

Bernard Shaw's *The Doctor's Dilemma*. Wright also showed that there are substances, which he called opsonins, in the blood which make the micro-organism more readily devoured by the phagocytes and he invented ways of measuring the quantity of opsonins present.

In general the antibodies are *specific*; that is to say they react only towards the species of germ which induced their formation in the first place. From this it follows that they can be used for diagnosis. Thus, if a patient's blood serum will agglutinate typhoid bacilli, we can conclude that he has, or has had typhoid fever (unless he has had antityphoid vaccine, which also produces 'agglutinins'). Conversely we can use sera to identify bacteria, just because of the specificity of the antibodies.

When the *bacteriolysins*, which disintegrate bacteria, act upon them, there is also removed from the blood a third substance called the 'complement', which is normally present in human blood. It is possible to test for the presence or absence of the complement in normal blood in which we have mixed the pathogenic germs with the serum we suspect of containing antibodies. The most famous of these complement-fixation tests is the Wassermann test for syphilis, which is of great help in diagnosis. The Kahn test and others are simpler to perform and it is believed that they all detect the same antibody. Unfortunately none of these tests are infallible. Continued efforts have been made to devise a single test which would give a specific and unequivocal result, because it became known that some tests gave a positive result in non-syphilitic conditions.

In 1949 two Americans, R. A. Nelson and M. M. Meyer demonstrated their Treponema Immobilization test. The spiro-chaetes (or treponemata), which are the causal organisms of syphilis, are obtained in pure culture by a rather elaborate process involving rabbits' tissues. To a sample of the liquid is added a portion of the patient's blood-serum. If the organisms become immobilized after overnight incubation, the patient has some specific antibody and the test is positive. This is a very accurate test and the most reliable one available, but the work involved is time-consuming, complicated and expensive.

For many years all attempts to produce immunity to tuberculosis had failed. When Robert Koch had discovered the tubercle bacillus in 1882 he had hoped that his work would be the key to a certain cure for tuberculosis. Enthusiasm ran high, but Koch was modest in his claims and cannot be held responsible for the mad rush of sick and dying to Berlin. Koch had prepared a non-living toxic substance from cultures of tubercle bacilli which he named 'tuberculin'. He had hoped to use this in the treatment of tuberculosis; but the results were very disappointing. None the less tuberculin has proved of great value in other ways.

If a very small quantity of tuberculin is injected into the skin of a new-born infant who has not been infected with tuberculosis, there is very little reaction. With a healthy adult who is not clinically tuberculous, but who has at one time been infected, there is more reaction. Any animal that has once been infected is, in fact, very sensitive to the toxin. It was found that ninety per cent of persons in big towns reacted positively to tuberculin. It seems that most people are, at one time or another, the victims of a slight infection with tuberculosis, that they recover and have some kind of resistance to the disease. This accounts for the fact that, in spite of the widespread possibility of infection, only a relatively small number of people develop obvious tuberculosis. This is corroborated by the fact that, in X-ray and in post-mortem examinations, old and healed tuberculous foci are often found in people who have no history of having suffered from tuberculosis. Thus tuberculin can be used in man and in animals to ascertain whether or not there has been any tuberculous infection in the past. In this way it is possible to test cattle and to collect herds of tested cows that are guaranteed to give milk free from all tubercle bacilli. In the United States, public health laws requiring periodical tuberculin-testing of dairy herds were found very effective in eliminating the spread of tuberculosis from milk. In England and Wales, before the Second World War more than two thousand children died every year from bovine tuberculosis, almost certainly acquired from milk. Since the war it was forbidden to sell any milk from herds that had not been tested, unless it was pasteurized or otherwise heat-treated to kill bacilli. Later still tuberculin-tested herds were built up throughout the country and bovine tuberculosis in Great Britain is now a rare event.

When it became clear that tuberculin was not a cure for tuberculosis, research-workers turned their attention to prevention rather than cure. Koch had shown that a guinea-pig which had been inoculated with tuberculosis shortly afterwards became immune to a second injection. The primary infection continued its normal course and finally the animal died. By contrast the second infection, after producing a marked local inflammation, rapidly healed. This became known as 'Koch's Phenomenon'. It was argued that, if a safe vaccine could be used for the primary infection, then any subsequent attack by tubercle bacilli would be repulsed. This idea was given powerful support by the observation that healed tuberculosis of the skin (lupus) or of the neck-glands (scrofula) seemed to give protection against pulmonary tuberculosis.

Many vaccines were prepared from dead tubercle bacilli in the hope of producing complete immunity, but the results fell so far short of the aim that the project was abandoned and it began to be widely accepted that only a live vaccine could succeed.

The discovery of B.C.G.—Bacillus Calmette-Guérin—like so many other medical inventions, began by a chance observation. A virulent bovine strain of tubercle bacilli, isolated originally from a cow in 1902, was being used by Albert Calmette and C. Guérin in Paris for experiments on calves. The culture was being grown in a liquid medium containing glycerine, bile and potato in saline solution. They found that repeated sub-cultures in this medium caused loss of virulence. This gave them the idea that if they went on long enough the bacilli might become harmless. So they went on, sub-culturing the bacillus at intervals of fourteen to twenty-five days for years and years. By 1908 they had shown that this bacillus, fatal at first, became innocuous to calves after thirty sub-cultures. Later it became harmless to monkeys. By 1919 it could no longer produce tuberculosis in such a highly susceptible animal as a guinea-pig. In 1924 Calmette proclaimed it a 'virus fixe', by which he meant that the attenuation of its virulence was immutable.

Two years earlier B. Weill-Hallé first dared to give B.C.G. to infants and, when no harm resulted, the use of the vaccine spread throughout France: but unfortunately, in the enthusiasm of the moment, mass vaccinations were carried out without any properly controlled experiments. The results, therefore, were received with considerable mistrust by scientists and accordingly they opposed the introduction of the vaccine into many other countries. In particular it was denied entry into Great Britain. Then came the ghastly affair at Lübeck in Germany, which set back the general use of this vaccine for years. In the winter of 1930–31 some two hundred and fifty infants were given the vaccine orally—*not* by injection. It had been prepared by sub-culturing organisms sent from Paris. Within three months sixty-eight of them were dead of acute tuberculosis and by autumn the death roll had risen to seventy-three. The question at issue was whether the B.C.G., for some unexplained reason, had become suddenly virulent, or whether there had been some blunder whereby a different and virulent strain of organism had been given in error. Criminal proceedings were instituted by the State against three doctors and a laboratory sister. After a long trial the verdict of the court was that contamination with a virulent strain of tubercle bacilli from Kiel had occurred in the laboratory, so that Calmette's vaccine was vindicated; but its prestige had received a damaging blow, from which it took years to recover.

Here it may be mentioned that the tuberculin-test is very valuable in deciding which individuals need B.C.G. A person who has had a primary infection and has recovered spontaneously will have acquired his immunity to further infection and will not need the vaccine. It is usual to test all candidates for vaccination and give the B.C.G. only to those who are negative to the test. The same test can be used to make sure that the B.C.G. has produced immunity, because six weeks after a successful inoculation the tuberculin reaction becomes positive.

Gradually B.C.G. has become accepted throughout the world, though its use in Great Britain was not allowed until 1950. Many mass vaccination campaigns have been carried out. For example the Danish Red Cross began work in several European countries where tuberculosis was rife as a result of the war and carried out 200,000 vaccinations within the year, and later this work was taken on by the World Health Organization. It has been estimated that by now the total of vaccinated people in the world has reached some 250 million.[1] There is no doubt that the widespread use of

[1] Hart, P. D'A., *British Medical Journal*, 1967, I, 587.

B.C.G. has been among the most successful campaigns in the history of preventive medicine.

In 1929 George W. M. Finlay and Edward Hindle at the Wellcome Bureau of Scientific Research began to produce immunity to yellow fever in monkeys by means of attenuated virus preparation. The following year Max Theiler discovered that he could get attenuated virus by inoculating the brains of mice. He passed the disease from mouse to mouse up to a hundred times and more and found that the virus became less and less virulent. The reason for this was not known, but the important point was that, though the virulence was reduced, the vaccine so prepared was fully effective in giving protection against yellow fever. More recently it has been possible to grow the virus in the developing embryo of the chicken.

In the war years from 1939 onwards millions of British and United States troops, stationed in parts of Africa where the disease was rife, were inoculated against yellow fever and remained free from the disease. It was found that this protection lasted many years.

The story of poliomyelitis vaccines is more recent still. There had been large epidemics of this disease, which used to be called infantile paralysis until it became obvious that no age was exempt. In 1916 there were about 27,000 cases in the United States, with 6,000 deaths. In 1921 Franklin D. Roosevelt developed the disease and it left him with nearly complete paralysis of both legs.

It was discovered that the disease is caused by a virus which infects the intestines of man, but it produces the crippling and often fatal nerve paralysis in some cases only. It was found necessary to use monkeys to grow the virus. Another difficulty arose when it was found that there were at least three different strains of virus.

Between 1949 and 1954 Jonas E. Salk of Pittsburg University elaborated his anti-poliomyelitis vaccine, which contained all the known strains, attenuated or inactivated by treatment with formalin. In 1954 a mass, controlled trial of the Salk vaccine was carried out by the National Foundation for Infantile Paralysis of New York, on some 650,000 children. This showed that the incidence of paralytic disease was four times as great in the unprotected children as in those who had been inoculated. Unfortunately there were a few disastrous cases of poliomyelitis among the vaccinated, because some batches of the vaccine had been inadequately inactivated. This set back the movement for wholesale vaccination for a number of years.

In 1956 Albert B. Sabin produced his attenuated *oral* vaccine, which he claimed produced resistance to infection in the intestinal wall and so protected the patient from the nerve paralysis. Sabin was so confident of his vaccine that he began his campaign by administering it to himself and his family. There has been much controversy over the relative efficacy and safety of the Salk and Sabin vaccines. The incidence of paralytic poliomyelitis in Great Britain has steadily declined since immunization with the Salk vaccine began in 1956 and the fall in new cases has been even faster after the introduction of the Sabin oral vaccine, which from 1962 has been distributed freely to general practitioners and Local Authorities. This trend could continue, provided a high level of immunization is maintained. Unfortunately there is good evidence to show that about 30 per cent of new-born babies go unprotected in England and Scotland at the present time.

(d) The Attack by means of Drugs

One of the most ancient methods of combating sickness has been the use of drugs. A hundred years ago there were very few preparations that had any direct action in curing disease. Most of the substances in the pharmocopoeia were useful only in removing symptoms. Thus morphia killed pain, but did not remove the cause.

Among the drugs which had a specific effect on the causal organism of sickness was quinine. This was imported into Europe from South America in the seventeenth century as crude Cinchona[1] bark. The plant was later grown extensively in Java. Until about thirty years ago quinine was the only drug which was effective in

---

[1] Used to cure herself of fever by the Countess of Chinchon in 1638 (*Murray's English Dictionary*). The plant was named Cinchona by Linnaeus in 1742: but the facts about the Countess are wrong (*British Medical Journal*, 1932, II, p. 212).

treating malaria. Its chief drawback was that it had little value as a prophylactic. Newer drugs, such as mepacrine, became of outstanding importance when the Second World War cut off our supplies of quinine. Its great advantage was that it was effective in *preventing* malaria, and by so doing it played a large part in the Allied victory. Even so malaria is very far from being under control. For one thing there has been a steadily increasing number of records of malarial parasites becoming resistant to the chief anti-malarial drugs; from places as far apart as Colombia, Brazil, British Guiana, Cambodia, Thailand and Malaya. What is now needed is a steady supply of new and cheap drugs. A search for new synthetic antimalarials is being carried out by the Walter Reed Institute of Medical Research.

The substance that had been most in vogue against syphilis had been mercury. Then in 1905 the causative organism, *Spirochaeta pallida*, was discovered by Fritz Schaudinn and a search began for some suitable killing agent. The invention of staining methods in the examination of organisms under the microscope had given rise to the hope that a dye could be found that would be poisonous and at the same time stain the germs more readily than the tissues of the host. The hunt for a poisonous dye to stain the spirochaete of syphilis led to the discovery of salvarsan by Paul Ehrlich in 1909. This drug was not found by chance, but by the systematic trial of hundreds of different chemicals. Salvarsan was announced as '606', the 606th arsenical substance tested, at the Congress for International Medicine at Wiesbaden in 1910. Apart from its effectiveness in treating syphilis, Ehrlich's discovery had shown that there was a scientific method which could be used in the search for drugs to be employed in what he was the first to call 'chemotherapy'. It seems surprising therefore that, apart from numerous variants in the arsenical compounds, not much further progress in chemotherapy was made for a further seventeen years.

In 1927 Gerhard Domagk, working in the laboratory of the I.C. Farbenindustrie, began to study a particular group of dyes containing the chemical group SO_2NH_2—the sulphonamides. Beginning with mice infected with streptococci he found convincing evidence of the curative value of sulphonamides and in 1935 he announced the invention of prontosil, the first of the 'magic bullets', that is to say drugs which could be aimed against specific organisms, just because they were dyes that stained them. Prontosil had enormous success in treating pneumonia and the streptcococcal diseases, in particular puerperal fever. Later it was found that prontosil was not thus effective in that it was a dye, but because it was a sulphonamide. As a result of this, numerous sulphonamide drugs were manufactured by different chemical companies all over the world, the one most commonly heard of in this country being 'M & B', the initials of the manufacturers. These drugs have saved many thousands of lives throughout the world. In fact they became our chief weapon against many lethal infections until the advent of the antibiotics.

(e) The Attack by Antibiotics

Alexander Fleming, the discoverer of penicillin, was a pupil of Sir Almroth Wright. Having seen the misery and suffering experienced by the soldiers with infected wounds in the 1914–1918 war, he was constantly on the look-out for something that would kill the germs of sepsis. In 1922 his first important discovery was made. When growing bacteria from nasal secretions on solid culture medium, he noticed that besides the bacterial colonies there were blank areas on the culture plates. He deduced that there must be some potent substance which prevented the germs from growing and he was able to prepare from nasal secretions and from tears as well, a solution which would destroy organisms in a liquid broth culture. Unfortunately these germ-destroying substances (which, at Wright's suggestion, he called lysozymes) were active only against germs that were non-pathogenic; but he was quick to see that the harmless bacteria were in fact non-invasive just because they were kept at bay by the lysozymes. Could he find something that would kill disease-producing organisms?

The next step came in 1928 when he found that one of his culture plates of staphylococci had become contaminated by a growth of mould and round one of these mould colonies there was a clear area where there were no staphylococci. He found that the mould itself was producing something which could stop the growth of the staphylococci. Here was something which, unlike the lysozymes, was active against pathogenic bacteria. The mould itself was identified by Thom, an expert American mycologist, as *Penicillium notatum*. Fleming went on to culture the mould by itself in broth which he then filtered and found in the filtrate the bacteria-inhibiting agent which he named penicillin. Moreover he was able to show that the new agent was not harmful to normal human tissues. Unfortunately his attempts to concentrate and purify it met with little success, because, as it turned out, penicillin is a chemically unstable substance. When the discoverer (who rightly predicted that penicillin would be of value in venereal diseases) gave a demonstration in 1936 at an international conference, no one seems to have grasped the supreme importance of this life-saving agent.

Shortly before the outbreak of the Second World War Howard Florey, an Australian working at Oxford, invited E. B. Chain, a refugee from Nazi Germany, to help him to isolate and purify Fleming's penicillin. By that time the now well-known process of freeze-drying had been invented and by this method they extracted from the filtrate of a penicillium culture a brown powder which they were able to purify by chemical means. They finally produced a substance, non-toxic to mice, but a million times as potent in its bacterio-static action as Fleming's original filtrate. These results were made possible by a generous grant of 5,000 dollars from the Rockefeller Foundation. At this time England was in a critical condition. It was in 1940. The Germans had broken through the Maginot Line, had overrun France and had driven the British Army into the sea at Dunkirk. Invasion of Britain seemed certain. None the less in the summer of that year the patient investigation went on. Florey and Chain were able to show, with carefully controlled experiments, that their new purified product could save the lives of mice which had been deliberately infected with deadly streptococci. In 1941 they treated an Oxford policeman who had staphylococcal septicaemia. He rallied, but the available penicillin ran out and the patient relapsed and died. None the less here was the beginning of penicillin treatment.

Clearly it was of vital importance that the new drug should be produced on a massive scale. This was not possible in England because every available man and factory was devoted to an all-out effort to rally the country. Accordingly Florey and Chain went to America in 1941. The Americans were able to produce huge quantities of penicillin by growing different species of penicillium in various media. Eventually two commercial firms were induced to take up the wholesale production of the new life-saving drug.

Penicillin is a powerful weapon in very many bacterial diseases, but it was found ineffective in certain other very common infections and, in particular, it had no action on the tubercle bacillus. The recent history of tuberculosis is told in chronological order in the ensuing section, but the present section must include the discovery of one more very valuable antibiotic, namely streptomycin. The discoverer was Selman Waksman, who had settled in the United States, a refugee from czarist Russia. He became deeply interested in microbiology and especially in the bacterial population of the soil. He noticed that disease-producing organisms (pathogens) were rare in soil and he wondered why this should be so, since the soil must be constantly restocked with such pathogens through animal and human excreta and the burial of corpses. Why did the pathogens disappear? Either the environment was unsuitable from physical or chemical causes or they were destroyed by other organisms. In 1932 Waksman was asked by the National Research Council and the American Tuberculosis Association to find out what happened to tubercle bacilli in the soil. By 1940 he began to discover antibiotic substances in the soil. The first was actino-mycin, derived from the ray fungus, actinomyces, but he found that it was far too toxic to have any medical use.

Waksman then set out to examine systematically every variety of soil organism that he could find, testing their power of inhibiting the growth of different pathogens, firstly when cultured in vitro and then when actually growing in the animal body. The amount of tedious work that this involved may begin to be realized when it is known that it was not until some 100,000 cultures had been set up, treated and examined that success at last came his way in 1943 with the discovery of streptomycin, the product of the mould *Streptomyces griseus*. In 1944 he showed that his new antibiotic could prevent the growth of tubercle bacilli on culture plates; but Waksman was a biologist, not a doctor, so he put his discovery into the hands of Drs Feldman and Hinshaw at the Mayo Clinic, Rochester, Minnesota, who showed that streptomycin could save the lives of guinea-pigs infected with tuberculosis. The next step was to cure human beings, but at this point it is important to note that, unlike penicillin, which was discovered by a lucky chance (though such an accident might have been overlooked by a less acute observer than Fleming), streptomycin was discovered by unremitting hard work. In other words Waksman found the antibiotic because he was looking for it.

Since the discovery of penicillin the hunt for newer and wider ranges of antibiotics has continued. This was necessary firstly because penicillin was not lethal to all species of bacteria and secondly because under treatment some strains of bacteria, previously sensitive, became resistant to penicillin. More recently, synthetic antibiotics were made and some are very effective. In particular there is the tetracycline group of drugs, which has proved invaluable in the winter respiratory diseases which are so prevalent in this country. More recently still, synthetic drugs of the penicillin type have been evolved to attack bacteria not sensitive to natural penicillin.

Unfortunately there is little doubt that ill-considered or inadequate treatment has been one of the main reasons for the development of drug-resistant strains of organisms. In some diseases it is possible to avoid this man-made disaster by giving two different antibiotics at the same time. This often delays the onset of drug-resistance, or even stops it altogether.

IV. TUBERCULOSIS

Among all the infectious diseases described in earlier chapters, tuberculosis merits special consideration. Throughout history it has been one of the most ubiquitous and persistent scourges. The bones of the ancient Egyptians clearly show its presence. A hundred years ago it was widely regarded as a non-infectious disease.

We have seen how Laennec, the inventor of the stethoscope, had put the study of lung disease on a firm basis. He had clearly differentiated between pulmonary tuberculosis and other chronic lung complaints. He had focused attention on the advanced and terminal stages of tuberculosis. It was left to his successors to attack the problem of early and curable disease.

It was fourteen years after Laennec's death from tuberculosis in 1826 that George Boddington, a general practitioner in Warwickshire, put forward the new idea that fresh air and sunlight were beneficial to consumptives. Before this the examples of Russell's establishment at Brighton and the Royal Sea-bathing Hospital at Margate had shown that certain complaints were better treated by a more spartan régime than was commonly practised. Boddington showed the great advantages to be gained by treating tuberculosis in the open air, with a nutritious in place of a lowering diet and by carefully graduated exercises. Here was the idea of sanatorium treatment. In England Boddington was voted a dangerous crank, but his methods were adopted enthusiastically in Germany where the success of sanatorium treatment for tuberculosis was first accepted by all. It was in Germany too that Peter Dettweiler, himself a patient, showed the importance of rest and the dangers of exercise in treatment. The plan of providing long periods of rest out of doors, with regular and nutritious food thus took shape; but the value of such treatment did not become widely accepted until the next generation, at the turn of the century.

In America the idea was taken up by Edward Livingstone Trudeau, one of the most heroic and beloved figures in modern medicine. After graduating as a doctor in 1871, he was found to have advanced pulmonary tuberculosis. He was advised to go south, live out of doors and ride horses; but this treatment did him no good. Instead he took himself to the Adirondack Mountains in 1873 and remained there for the rest of a long and useful life. Having come across an article describing Dettweiler's sanatorium and rest cure, he decided to try it on himself and his patients and conceived the idea of developing a 'sanitarium' at Saranac Lake. This was the beginning of one of America's most important medical institutions. Among the many famous people who came to Saranac Lake to be under Dr Trudeau's care was Robert Louis Stevenson, who spent the winter of 1887–8 there. When he left he inscribed a copy of *Dr Jekyll and Mr Hyde* to Trudeau, with the following couplet:

Trudeau was all winter at my side;
I never spied the nose of Mr Hyde.

Trudeau lived until 1915 and saw the triumph of his ideas. He wrote the story in a moving autobiography,[1] a book which every student of tuberculosis should read.

In 1865, Jean Villemin, a French Army surgeon, startled the medical world with his proof that tuberculosis was indeed a communicable disease. It could be readily passed from a human being to a rabbit by inoculation with tuberculous material. His results were soon confirmed in England. When Koch announced his discovery of the tubercle bacillus in 1882, it was hoped that victory was in sight. The unsuccessful attempts to treat tuberculosis with Koch's tuberculin was a major set-back, but now that the infectious nature of the disease had been proved, public opinion was aroused to the necessity for action. Voluntary efforts began the campaign. Sanatoria were opened at Frimley and Midhurst. Later it will be seen how large a part State Medicine played in the battle against tuberculosis. Here the actual treatment of the disease will be traced through the three main phases which followed the first important one just described.

Chest X-rays in the detection of pulmonary tuberculosis have proved one of the most valuable diagnostic weapons. Francis H. Williams of Boston began to examine lungs by X-rays as early as 1896 and the following year he claimed that it was possible to diagnose pulmonary tuberculosis which was not detectable by any other means; but it took another fifteen to twenty years before regular chest X-ray became a routine procedure in the examination of the lungs. Today it is universally accepted that the X-ray is the best means of diagnosis and gives more information about the course and prognosis of the disease than any of the older methods of examination.

The second phase in the treatment of tuberculosis is generally referred to as 'collapse therapy'. About 1880 a number of observers called attention to the fact that tuberculous patients in whom pneumothorax developed spontaneously were sometimes strikingly benefited. (Pneumothorax denotes the presence of air between the

[1] Trudeau, E. L., *An Autobiography*, New York, 1916.

chest-wall and the lung.) In 1882 Carlo Forlanini of Naples suggested the use of artificial pneumothorax in the treatment of tuberculosis, but he waited ten years before he dared to attempt it. This he did by means of repeated small injections of nitrogen. Gas or air has to be injected into the chest, between the chest-wall and the lung, so compressing and collapsing the affected lung. This provides rest to the lung and, by altering the pressure of the injected air, it is often possible to close tuberculous cavities. This treatment was at first ridiculed, but after Forlanini's publication of the results of fourteen years' work in 1906, the method was quickly recognized and adopted by tuberculosis specialists all over the world. The refills of gas (or air) had to be repeated at intervals of one to three weeks for a number of years to effect a cure. In every large town in England and in every civilized country clinics were set up to provide this regular refill treatment. An alternative method was to inject air into the abdominal cavity, having previously produced paralysis of the diaphragm on the side of the affected lung. In this way the lung was compressed by pushing up the diaphragm from below—the so-called artificial pneumoperitoneum treatment.

In a proportion of cases of artificial pneumothorax the lung is prevented from collapsing by bands of adhesions, sticking the lung to the chest-wall. In 1910 Hans Christian Jacoboeus of Stockholm worked out a method of cutting these adhesions, using an instrument similar to a cystoscope, inserted through the chest-wall. In this way he could see the actual adhesions and was often able to divide them with an electric cautery and so bring about a satisfactory collapse of the lung.

The next phase was the surgical one. Surgical methods were used for collapsing the lung when artificial pneumothorax had failed. Large portions of the ribs on the affected side were removed, allowing the whole chest-wall to fall in and so compress the lung. This procedure, known as thoracoplasty, was a drastic one and caused a good deal of deformity, but it undoubtedly saved a large number of lives. This gross deformity always followed the operation until it was recognized that it could be largely avoided if intensive and regular physiotherapy was started immediately after the operation.

Other surgical methods included removal of smaller or larger parts of a lung, or sometimes of the whole lung, if it was completely destroyed by disease; but these resection operations could not be undertaken with safety until the advent of the new antituberculous drugs.

The last phase of treatment is the chemotherapeutic one and it is now the standard practice, to the exclusion of all other methods.

The discovery of streptomycin by Waksman has already been described. It first became available for general treatment outside hospitals in the United States in 1947. Streptomycin was very powerful in inhibiting the growth of the tubercle bacillus, but it killed the organism only very slowly. Another drawback was that prolonged treatment with streptomycin was liable to produce drug-resistant forms of tubercle bacilli. Yet another disadvantage was that the drug often produced unpleasant side effects, mainly on the ear, causing giddiness and sometimes deafness. An intensive search was therefore made for other drugs. J. Lehman tested a variety of benzoic and salicylic compounds and finally the salts of para-amino-salicylic acid (known to patients as P.A.S.) were found to be very effective. Later still the compound isoniazid, which had been first made in 1912, was tried in the laboratories of three different drug manufacturers (Bayer, Hoffmann Laroche and Squibb) all independently and at about the same time and was found most effective against the tubercle bacillus. Furthermore this drug, unlike streptomycin, could be given orally. Besides this, when given in doses of only 100 milligrammes, isoniazid appeared within a few hours in the blood plasma and in the cerebrospinal fluid in concentrations more than twenty times that required to inhibit the growth of tubercle bacilli.

It was found possible to avoid the development of drug-resistant forms of organisms by giving at least two, and sometimes all three of the new drugs simultaneously. The results were striking indeed, once the correct principles of treatment had been worked out. It has been shown that if patients can and do take the prescribed drugs regularly and faithfully, then, between the third and the sixth month of treatment 100 per cent of them find their sputum free of tubercle bacilli. To guard against a relapse chemotherapy is often continued for a full two years.

This chemotherapeutic phase has had widespread success in this and many other countries. The death-rate has fallen rapidly and the incidence of new cases has likewise declined. Moreover the patients are now eager and anxious for early treatment, which they are confident can effect a rapid and lasting cure. One of the most gratifying features of the decade 1950–60 was the change in the atmosphere among patients in tuberculosis hospitals. Whereas before all had been gloom and alarm, with the recurring fear that rest and 'collapse' treatment would fail, or that major surgical operations loomed ahead and with the depressing spectacle of their fellow-sufferers dying in the wards; in a few short months the atmosphere changed to one of hope and confidence and the certainty that cure was near.

With all this success in Western Europe and America, there is no room at all for complacency about tuberculosis. There are large areas in the world, in India and in the under-developed countries, for example, where the disease is rife and still an important cause of death and disability.

CHAPTER SIX

SOME LARGER PARASITES

WE must not leave the subject of the living causes of disease without mention of some of the larger animal parasites. The bacteria belong to the vegetable kingdom, while the parasites of malaria, sleeping-sickness and amoebic dysentery are members of the single-celled and primitive animal group known as protozoa. There are, however, some very much larger internal parasites which are extremely worthy of note, not only because they cause considerable damage to human life in many parts of the world, but also because of the great interest attaching to their remarkable life-cycles. The existence of many of these creatures must, in the nature of things, have been noted long ago, but it is only in the last hundred years that their strange habits have been fully disclosed.

The first large group contains the flukes. In many tropical and subtropical parts of the world, various forms of fluke-infection are found. The symptoms are irritation of the bladder with haemorrhages, fever and other disturbances. The first of the flukes was discovered by a German, Theodor Bilharz in Cairo in 1851. Patrick Manson found a different species in 1903 and a third kind has been found in Japan.

These schistosomes, as they are called, are small flat worms about half an inch in length. The larvae are tiny swimming bodies which can pierce the skin or lining of the mouth or throat of a man washing in or drinking infected water. They travel in the blood to the liver where they mature into adult worms and conjugate. They then travel towards the bladder where the female discharges eggs which appear in the urine. It is in passing through the bladder-wall that the eggs cause the chief symptoms.

In 1870 Cobbold showed that the eggs hatched in fresh or salt water and that certain snails acted as essential intermediate hosts for the parasite. This requirement is fortunate, for it provides an obvious method of preventing the disease, namely by exterminating the snails, by drying up the pools in which they live, by poisoning them, or by getting ducks to devour them. Human beings must drink filtered water and avoid washing in water where the snails are found. In addition it is important to prevent water supplies from being polluted by human excreta. Once infected, humans can be cured by chemotherapy. In particular a very effective new drug, called ambilhar, was introduced in 1960. Total eradication of the disease may be possible, but there are many difficulties; for example baboons and other animals may act as alternative hosts to Manson's fluke and in China domestic animals can carry the Japanese fluke.

In the United Kingdom there is a common fluke, *Fasciola hepatica*, which is primarily the cause of a disease of sheep, known to farmers as 'sheep-rot'. The parasite invades the sheep's liver where the eggs are laid and pass via the bile to the faeces. They hatch in water and here again there is an intermediate host, a mollusc. The embryos leave the mollusc and attach themselves to blades of grass and so become eaten by other sheep, or by man if he is given to chewing grass. Sheep-rot can be prevented by exterminating the molluscs.

The tape-worms are the largest of these animal parasites. One species can attain a length of up to thirty feet. Each worm consists of a head, which fixes it to the wall of the intestine and a great number of segments, those farthest from the head being the most mature. The ripe segments fall from the worm and are discharged in the faeces and the eggs become free. They are eaten by an intermediate host and the embryos burrow into its muscles, where they remain until eaten, in a raw or partially cooked state, by another person. The three intermediate hosts for the three largest species are respectively the pig, the ox and certain fish, such as trout, grayling or pike. Tape-worm infection has been widespread wherever pig products are eaten. In Abyssinia at one time the infection was regarded as normal because the entire population was infected. By contrast, strict Jews and Moslems are not affected in this way because they do not eat pig-meat. In the middle of the nineteenth century it was rife in London. In 1864 the Privy

Council commissioned a London doctor, J. L. W. Thudicum, to inquire into the extent of the infection in the London meat markets and slaughter-houses. There he found conditions of filth 'of which no conception can be found apart from ocular inspection', in fact widespread infection with tape-worms can only occur under revoltingly insanitary conditions. The extract of the male fern is an effective means of destroying the worms in the human intestine.

There is another tape-worm which is much smaller and which normally lives in the intestine of the dog. If living eggs are swallowed the embryos burrow into the tissues of their host and frequently lodge in the liver. Here they may form cysts which can grow as big as a coco-nut or even larger. These are called 'hydatid cysts' and are very common in Australia and in Iceland, but may occur in any community that keeps dogs. The prevention of this infection is to stop the dogs from becoming infected, which they often do from eating raw meat in slaughter-houses, and also to stop them fouling food or water intended for human use.

Another group contains the round worms, the commonest of which, *Ascaris lumbricoides*, looks like a very long and pale earth-worm. This worm has no intermediate host, but none the less has a curious life-cycle. The worm lives in the human intestine and the eggs pass out in the excreta. If, through insanitary conditions, the eggs become eaten, they quickly hatch and the embryos pierce the gut and are carried round by the blood to the lungs, travel up the windpipe into the throat and are swallowed. Here is an extraordinary roundabout way for a worm to travel, only to find itself in the place where it began life as an egg. If a massive dose of eggs is swallowed, pneumonia-like symptoms may arise as the embryos travel through the lungs.

The hookworms are perhaps the most damaging of all these parasites, because they cause very severe anaemia. There are two species, *Ankylostoma duodenale* and *Necator americanus*, found mainly in the northern and southern hemispheres respectively. In 1853 Griesinger and Bilharz showed that Ankylostoma (discovered ten years earlier by the Milanese, Angelo Dubini), was often the cause of severe and sometimes fatal anaemia. It can occur in temperate climates, but is then confined to sheltered places such as tunnels and mines. In 1880 it attacked the men engaged in the construction of the St Gothard tunnel under the Alps. In 1902 it was shown to be the cause of the severe 'miners' anaemia' among the workers in the Cornish mines. The Sanitary Commission of the Rockefeller Foundation investigated this condition in the island of Puerto Rico in the West Indies, where it was said that a third of all the deaths was from hookworm infection. As in all outbreaks of this disease, the worm was transferred to man by insanitary habits. The worm, which lives in the upper part of the human intestine, discharges its eggs into the excreta. In warm and moist places the larvae develop into sharp, needle-like bodies, about 0·5 millimetres long, which can pierce the bare skin of man and so pass by way of the circulation to the lungs, then they travel up the air tubes and finally reach the intestine, where they grow into adult hookworms. When the larvae pierce the skin they may cause a rash, known as 'ground itch,' but the chief damage is the anaemia which the adult worms can cause. Preventive measures are segregation of the infected, provision of adequate latrines and washing facilities and, most important, persuading people to use them. Stout boots impregnated with oil will protect the feet from the piercing larvae. Those already infected can be cured by suitable anthelmintic drugs. Thymol was used for this purpose as early as 1880, but more recently carbon tetrachloride or tetra-chlorethylene have been found very effective.

The last worm that there is space to mention here is the thin thread-like filaria which is the cause of elephantiasis—a hideously deforming disease which is prevalent in Africa, Asia, the West Indies, South America and some parts of Australia. Patrick Manson showed that the enormous dropsical swellings which characterize the disease were due to the blocking of the lymphatic channels by the actual filaria, now called *Wucheria bancroftii*. Manson proved that the disease was carried by a mosquito, *Culex fatigans*, which takes up the embryos from the superficial blood and conveys them to another person. Incidentally it was this proof of the transmission of filaria by mosquito bites that led to the conception of insect vectors of disease and so to the magnificent discoveries already described.

Extermination of the particular mosquito offers the best method of prevention, but this is by no means a simple task. Mass poisoning may destroy beneficial insects as well as the mosquito. All the methods that have been used against malaria can be used, but it may well be that eventual success will come from the use of some biological (genetical) control. Professor H. Laven of Mainz University, a World Health Organization consultant, has introduced a new method in Burma.[1] The W. H. O. brought in a foreign strain of mosquito and bred them in the filariasis research unit in Rangoon. Professor Laven chose Okpo, an isolated village, for his experiment which is based on his discovery that male mosquitoes of one region cannot reproduce with females of another region. He organized the daily release of 5,000 laboratory-bred males. They mated with the local females, who mate once only in a lifetime, and, because of the incompatibility, these females lay only sterile eggs. In this way the native Culex is expected to die out. The research unit later plans to release more and more foreign males all along the Rangoon river.

[1] *The Times*, 13.5.1967, p. 5.

CHAPTER SEVEN

THE HORMONES

THE conception of the control of the body by chemical agents has provided medicine with a whole series of new therapeutic weapons. The history of chemical messengers, or hormones, as they are called, began in 1855 when Thomas Addison of Guy's Hospital published his work *On the Constitutional and Local Effects of Disease of the Suprarenal Capsules.* He described a disease which is characterized by progressive loss of strength, anaemia, low blood-pressure and an enfeebled heart, together with curious patchy pigmentation of the skin. The oddest part of his discovery lay in the fact that in every case of this disease he found that the little gland perched on the top of each kidney (the suprarenal 'capsule') was degenerated. If the failure of these little glands was the cause of the other changes, then here was something quite new: that a minute disturbance in a special organ could cause such profound and widespread changes. At the time of the discovery its full significance was missed and for a long time the matter remained a pathological curiosity.

A further step in solving the mystery was taken by Charles Edouard Brown-Séquard, the Americo-Frenchman who succeeded Claude Bernard at the Collège de France. Brown-Séquard cut out the superarenal capsules from animals and they rapidly developed symptoms of Addison's disease. Here was the proof that failure of the suprarenal glands was the cause and not one of the many effects of the condition. It should be noted that this experiment was conducted by operative surgery; for much of our knowledge of hormones has been gained by procedures such as this. In other words Brown-Séquard had invented a new method of investigating certain diseases.

Enlargement of the thyroid gland, associated with other serious disorders had been described earlier, but in 1835 Robert Graves, a

146

Dublin physician, put forward his classic account of the disease which now bears his name.[1] The patient—generally a woman—is 'highly strung' and has an enlarged thyroid gland, fine tremors of the hands, rapid heart-beat and protruding eyes. Graves's *description* of his disease preceded that of Addison, but it was many years before the *cause* of either disease became known.

In Graves's disease there is excessive thyroid activity, which is the cause of all the other symptoms. By contrast there are other diseases where the thyroid function is deficient. In 1850 T. B. Curling described a condition of absence of the gland, accompanied by defective brain development and swellings at the sides of the neck. This condition called *myxoedema*, is caused by degeneration of the thyroid in adults. In a fully developed case there is great increase in bulk, the skin becomes puffy while the features become coarsened, with thick lips and enlarged nostrils and the hair falls out. There is marked mental sluggishness and the memory begins to fail.

Closely allied to this condition is that of cretinism which is due to absence or deficiency of normal thyroid activity in children. It occurs particularly in certain valleys in Switzerland, the Tyrol and the Pyrenees and, in England in Derbyshire. Though apparently normal at birth, when about eighteen months old it becomes apparent that the child's intelligence is sadly lacking, its growth below normal and its general shape characteristically deformed. The bones fail to grow normally, the skin becomes doughy and hangs in folds around the joints and on the abdomen and the hair is coarse and thin. The child fails to walk at the right time and may never be able to perform anything better than a clumsy waddle. Its speech, if it comes at all, arrives late and is often almost unintelligible. The child seldom grows to more than four feet high and its mentality may remain that normally found in a child of three.

The actual proof of the cause of myxoedema came from two sources, both observers using operative surgery. Moritz Schiff of Frankfort-on-Main first of all showed that complete removal of the thyroid was fatal to a dog. Later J. L. Reverdin at Geneva

[1] Graves, R., *London Medical and Surgical Journal*, 1835, Part 2, pp. 516, 517.

proved that partial removal of the gland led to an experimental disease closely resembling myxoedema. Schiff went a step further when he demonstrated that the fatal results of his former experiments did not occur if he grafted a piece of thyroid gland elsewhere in the dog, before removing the gland from the neck. Evidently the thyroid acted by giving out some substance into the blood, since the actual position of the graft made no difference. The fatal result could also be postponed by injecting the juices of thyroids into the dogs.

George Murray of Manchester saw the importance of these discoveries and in 1891 he announced that the hypodermic injection of extract of animal thyroid was very beneficial in cases of myxoedema. Directly following this Howitz of Copenhagen and other independent observers began to try the effect of giving patients thyroid to eat. Unexpectedly it proved as effective as the injections. The patients recovered steadily and almost completely. The same remedy was tried on cretins with great success. If treatment is started early enough the child may even grow up into a normal healthy adult. The treatment must be continued throughout the patient's life.

More recently, in 1915, the American chemist E. C. Kendall was able to extract from thyroid glands pure chemical substances, thyroxine in particular, which perform most of the functions of the normal human gland. These compounds contain iodine which is essential to the regular working of the human body. It is significant that in certain localities where simple goitre is endemic this is often associated with a deficiency of iodine in the water or soil. Giving small doses of iodides has helped in the prevention of this disease.

In 1902, while inquiring into the way in which the various digestive juices were poured into the stomach and intestine, W. M. Bayliss and E. H. Starling made a surprising discovery. It was thought that the pancreas gave out juice when the food reached the opening of the pancreatic duct and that the mechanism was a local one. Bayliss and Starling found that if they ground up a piece of the stomach-wall with some acid and then injected it into the circulation of an animal, a powerful flow of pancreatic juice resulted. Evidently a substance contained in the acid stomach juices is normally absorbed into the blood-stream and so conveyed to the pancreas, which is stimulated thereby to pour its juice into the intestine. The discoverers called this hypothetical substance *secretin.*

The discovery of secretin started the theory of the control of the organism as a whole—apart from interference from the nervous system—by hormones. There are very many of these and the behaviour of the body depends largely on a delicate balance between these hormones, each tending to produce some different effect.

The suprarenal, or adrenal gland as it is now called produces hormones other than that concerned with preventing Addison's disease. The gland consists essentially of two different organs, the outside crust (or cortex) and the core (or medulla) and each has very different functions. Historically, the effect of the medulla was discovered first. In 1896 George Oliver and Edward S. Schäfer found that, if they injected a watery extract of adrenal glands into animals, there was a great and rapid rise of blood-pressure. Seven years later Jokichi Takamine succeeded in isolating in pure crystalline form the substance adrenalin which is responsible for this effect. Besides the rise in blood-pressure (which is caused by constriction of the blood-vessels in the skin and viscera) adrenalin causes relaxation of the muscles in the bronchi and mobilization of sugar stored in the liver. The constricting effect on the blood-vessels in the skin can be used to stop bleeding by local application. Furthermore, in local anaesthesia, the addition of adrenalin to the injection prevents the anaesthetic from diffusing rapidly away from the site of injection. Adrenalin is useful in the treatment of shock because it raises the general blood-pressure and in asthma because it abolishes the spasm of the muscles of the bronchi and so widens the breathing tubes.

The cortex of the adrenal gland serves a number of different functions by the action of the various hormones it makes. In general these hormones enable the body to cope with adverse internal chemical stresses, by regulating the general metabolism of carbohydrate, protein and fat. As will be seen later, there is evidence to show that the pituitary gland is the main seat of the chemical government of the body. Certainly it produces the hormone corticotrophin which controls the activity of the activity of the adrenal cortex.

The pituitary gland lies hidden away inside the skull, attached to the base of the brain by a short stalk. This gland, like the adrenals, is actually formed from two different kinds of tissue which have different functions and are derived embryonically from different organs. Nearly seventy years ago it was found that an extract of the hinder (posterior) part of the gland when injected into animals caused a large and prolonged rise of blood-pressure. The hormone causing this was named vasopressin, but it is doubtful how far this is a normal function of the posterior pituitary, because the effect is only produced with very large doses. Two other important hormones are made by this part of the gland, namely one which controls the secretion of urine by the kidneys (the antidiuretic hormone) and *oxytocin* which is concerned with breast-milk and also causes strong contraction of the muscles of the womb and doubtless has a useful function in the mechanism of parturition.

The front (anterior) part of the pituitary gland has many different functions, one of the most important being the control of growth. Removal of this part from young animals stops their growth at once and injection of a hormone prepared from the anterior pituitary gland can restore the rate of growth. It was found that certain giants and dwarfs had deranged pituitary glands. In some cases it is possible to show by X-rays that the bony cavity in which the gland is lodged has become much larger than normal. Such enlargement can be caused by a tumour of the anterior or posterior parts. In the former case there will be an excess of growth hormone. If this happens to a person before he is fully grown, then growth of the long bones continues, so that the adolescent becomes a giant. Most giants of seven or eight feet are victims of this disorder. If the excess of growth hormone occurs in adults the disease known as *acromegaly* results. This comes on insidiously. The bones of the limbs and head begin to enlarge, the first symptom often being that the patient finds he has to buy larger and larger shoes or hats. The features become broader and coarser and the lower jaw more and more prominent until the sufferer assumes so characteristic an appearance that he may well be taken for a blood-relation of anyone with the same disease.

Other important hormones originate in the anterior pituitary gland. There is one which raises the sugar content of the blood, producing an effect opposite to the hormone *insulin* which is described below. Other anterior pituitary hormones are concerned with sex development, since removal of the gland before puberty prevents the testes or ovaries from developing, whereas if this is done in an adult, it causes impotence in the male and sterility in the female. Thus we see that the pituitary gland has a controlling influence which is widespread throughout the body; but what has yet to be discovered is what controls the pituitary gland.

The experimental investigations into diabetes hardly progressed at all from the time of Claud Bernard until 1889, when Oskar Minkowski, a Russian physician working at Strasbourg, found that complete removal of the pancreas of a dog resulted in an artificial diabetes, characterized by intense thirst and increased sugar in the blood. The pancreas evidently had another function besides that of digestive juices.

The next step was made in 1900 by Eugène L. Opie, then a young instructor in pathology at Johns Hopkins Hospital, Baltimore. Studying microscopic sections of the pancreas of a girl who had died of diabetes, he saw that certain peculiar 'islets' of tissue, the so-called islets of Langerhans (named after the man who discovered them in 1869)[1] were completely degenerated; that is to say their normal microscopic structure had disintegrated. No one had suspected the function of the islets until then, but Opie's observation led Edward Schäfer, in 1916, to put forward the theory that these special cells produced some form of 'internal secretion' that controlled the metabolism of sugar. The islets, like other hormone-producing glands, had no ducts to drain off any secretions they might make. Such secretions found their way into the general circulation from what came to be known as the 'ductless glands'. Since 1913 they have been called endocrine glands.

All attempts to extract the active hormone from pancreatic tissue had failed, because the digestive juice, also present in the pancreas, destroyed the hormone as soon as extracts were made. In 1920 Frederick G. Banting, a Canadian then working as a demonstrator

[1] Langerhans, P., *Berlin Dissertation*, 1869.

in anatomy and physiology at the Western Ontario Medical School, began to see how the problem could be solved. He happened to read a report of a rare case of stone in the pancreatic duct, in which the blockage of the duct had caused atrophy of all the pancreatic cells *except those of the islets of Langerhans*. Here was a method of preparing an extract of the cells of Langerhans without interference by the digestive juices. Banting got up at two in the morning to write these three memorable sentences in his note-book: 'Ligate pancreatic duct of dog. Wait 6 to 8 weeks for degeneration. Remove the residue and extract.' He communicated his idea to Professor J. J. R. Macleod of Toronto University, who wisely gave him laboratory accommodation, ten dogs and the valuable assistance of Charles Best, a second-year medical student who was a trained chemist.

Soon Banting and Best were able to show that the juice of the artificially degenerated pancreas could temporarily save the life of a dog whose pancreas had been totally removed. They had found a way of preparing the active principle. They then worked out methods of improving and concentrating the substance which they named 'isletin'. They then discovered that the substance could be prepared without the preliminary operation and waiting period, if they extracted adult cow's pancreas with alcohol rather than with salt-solution. The alcohol inactivated the digestive juices and so stopped their destructive action upon the hormone from the islets. Now they had an unlimited and easy source of 'isletin'. It was Macleod who suggested that the new hormone should be called 'insulin'.

Banting's first human patient was a close friend, Joe Gilchrist, a Toronto physician, who was going downhill with diabetes in spite of the most careful dieting. The insulin was at once effective in lowering the level of the sugar in the blood and in keeping it so.

Much work has been done towards elaborating the commercial production of pure insulin, which can now be bought quite cheaply in standardized units. When first on the market it cost as much as twenty-five shillings for a hundred units, a prohibitive price for any but the very rich (the injections have to be continued throughout the life of the patient); but in the last decades commercial competition has brought the price as low as five shillings for a phial of forty units.[1]

There are many other hormones in the human body. Here we must content ourselves with a brief mention of just a few, those being chosen which have the most striking effects. There is one made by the parathyroid glands, which indirectly controls the amount of calcium in the blood. This is an important function, because too little calcium gives rise to a condition called tetany, in which cramp-like spasm of the muscles of the hand, face and larynx occurs. Accidental removal of the parathyroid glands in the course of extensive excision of the thyroid gland (in cases of goitre) has occurred in man and has been followed by tetany. This can be relieved temporarily by injecting parathormone (as the active principle of the parathyroid is called).

A further important group of hormones are those connected with the reproductive system, in particular those produced by the testes and ovaries. The testes, besides producing spermatozoa, have certain cells which produce testosterone and other 'androgens', as these male hormones are called. Testosterone is responsible not only for the development of the accessory male organs of reproduction, but also for the secondary male sex characteristics which occur in a boy at puberty, such as growth of hair on the face, trunk and axillae, the 'breaking' of the voice and general increase in muscle bulk. It seems that the activities of the testes are ultimately controlled by hormones from the anterior pituitary body.

In the human female the monthly ovarian cycle is also controlled from the anterior pituitary body, but the ovary itself produces important hormones of its own. These belong to the powerful steroid class of hormones which were extensively investigated in the late thirties and early forties. The first group to be isolated were the oestrogens, which play a large part in the control of the menstrual cycle.

One of the pioneers in the study of the ovarian hormones was Gregory Pincus, who became research director of the Worcester Foundation for Experimental Biology. He showed how another

[1] Of course it became free on prescription under the National Health Service Act, from 1948 onwards.

steroid hormone, *progesterone*, produced by the ovary, was present in much increased quantities during pregnancy and that it was this substance that prevented further ovulation so long as the pregnancy lasted. He went on to prove that this hormone could prevent ovulation when injected into non-pregnant animals. From 1950 onwards powerful new hormones of the progesterone type began to be synthesized and some of these were found to be active when taken orally. Here was the vital clue which Pincus saw was the key to the development of the famous contraceptive pill. He and his colleagues at the Worcester Foundation, Shrewsbury, Massachusetts set about testing more than 200 different compounds for their power to prevent ovulation. They then chose the three which seemed most likely to be fit for human use. In 1954 Pincus and John Rock began clinical trials and were soon able to prove that the new method was outstandingly successful in preventing conception. It also had obvious advantages, socially and aesthetically over the older methods—the mechanical devices and spermicidal chemicals.

The overwhelming importance of this invention cannot be too strongly emphasized. Not only was this a new scientific method of birth control, but at the first trial, it was practically 100 per cent effective. It was a discovery unparalleled in the whole history of medicine. To prove that the continued administration of these potent drugs over long periods was quite harmless was the next requirement. This has been fully investigated and, while some have claimed that the pill may slightly increase the risk of cardiovascular disease, on the whole it seems that the majority of women suffer no harm. The revolutionary impact of the Pincus pill is already being felt in many parts of the world and it may well go far towards preventing the disasters of 'population explosions' which threaten the well-being of the whole world. Pincus should be recognized as one of the greatest benefactors of his age.

Among the new artificial oestrogens that have been synthesized in the laboratory is one called *stilboestrol*. This is much more stable than naturally-occurring oestrogens, which, when given by the mouth are rapidly destroyed in the liver. Stilboestrol is not only effective when swallowed, but it has the additional advantage that it can be manufactured cheaply. It has been found of great value in controlling the spread of cancer of the prostate gland. Thus a female hormone is used to control an exclusively male disease. It does this because it antagonizes the male hormone testosterone, on which the malignant prostatic cells appear to be dependent for their growth.

From these few examples can be envisaged the tremendous complexity of the chemical government of the body. It is probable indeed that every organ gives out some form of chemical agent which has some effect in more distant parts of the body. This idea is by no means a modern one. In the eighteenth century Theophile de Bordeu had stated his opinion that 'every organ—not merely the glands—serves as a factory of specific substance, which enters the blood-stream and that these substances are of the greatest importance for the integrity of the organism'.[1] Some writers have gone further and have suggested that hormones control the actual mental make-up of a person. There is little doubt that the character of a man may be considerably influenced by his internal chemistry, but many will be perturbed at any attempt to explain the whole of human mental activity in such terms, and there will always be many to fight the suggestion that:

> 'Courage now is mere hormonogen
> And loyalty entails some ductless gland.[2]

[1] *Oeuvres Completes*, II, p, 942. Cited by Max Neuberger, *Essays in the History of Medicine* (translated), New York, 1932, p. 109.

[2] H. S. Mackintosh, *One Hundred and One Ballades,* London, 1931, p. 69.

CHAPTER EIGHT

THE RÖNTGEN RAYS

OF all the new physical aids to diagnosis none was so unexpected, unhoped-for and consequently unlooked-for as the Röntgen rays. This discovery, like so many others, had its beginning in an accident. In saying this we have no wish to detract from the genius of the inventor; for had not Wilhelm Conrad Röntgen been a physicist of exceptional ability, the new rays might so easily have been overlooked. Indeed it is certain that the rays had been produced previously in many physical laboratories all over the world; but their existence had remained unrecognized.

Towards the close of the last century almost every well-equipped physical laboratory possessed, in what is known as a Crookes tube, a potential means of producing the rays. These tubes were made of glass and contained various gases at very low pressures. By means of wires sealed into the glass, high-voltage electrical discharges could be passed from an induction-coil through the gas in the tube and the extraordinary phenomena which occurred could be studied.

Heinrich Hertz and P. Lenard had made brilliant experiments with a new kind of ray which, under certain conditions, they found emanating from the negative wire inside the tube. It was while experimenting with these so-called cathode rays that Röntgen, professor of physics at Würzburg, made his startling observations on November 8th, 1895.

Working in the dark, with the Crookes tube completely enclosed, he noticed that a small piece of paper coated with barium platinocyanide shone brightly while the electrical discharge was taking place. This may not seem a very striking observation, but it was to have far-reaching effects. Röntgen told no one of his discovery, but with immense energy set out on truly scientific lines to investigate the phenomenon.

The Röntgen Rays

Some weeks passed before he had convinced himself that the unlikely results he had obtained were indeed facts. He had worked out pretty completely the fundamental character of the new rays when, on December 28th, with some hesitation he presented his astonishing communication *On a New Kind of Ray*[1] to the Physical Medical Society of Würzburg. 'Now there will be the devil to pay,' he observed.

The paper showed at once how thorough Röntgen had been. He proved that the rays emanated from the point where the cathode-rays struck the wall of the glass tube. The most surprising objects, a book for example, seemed transparent to the rays, and objects varied in their degree of transparency according to their thickness and their density. Other substances besides barium platinocyanide fluoresced in the path of the rays. A photographic plate was sensitive to the rays, but the human eye was not. The behaviour of the rays differed in many ways from that of light-rays, in that the former could not be reflected by any substance nor deviated by a prism, nor could he produce 'interference' effects nor polarize the rays by any of the ordinary methods. Yet the rays seemed to travel in straight lines, for the shadows cast by a dense object were sharp. They differed too from the cathode-rays in that the new rays travelled much farther through the air and, unlike the cathode-rays, could not be deflected by a magnet. Röntgen illustrated his paper with some photographic shadow-pictures, including one of a human hand showing the bones. Since the inventor admitted that he was unaware of the true nature of the rays, he proposed to call them the X-rays and he put forward the suggestion, which was subsequently disproved, that they differed from light in being longitudinal (as opposed to transverse) vibrations in what was then called the luminiferous ether. After a demonstration before the Physical Medical Society it was decided that the rays should be called 'Röntgen's rays'. However, in most parts of the world they are more commonly known as X-rays.

Unlike so many great men who have had to fight desperately for the recognition of their discoveries, Röntgen became famous at once (although it should be added that, scientifically speaking, he

[1] *Eine Neue Art von Strahlen.*

would have been considered a great physicist even if he had not made this discovery). When the news became known there was great excitement all over the world and, since almost every laboratory possessed or could obtain a Crookes tube, the existence of the rays was soon confirmed.

The immense value of the new discovery to medical diagnosis was quickly seen and it was not long before surgeons began to take shadow-pictures of fractures and dislocations. Shot or other foreign bodies showed up well on the plates and photographs were also taken of teeth and stones in the kidney. The bony changes which occur in gout, rickets and other conditions began to be examined by the same method, while the heart and lungs, though not so dense as the bones could also be photographed with a suitable length of exposure.

The new discovery was fortunately given active encouragement by educated opinion and was patronized by many persons in high places. The German Emperor, for instance, before whom Röntgen demonstrated his rays as early as January 1896, was sufficiently impressed to have a picture taken of his crippled left arm with the object of determining the nature of the deformity.[1] Queen Amelia of Portugal is said to have had X-ray pictures made of several of her court ladies in order to demonstrate to them the evils of tight-lacing.[2] So Röntgen's fame spread and messages of congratulation began to reach him from all over the world. In 1901 he was awarded a Nobel prize.

Here too was something to interest the public. The popular press took up the subject, but, as so often happens, it failed to appreciate the true nature of the new scientific discovery. It mis-understood the 'invisible light' which could penetrate where the eye could not. In general people did not properly grasp the fact that the new photographs were merely shadows and not focused pictures. One periodical wrote of the 'revolting indecency' of an invention that would make privacy impossible. In London adver-tisements appeared offering X-ray-proof underclothes, while in America in 1896 an Assemblyman of New Jersey introduced a bill in the state legislature to prohibit 'the use of X-rays in

[1] Glasser, O., *Wilhelm Conrad Röntgen and the Early History of the Rontgen Rays,* London, 1933.   [2] Ibid.

opera-glasses in theaters'. The subject of the new rays was a favourite one with contemporary cartoonists.

Attempts were made to discredit Röntgen, including the allega-
tion that his discovery was really that of a junior assistant. There
have been many other claims to priority, but all have been carefully
scrutinized and not one could be substantiated. Such recriminations embittered the inventor, who was a modest and retiring man.
He was wounded by the vituperation of a few and, retiring into
private life, he died in 1922, lonely and neglected.

The uses of Röntgen-rays in medicine and surgery have multiplied a hundred times in the decades since the discovery. It was
realized that if certain hollow organs in the body, not ordinarily
seen in an X-ray picture, were filled up with some substance
opaque to the rays, then a picture could be taken showing the shape
of the inside of the organ in question. A beginning was made in
1896 when W. Becher of Berlin photographed the stomach of a
dead guinea-pig after filling it with a solution containing lead.
Soluble lead is very poisonous, so that in order to apply the same
process to human beings it was necessary to find something that
should be at the same time both opaque and non-toxic. The
problem was solved by Walter Cannon, later professor of physiology at Harvard, but at the time a medical student. In 1896 he
began to feed small animals with bismuth subnitrate and to follow
the opaque meal down the gastro-intestinal tract with the aid of a
fluorescent screen. Cannon was thus able to describe the normal
movements of the stomach and intestine during the digestive
processes in various animals.

Soon afterwards several independent scientists started to study
the alimentary tract in man and in a few short years the method
became and has remained one of the standard routine procedures
in the examination of the stomach and intestine. The patient drinks
a glassful of a mixture containing barium sulphate (also introduced
by Cannon as being less dangerous than bismuth) and this is
photographed at intervals during its passage through the body. In
this way tumours or ulcers can often be seen and a diagnosis made
with certainty.

Other opaque materials have been used to examine other organs.
The bladder, the ureters and kidneys can be studied by injecting

sodium iodide solution into the urinary tract. Photographs taken in this way are called pyelograms and they show up abnormalities in the cavities inside these organs. More recently, by injecting into the blood-stream a solution containing a special organic compound containing iodine, which is excreted by the kidneys, it is possible not only to see the anatomical abnormalities, but also, by timing the appearance of the opaque solution in the pelvis of the kidneys, to estimate the function of each kidney separately. Photographs such as these are called 'intra-venous pyelograms.'

An ingenious method of obtaining an X-ray picture of the gall-bladder was devised by E. A. Graham and W. H. Cole of St Louis in 1924. They found an opaque compound (again one containing iodine), which, when swallowed, appears later in the bile stored in the gall-bladder. An X-ray picture of this may show little holes, as it were, in the shadow of the gall-bladder if there are gall-stones present; for these are often more transparent to the rays than is the iodine compound. In this way one can detect stones which might not be seen at all in a 'straight' X-ray picture.

More recently it was found safe to inject radio-opaque materials into the blood-stream. Suitable preparations with a high iodine content are used and in this way satisfactory X-ray pictures can be obtained of the arteries and of the interior of the heart itself.

Great advances in knowledge of lung diseases have also been made by X-rays. Tuberculosis can be detected at a very early stage. In addition to the ordinary X-ray pictures of the chest, it has been found possible to fill up the living lung-spaces with non-irritating opaque substances and show up abnormalities by means of X-ray pictures, called bronchograms.

Much work has been done to improve the quality of radiography. In the early days very long exposure were necessary to secure good pictures. Soon better and better tubes were devised. A target of platinum was found to be a better source of the rays than the glass wall of the tube. In 1913 the American physicist William A. Coolidge produced the improved form of tube which bears his name. Photographic plates, too, were improved very much in quality and sensitivity. Nowadays films have superseded glass plates. The superiority of the films lies not only in the convenience of storage, but also in the fact that they are sufficiently thin to allow a sensitive coating to be applied on both sides without too much blurring of the picture. In this way the exposure time is halved and, by placing on each side of the film a sheet of paper coated with material that shines in the path of the X-rays, the speed is still further increased. By using these intensifying screens the actual picture is taken partly by the fluorescence of the coated paper as well as by direct effect of the rays on the film.

Apart from considerations of convenience, it was found highly important to reduce the exposure-time to the minimum because of the damaging effect of the rays. Unfortunately the Röntgen rays were not an unmixed blessing, for gradually among the X-ray pioneers came the distressing and disastrous effects of X-ray burns. Redness and brown pigmentation of the skin, dropping out of the hair, superficial ulceration and even skin cancer—all these followed insidiously and relentlessly in the wake of prolonged exposure to the rays. There were many workers who lost limbs and lives in this horrible way. Twenty-eight American martyrs to Röntgen rays have been listed by Brown in his book on the subject.[1] Now that the danger is recognized every worker with X-rays protects himself, his neighbours and his photographic films with walls, screens, aprons and gloves heavily impregnated with lead. Professor Röntgen himself escaped without harm because, though he did not foresee the damaging effect of the rays on the skin, for the sake of convenience he worked almost entirely inside an enclosed and metal-lined cabinet with only one window through which the rays were admitted from the Crookes tube outside.

Once it was known that the X-rays had a destructive effect on the skin, it was natural that empirical attempts should be made to destroy cancerous growths in the same way. The rays were turned from diagnostic to therapeutic use. They have certainly proved useful in controlling certain types of cancer and in the actual cure of other types, for example rodent ulcers of the face. X-rays are also used with the object of preventing a recurrence of a cancer after it has been removed by surgery. Deep internal tumours have also been attacked by the rays, but since the radiation cannot be

[1] Brown, P., *American Martyrs to Science through the Roentgen Rays*, 1936, Springfield, Ill.

focused, there is grave danger that the skin over the tumour may be burned before the tumour is destroyed. This can be avoided to some extent by giving multiple short doses directed at the tumour from various angles outside, so that no single area of skin receives more than a small dose, but the tumour receives them all.

Radiotherapy, as treatment by X-rays is called, has grown up into a specialized branch of medicine, which now includes treatment by radioactivity as well. This will be discussed more fully in the ensuing chapter.

CHAPTER NINE

RADIUM AND RADIOACTIVITY

THE revolutionary effect of the discovery of radium on the basic science of physics completely outweighs the medical value of the new substance. The study of radioactive elements has changed our fundamental ideas about the constitution of matter. It has given rise to the conception of intra-atomic energy and, not only has it made a reality of the ancient belief in the transmutation of the elements, but it has provided proof that matter is spontaneously changing into energy.

After the discovery of X-rays it was suggested by Jules Henri Poincaré, a French physicist, that it might be rewarding to try whether any of the known fluorescent or phosphorescent substances gave out invisible rays. His colleague Henri Becquerel undertook a systematic investigation of such substances by placing them on photographic plates wrapped in black paper. After a number of negative results he was able to report to the Academy of Sciences in 1896 that salts of uranium gave out rays which affected a photographic plate. The rays arose quite spontaneously and the magnitude of the effect depended solely on the quantity of uranium present.

Two years later Marie Sklodowska, the Polish wife of the physicist Pierre Curie, began to investigate the Becquerel rays, measuring their intensity with an electrometer designed by her husband. In a search for other radioactive elements she found that thorium also gave out rays. She then began to examine systematically every kind of metallic substance. She noted that certain ores containing uranium were far more active than could be accounted for by their content of uranium and thorium alone. From this she inferred that such ores must contain a small amount of something many hundred times as potent as uranium.

The mystery had now become so fascinating that her husband

joined her in her work. Together they set out to isolate this hypothetical substance by purely chemical means. More than a ton of pitchblende (the active ore) was given by the Austrian Government and after two years of immense labour the two savants succeeded in extracting a few thousandth parts of an ounce of pure chloride of radium—the name they gave to the new element.

They found that this new stuff possessed truly remarkable properties. It gave off light, heat and electricity continuously without suffering any apparent change. We know now that the element is spontaneously turning part of its own substance into energy and is in fact slowly losing both weight and radioactive power. A definite small fraction of all the atoms of radium undergoes disintegration in any given interval of time. The process is so slow that it would take some 1,600 years for a mass of radium to lose half its radioactivity. This concept of the 'half-life' of a radioactive element is of great importance in the use of these materials in medicine. No known chemical or physical process was found to influence the rate of radiation and disintegration which proceeded continuously and inevitably.

From the unlucky circumstance of receiving a burn from some radium that he was carrying in his waistcoat pocket, Becquerel was able to draw attention to the strange physiological properties of the element. Pierre Curie confirmed this by producing on himself in a few hours a burn which took months to heal.

The Curies were awarded a Nobel prize and a special professorial chair was created for Curie to continue his important work; but in 1906 the scientific world was shocked to learn that he had been crushed to death under the wheel of a two-horse dray in the streets of Paris. Fortunately his widow lived for many years to carry on her investigations. She died in 1934 from anaemia which was almost certainly due to the destruction of her blood-forming bone-marrow by the relentless action of the rays with which she worked.

As soon as it had been shown that skin burns could be caused by radium, doctors began to try if malignant growths of the skin could be destroyed by the same agency. The first results of treating cancer were published in 1904 by H.-A. Danlos, a dermatologist at

St Louis Hospital in Paris. Skin cancers were also treated about the same time in St Petersburg and in New York.

The biological Laboratory for Radium was set up in 1906. Its staff included the physicist Jacques Danne, the physiologist Henri Dominici and the doctors Louis Wickham and Degrais, both dermatologists. The most fundamental contributions to the new science of radiotherapy were made by Dominici. Radium emits three types of rays, all invisible, called alpha, beta and gamma rays respectively. The first two types do not possess much power of penetration, though they do enter the skin deeply enough to cause severe damage. Dominici showed how to exclude the alpha and beta rays by suitable metallic screens, leaving only the gamma rays (which are a kind of X-ray with very short wavelength) to pass out. In 1908 he used gamma radiation to treat deeply seated tumours and found that the overlying tissues were hardly damaged, while the tumour tissue regressed. This process of filtering out unwanted and damaging fractions of a complex beam of radiation is one which has had many applications in radiotherapy. Dominici, like so many pioneers of radiation, died in 1919 from exposure to the rays.

Many different methods of applying radium were devised. The radium salt was put into glass tubes, sealed and enclosed in an outer tube of silver or platinum which acted as a filter. Such tubes could be inserted into the natural cavities of the body, such as the uterus or the oesophagus or, as needles, at strategic positions into and around a tumour, so that a complete barrage of rays reached every part of the growth and the neighbouring lymphatic drainage system along which malignant cells could spread.

The technique of placing the needles properly called for a high degree of skill. It required, too, great experience to decide which cases were suited for radiotherapy, because certain growths, by reason of their inaccessibility, nearness to dangerous areas or other cause, could not be so treated. One of the most useful expedients was devised by Giocchimo Failla of New York. Radium, in the process of disintegration, goes through several stages and gives out a gas called radium emanation (or radon). The breaking down of the radon is largely responsible for the healing gamma rays. Radon decays comparatively quickly, having a half-life of rather under four days. Furthermore, being a gas, it can be pumped off from the parent radium. In 1924 Failla sealed radon in small lengths of fine gold tubing. These 'radon seeds' were used just like radium needles, but by contrast they could be left permanently in place, because their radioactivity rapidly became negligible after a few days.

We must now enter briefly and in a much over-simplified way into the mysteries of artificially induced radioactivity, as this has had an increasing importance in medicine in both diagnosis and treatment. In doing so it will be necessary to use some of the technical terms employed by the physicists, without having space to explain their exact meaning. In brief the alpha rays consist of rapidly moving, positively charged nuclei of helium atoms. The beta rays are streams of high-speed electrons, negatively charged. In 1919 Ernest Rutherford, in the Cavendish Laboratory at Cambridge, used alpha particles from radium to bombard thin layers of matter and found that the nuclei of nitrogen atoms could have hydrogen nuclei knocked clean out of them. This was the first proof that the atom (previously thought to be an indestructible and fundamental unit of nature) could be split. Later Cockcroft and Wilson in the same laboratory produced similar atom-splitting effects by purely electrical means (i.e. without using radioactive substances). This they did by using hydrogen nuclei (positively charged protons) as bullets, accelerating them to enormous speeds by electrical forces.

Three years later came the first artificial radioactive elements, produced by bombarding various light elements with alpha particles. By 1931 machines had been specially designed to accelerate charged particles—either hydrogen, heavy hydrogen (deuterium) or helium nuclei—to speeds high enough to penetrate the nucleus of any atom and cause it to split up and in some instances to form artificial radioactive elements. The cyclotron, built in 1931 by Lawrence and Livingstone in America, was the first effective machine to produce these new substances. In this machine the charged atomic particles are passed, in a near vacuum, through a magnetic field engendered by a very powerful electromagnet. By reversing the magnetic field at pre-determined intervals the particles can be made to fly round the machine at ever-increasing speeds. These fast-moving bullets are fired into suitable targets of inert and normally stable substances placed in their path, and so some of the bullets penetrate the nuclei of the target. When this happens the charged particle either adds itself to the target nucleus or else knocks part of the nucleus clean out. In either case fresh elemental nuclei are produced and these are generally radioactive.

These new substances are 'isotopes' of known elements. They have chemical properties indistinguishable from the corresponding elements, but they have different atomic weights, because they carry extra matter (in the form of neutrons) which makes them unstable. Thus they continually 'decay', transforming themselves at a constant rate into lighter elements with the emission of radiation. Each different isotope has its own half-life, which may be a few minutes, a few days, a few years or even thousands and millions of years. It is the isotopes with half-lives of a few days that are likely to prove of the greatest use in medicine today.

We have space to consider only a few of the many medical uses of isotopes. The so-called 'tracer-techniques' consist in using radioactive elements to replace in part the normal elements in the body. For example, by using radioactive iron it is possible to study the fate of the iron normally contained in the haemoglobin of the blood. Such radioactive iron can be 'traced' with suitable machines which pick up and measure the radiations it gives out. A radioactive iodine, with a half-life of 13 days, or another one with a half-life of 8 days can be used in research into the metabolism of the thyroid gland. For example a measured amount of radio-iodine is swallowed and, by means of a gamma-ray-counter applied to the neck, the rate at which the iodine is taken up by the thyroid can be measured. Other radioisotopes which have been used are cobalt in the study of Vitamin B_{12} and so in the diagnosis of pernicious anaemia, arsenic in the location of brain tumours and phosphorus in measuring the volume of the circulating blood.

However, it is in treating cancer that radioisotopes have been more generally used. As with X-rays, it is necessary to irradiate deep-seated tumours from different directions, so that the overlying tissues are not too badly damaged by the gamma rays. The radioactive isotope Cobalt-60 is now widely used, as it is an effective substitute for expensive and cumbrous X-ray machines. Furthermore it can be made fairly cheaply as a by-product of the giant nuclear reactors. (Not that a nuclear reactor is a cheap thing to build; but once it has been set up, with the prime purpose of turning nuclear forces into electricity, many different isotopes can be prepared on a commercial scale as a kind of sideline). Cobalt-60 has a half-life of 5·25 years, so that not only does it have to be replaced from time to time, but, in regulating the dose of radiation, allowance has to be made for the gradual falling-off of radioactivity. As we have seen, radium was the first substance to be used for radiotherapy and, with a half-life of 1,600 years, it may be regarded for practical purposes as inexhaustible. But radium is very scarce and laborious to extract, so that it is correspondingly extremely expensive. The introduction of artificial radioisotopes has largely overcome these difficulties.

Obviously it would be a big step forward if we could introduce into the body radioactive substances having a direct affinity for malignant cells, that is to say acting like dyes which stain different kinds of cells selectively. In this way we could use selective isotope radiotherapy, choosing the appropriate isotope, with a short half-life, as a 'magic bullet' fired at the tumour alone. Work has been done and undoubtedly will be continued on these lines, but so far success has been very limited.

There are many ways of using radioactivity in industry but one of the most useful to medicine is the sterilization of 'disposable' surgical kits and plastic syringes and hypodermic needles (for use once only) by means of gamma rays. Since Lord Lister's day sterilization of surgical gear has been one of the most expensive and time-consuming procedures in all medicine. A central sterilizing unit (an autoclave) in a hospital costs several thousand pounds, to say nothing of the maintenance costs and the salaries of the persons using it. On the other hand disposable instruments are safely and completely sterilized by gamma rays in the factory and are sent to the ward or theatre wrapped in plastic foil. It can be readily seen that the extension of this practice to all hospitals and surgeries is going to save the health service enormous expenditure of time and money.

CHAPTER TEN

THE VITAMINS

AFTER the discoveries of the great nineteenth-century chemists and physiologists it seemed that knowledge of the essential constituents of food was fairly complete. None the less an adequate diet could not be built up from chemically pure substances. This was first discovered in 1880 by Niko ai Lunin, a Russian chemist working at the University of Basel. He fed mice with a synthetic diet of pure casein (milk protein), fat and cane-sugar and they did not survive beyond three weeks, although this was a mixture which should have been adequate in the light of all the accumulated chemical knowledge. On the other hand, if he gave the mice powdered milk alone, then they lived for months, so that evidently milk contained some unknown substance essential to life.

A comparable discovery was made in human beings in connexion with the disease beriberi which was very prevalent in the East. The Japanese Navy had suffered severely from this. In 1882 Takaki proved that it was due to faulty diet. He changed the rice diet to one containing meat, bread, fruit and vegetables and beriberi disappeared.

Ten years later Christian Eijkman, a Dutch medical officer working in the East Indies, discovered the cause of beriberi through a curious accident. Having run out of food for his laboratory chickens, he gave them polished rice from the hospital and they developed an illness very like human beriberi. He found he could prevent this by adding rice-polishings to the food. There was an anti-beriberi factor in the husks. Human beings took the disease by eating only rice or beans which had been polished, a process which removed the husks. Unpolished rice was the remedy.

Thus began the hunt for these essential factors which we know today as vitamins. The name 'vitamine' was originally proposed by Casimir Funk who applied it to the anti-beriberi substance in the rice-husks. He believed, erroneously as it turned out, that it belonged chemically to the class of nitrogen-containing compounds known as amines; but though the idea was wrong, the name has survived. The vitamins are classified alphabetically (vitamin A, B, C, etc.), corresponding to the order in which they were discovered, though the simplicity of this arrangement has been vitiated by the fact that vitamin B has been found to be a highly complex substance containing about a dozen different factors. None the less it is in alphabetical order that they can best be described.

Vitamin A. This is the growth-promoting factor. In 1912 the English biochemist Frederick Gowland Hopkins fed groups of rats on pure casein, carbohydrates and salts. At the same time other groups were fed with exactly similar food with the addition of a small ration of fresh milk. The rats who had no fresh milk failed to grow although they ate just as much as the others. Later their appetites failed, but the important point was that they ceased to grow before they ceased to eat. The synthetic diet was wanting in some factor which is found in fresh milk and which is essential to growth.

The matter was pursued by E. V. McCollum and others at the University of Wisconsin. In 1913 they proved that the growth-promoting factor was contained in certain fats, particularly butter-fat and egg yolk. At about the same time it was discovered at Yale that cod-liver oil was a rich source of this vitamin, which became known as 'fat-soluble A'.

In 1919 Harry Steenbock, also at Wisconsin, proved that vitamin A was somehow derived from the yellow pigment in certain vegetables such as carrots and, nine years later, it was discovered by Thomas Moore at Cambridge that this yellow pigment is converted in the body to the colourless vitamin A found in liver oil. The chemical structure of the vitamin was fully worked out in Switzerland by 1931 and not long afterwards it was synthesized in the test-tube at the University of Illinois.

In brief this essential factor is found in nature in milk-fat, and therefore in butter and cream; in eggs; in huge amounts in liver-fat, especially in cod-liver oil and in even larger concentrations in halibut-liver oil. Vitamin A is absent from purely vegetable oils, such as olive-oil or coconut-oil and consequently is not found in purely vegetable margarines; but since 1940 vitamins A and D have been added to all margarine sold in Great Britain.

Vitamin B. As has been told the story is bound up with that of the disease beriberi. This anti-beriberi factor became known as the antineuritic vitamin, because of the degenerative changes in the nervous system caused by lack of it. In 1916 McCollum called it 'water-soluble vitamin B.'

About the same time Joseph Goldberger, working for the U.S. Public Health Service, proved that vitamin B contained a quite separate component, the lack of which caused the disease pellagra. This is characterized by soreness of the mouth and tongue, a rash on the hands, face and neck, and ultimately to degeneration of the nervous system. For hundreds of years it had been known to affect peoples living mainly on corn. In 1915 there were over 10,000 deaths from this disease in the United States, chiefly among the rural poor and in orphanages and asylums. In 1914, by adding milk and a daily egg to the diet Goldberger abolished pellagra from two Mississippi orphanages in which there had been 200 cases the year before.

Today the water-soluble B is known to contain, in addition to the antineuritic factor (thiamin) and the antipellagra substance (nicotinic acid), other vitamins essential to well-being, but too numerous for consideration here. The story of vitamin B_{12}, the cobalt-containing factor, which plays an essential part in the normal development of blood, is told later in connexion with pernicious anaemia.

Vitamin C. Scurvy made its appearance as soon as the fifteenth-century navigators began to make really long voyages. In the sixteenth century Sir Richard Hawkins estimated that it had killed 10,000 men during his twenty years at sea. An excellent description of the symptoms can be found in Hakluyt's account of Jacques Cartier's voyage to Newfoundland in 1535. '. . . the said vnknowen sickness began to spread itselfe amongst us after the strangest sort that euer was eyther heard or seene, insomuch as some did lose all their strength, and could not stand on their feete, then did their legges swel, their sinnowes shrinke blacke as any cole. Others also had their skins spotted with spots of blood of a purple coulour; then did it ascend vp to their ankels, knees, thighes, shoulders, armes and necke; their mouth became stincking, their gummes so rotten that all flesh did fall off, euen to the rootes of the teeth which did almost all fall out'. In Anson's famous voyage round the world in 1740–44 he lost four-fifths of his crew from scurvy. However, the disease was not confined to seamen. It has followed regularly in the wake of war and famine.

We have seen how Lind had rid the Royal Navy of Scurvy. He did this in 1753 by adding orange and lemon juice to the diet. But it seems certain that long before that time the knowledge was available, had men chosen or been able to use it. Francis Bacon in his *New Atlantis*, published in 1627, the year after his death, wrote these uncompromising words: 'Besides, there were brought in to us a great store of those scarlet oranges for our sick; which (they said) were an assured remedy for sickness taken at sea.'

Although it was easy to prevent scurvy in practice, all attempts to isolate the vitamin chemically were for long unsuccessful because vitamin C is so easily destroyed by chemical reagents. The problem was solved in 1932 by Charles G. King of Pittsburgh University, who after years of work succeeded in isolating it in pure crystalline form from lemon-juice. Its chemical identity was established in Switzerland and in Hungary as ascorbic acid. In 1934 A. Szent-Györgyi of Szeged University developed a method of manufacturing vitamin C on a large scale from the fruit of the 'noble pepper' (*Capsicum annuum*), a vegetable used ordinarily to make paprika. Chemical synthesis followed soon after and today synthetic ascorbic acid is available and cheap.

Vitamin D. Rickets is a disease of infancy and it is all too common today. It produces the well-known bony deformities which are particularly noticeable in the legs, arms, chest and head, due to faulty deposition of lime-salts in the growing parts of the bones. In 1908 L. Finlay succeeded in producing the disease in puppies by feeding them on a diet deficient in raw milk. In 1918 Edward Mellanby found that the disease could be prevented by the addition of a variety of substances rich in vitamin A, notably butter, cod-liver oil and animal fats. At first this effect was attributed to vitamin A, but Hopkins in England and

McCollum in the U.S.A. invented methods of destroying the vitamin A, yet the cod-liver oil retained its power to prevent rickets. There must be a fourth factor, which was accordingly named vitamin D.

In the nineteenth century it had been pointed out by Theobald Palm, an English medical missionary in the East, that the one factor common to all countries where rickets was unknown was an abundance of sunlight; but his message went unheeded. It was not until 1916 that Kurt Huldschinsky, a German pediatrician, showed that ultra-violet light could prevent or cure rickets in children. Later still Harry Steenbock at Wisconsin University made the surprising discovery that the antirachitic effect occurred whether the animal itself or its food was treated with the light. This was explained later by the proof that a substance called ergosterol (named from the plant ergot from which it was first prepared), which is widely distributed in plants and animals, is activated into vitamin D by the action of ultra-violet light. In this way the vitamin is made commercially by dissolving irradiated ergosterol in oil. It is sold under the name calciferol.

Besides the influence on the development of the bones, it seems that vitamin D plays a big part in protecting the teeth from decay. When the vitamin D content of the diet is deficient and, especially when there is also an excess of cereals and a shortage of calcium, the teeth are poorly developed and readily decay. This is over-simplifying matters, because in some parts of the world where there is gross rickets, the children's teeth are good, whereas in England today children with well-developed bones have many bad teeth.[1] Cleaning the teeth regularly certainly helps by removing particles of fermenting food which cause decay, but here again we can point to the perfect teeth of some people for whom oral hygiene hardly exists. In 1932, on a visit of H.M.S. *Carlisle* to Tristan da Cunha, some 156 of the inhabitants were examined and 131 were found to be completely free from dental caries, and the oldest man, aged seventy-five, had a complete set of teeth. These islanders, it was said, lived mainly on potatoes, fish, milk and eggs and *they never cleaned their teeth*. It must be added that they were all breast-fed and were compelled to live on a diet without cereals,

[1] See below, p. 352 *et seq.*

for in 1885 rats were introduced on the island and thereafter prevented the growth of grain.[1]

Light was shed on all this by May Mellanby's discovery that vitamin D has this influence on the proper growth of the teeth and that normal teeth are more resistant to decay than those imperfectly formed. Mellanby went on to show that a diet containing much cereal, and oatmeal in particular, was associated with rapid decay of teeth in children. Apparently cereals contain something which counteracts the effect of the vitamin.

Dental decay is very prevalent in this country today. Mellanby has pointed out that the natural foods which are rich in vitamin D—eggs, milk, suet, butter and cheese are expensive compared with cereals and carbohydrates. The vegetable oils, as bought in shops, are generally no good as a source of the vitamin. The cheap cereals hinder the action of vitamin D, so that big consumers of the former need extra supplies of the latter.

Other vitamins have been discovered, for example the so-called fertility vitamin E, which was shown to be essential to the reproduction of rats. However, it must be admitted that no disease due to the absence of this vitamin has been demonstrated in man. Vitamin K, widely distributed in nature, is indispensable in the defensive mechanism of blood-clotting.

Vitamin B_{12}. Yet another dietetic success must be mentioned here. It concerns the disease pernicious anaemia, or Addisonian anaemia, called after Thomas Addison of Guy's Hospital, who first clearly differentiated it from other anaemias in 1849. It is (or was) a fatal disease in which the patient becomes progressively more and more bloodless. For its victims the road to death was long and hard, being often marked by curious remissions, followed always by recurrence of the symptoms.

An American, William Pepper, noticed that in pernicious anaemia the red marrow of the bones is much altered. This marrow, which normally manufactures the red blood-corpuscles, becomes unable to make or to supply perfect red cells, so that immature cells are found both in the blood-stream and also heaped up in the marrow. Pernicious anaemia is essentially a disease of the blood-forming organs.

[1] *British Medical Journal*, 1932, I, p. 538.

The Vitamins

In 1922 George Whipple at the University of Rochester, had done a series of experiments on dogs made anaemic by bleeding and had found that a diet containing fresh uncooked liver had a powerful effect in restoring the blood to normal. In 1923 George R. Minot, an American physician, began to treat patients with pernicious anaemia with a regular diet of liver and by 1926, he and his colleague William Murphy began to publish excellent results. Within a week of beginning treatment their patients began to mend and the improvement not only continued, but was maintained for a year.

The daily dose of liver was generally as much as half a pound and this was one big difficulty about the treatment. After a long course, patients faced with unending large amounts of liver sickened to the point of revolt. The next task of Minot and Murphy was therefore to prepare a concentrated extract of the blood-building factor. This was difficult because the chemical nature of the substance was unknown. They succeeded eventually in producing a fairly potent preparation which was effective when taken by the mouth. Later chemists all over the world attacked the problem and made extracts that could be given by intramuscular injection. Rather surprisingly it was found that these extracts, when injected, were from 30 to 50 times as potent as when given by the mouth.

In 1928 William Castle, working in Minot's laboratory, found that the stomach produced a curious 'intrinsic factor' (as he called it), which was essential to the proper absorption of the blood-forming agent from the food. Pernicious anaemia occurred when there was a deficiency of this factor, however much of the new vitamin there might be in the food. In Castle's own words 'the disease would not occur if the patient could daily effect the transfer of a millionth of a gram of vitamin B_{12} the distance of a small portion of a millimeter across the intestinal mucosa into the blood'.

There is a progressively paralysing complaint known by the cumbrous name of 'sub-acute combined degeneration of the spinal cord'. This occurs in people from middle-age onwards and, because of the severe anaemia of the Addisonian type which always accompanies it, it was thought to be a late sequel of pernicious anaemia. It is now certain that this is so, because the disease yields to the same treatment.

175

The natural sources of vitamin B_{12}—which contains cobalt—are chiefly liver, kidney, muscle, yeast, eggs and milk, but for treatment purposes this vitamin is now produced from cultures of the mould *Streptomyces griseus*, the same organism which makes the antibiotic streptomycin.

The actual quantities of vitamins needed for the maintenance of health are very small indeed in terms of weight. They are therefore more usually measured in artificially defined International Units. Thus the vitamin A requirement is about 5,000 I.U. of carotene or perhaps 6,000 for a growing child or at puberty. Damage can be caused by overdoses of this vitamin if taken in enormous excess of the natural needs. Of the vitamin B complex 2 milligrammes or less of thiamin and perhaps 10 to 15 milligrammes of nicotinic acid represent the optimal daily amounts required. With vitamin C. 10 mg. of ascorbic acid daily will give complete protection from scurvy and this amount is contained in one orange, half a grape-fruit or a generous helping of properly cooked green vegetables. Babies who are bottle-fed need supplements of orange or black-currant juice. Unlike vitamins A and D, excessive dosage of Vitamin C is not harmful, because ascorbic acid is readily excreted by the kidneys. Finally vitamin D is required in extremely small amounts. 250 I.U. per day are undoubtedly enough and this quantity is contained in a few thousandths of a milligramme. Here gain over dosage may cause serious damage with nausea, vomiting and deposits of calcium compounds in the heart, lungs and kidneys, the last of which may be fatally damaged.

It is unfortunate that vitamins should have been so shamelessly exploited by commercial firms. Excess of any vitamin over the normal needs can do no good at all and undoubtedly most of the money spent by the public on vitamin preparations is frankly wasted. It cannot be too plainly stated that, given a limited amount of money, it is better spent at the grocer or the green-grocer than at the chemist's shop.

CHAPTER ELEVEN

THE DEVELOPMENT OF MODERN SURGERY

IN this chapter it is not proposed to describe all the various surgical operations which have been devised for the relief of human suffering, but rather to point out the main discoveries which lie at the root of all the major advances in surgical technique.

The earlier stages in the conquest of infection have already been related in the section on Lister and the Antiseptic Method. Lister's ideas were widely adopted in Germany and it was there that the antiseptic method was improved in many respects between 1880 and 1890. First of all Koch and others identified the actual species of bacteria which caused wound infection: for example, in 1883 Friedrich Fehleisen of Berlin proved by inoculation experiments on animals and man that streptococci were the cause of erysipelas. It then became evident that bacteria normally present in air were comparatively harmless, so that Lister's carbolic spray was not really doing what was intended. It became clear, too, that disease-producing bacteria were being conveyed to the patients by the surgeons and nurses by means of direct contact or by the use of imperfectly sterilized instruments or dressings. Hugo Davidsohn, working in Koch's laboratory, was able to prove, in 1888, that boiling instruments for five minutes was enough to destroy all bacteria and their spores.

There still remained the problem of disinfecting the skin of the patient as well as that of the surgeon and the nurses. Carl Eberth, professor of bacteriology at Zürich, had shown as long ago as 1875 that the skin normally harbours millions of bacteria and that these hide deep in the glands and are brought to the surface continually in the sweat. Later Hermann Kümmell at Hamburg demonstrated, rather surprisingly at the time, that prolonged and thorough scrubbing of the skin with soap and water was more effective in removing bacteria than any of the chemical disinfectants then in use. This indeed is the essence of modern surgical technique, namely meticulous mechanical removal of all living bacteria from the skin, rather than their destruction by chemical agents. Antisepsis gave place to asepsis. The aseptic method was described in great detail by Carl Schimmelbusch in 1892 in his book *Anleitung zur aseptischen Wundebehandlung* (The Aseptic Treatment of Wounds). Unfortunately, apart from Germany, the new technique met with little or no enthusiasm. In 1876 Lister toured the United States and found that hardly anyone was using his methods. As late as 1883, in a discussion before the American Surgical Association, leading surgeons, almost to a man, condemned Lister's methods, which they said they had tried without success. The truth was that they had failed in the essence of the matter, namely painstaking attention to detail. One of America's greatest surgeons, J. M. T. Finney, wrote an account of the 'antiseptic' technique at the Massachusetts General Hospital in 1888, which shows only too plainly why it had failed to reproduce Lister's results. The surgeons wore the old frock-coats they had always done. The instruments had wooden handles which at best were merely wiped with carbolic lotion. The operation wounds were dabbed with old sponges which were used over and over again. The aseptic lesson had not been learnt.

A younger generation of American surgeons, who had seen Lister's methods succeeding in Germany, brought the proper use of asepsis and sterilization by heat into effective use in the United States. Unfortunately it has to be admitted that Lister's own country was almost the last to recognize and practise his methods. The American surgeon Halsted put the matter in a nutshell when he said that America had learned antisepsis from Germany and that England had learned it from America.

The chemical control of wound-infection continued to be an ideal; and men were always looking for substances which would kill bacteria without doing too much damage to the tissues of the patient. Mercurochrome was introduced with some measure of success by Hugh Young at Johns Hopkins Hospital to control the inevitable infection which followed operations on the prostate gland. In the thirties the discovery of highly efficient bactericidal agents such as the sulphonamides, gave further high hopes that sepsis could be prevented or cured by chemical means. The advent of penicillin during the Second World War provided a means of control far more effective than anything that had gone before.

In spite of all this, even today the problem of wound-infection has not been wholly solved. Infections still occur from time to time. The trouble is usually due to certain types of staphylococci which are resistant to penicillin. These organisms actually produce an enzyme (or ferment) called penicillinase, which destroys penicillin. Fortunately this problem of staphylococcal infection, though it has still not been completely solved, has at least been made more manageable in recent years by the invention of some semi-synthetic penicillins which are not destroyed by penicillinase. None the less there seems little doubt that when these disastrous infections do occur in operation wounds, it shows that too much reliance has been placed on chemical antiseptics and antibiotics and that the teaching of Lister has been neglected. There is no doubt that even today meticulous cleanliness and sterilization by heat (or other physical means such as gamma rays) must continue to be the chief bulwarks in the defence against sepsis.

When pain had been overcome by anaesthesia and infection by asepsis, the chief problem confronting the surgeons was the control of haemorrhage. Excessive bleeding not only weakens the patient but also, by flooding the site of the operation with blood, makes it difficult or impossible for the surgeon to see what he is doing. The tourniquet is said to have been invented at the siege of Besançon in 1674. In the eighteenth century ligatures of waxed silk or linen threads were used for tying the larger blood-vessels during amputation operations.

In the following century when surgery had enlarged its field into the abdomen, complete control of haemorrhage was seen to be essential, not only to enable the surgeon to see what he was about, but also to guard against any internal haemorrhage after the operation wound had been closed. Delicate artery clamps, which would lock firmly after they had been applied, were the answer to this problem. Jules Péan in Paris in 1862 and Spencer Wells in London in 1872 devised such clamps which are very like those in use today, with ring handles and ratchet locks. Nowadays very many of such instruments are used in every surgical operation, to pick up each bleeding point as it occurs and so keep the field of operation dry and visible. It is not unusual for a surgeon to use scores or even hundreds of artery clamps in an extensive operation, and their value can hardly be over-estimated. In a wound that is dry and where the tissues are never allowed to be covered in blood, the operator may work calmly and for hours without undue fatigue. The control of haemorrhage in fact engenders calmness and clear thinking.

Following the conquest of pain, infection and haemorrhage, the next enemy to be reckoned with was surgical shock. This is a condition of general collapse which may follow any severe injury or wound and may prove fatal. Military surgeons had long been aware of this hazard, because severe wounds, often followed by hours of neglect on the battlefield, always led to shock. In 1740 Henri François le Dran,[1] surgeon to Louis XIV, had described shock, or 'commotion' as he termed it, in his book on gunshot wounds.

It was nearly a century later that a further important contribution to the subject was made by Benjamin Travers of St Thomas's Hospital, London. In 1836 he published his book *An Inquiry Concerning that Disturbed State of Vital Functions Usually Denominated Constitutional Irritation*. He summarized the symptoms thus: '. . . universal pallor and contraction of surface, shuddering, very small rapid pulse, astoundment of the mental faculties, generally a dilated pupil, shortened respiration, dryness of tongue and fauces . . . at length cessation of the pulse at the wrist, oppressed and noisy respiration, coldness of the feet and hands, involuntary twitchings, relaxation of the sphincters, confirmed insensibility, stertor and death'. Travers recommended brandy as treatment and warned of the dangers of blood-letting and purging which were so widely used at the time.

None the less as late as 1855, G. J. Guthrie, the great exponent of military surgery, was still advising bleeding in the treatment of shock in his *Commentaries on the Surgery of War in Portugal, Spain, France and the Netherlands, from the Battle of Roliça in 1808 to that of Waterloo in 1815 : with additions relating to those in the Crimea in*

[1] Le Dran, H. F., *A Treatise, or Reflections Drawn from Practice on Gunshot Wounds*, translated from the French, London, 1743.

1854–1855. He quotes the case of an officer shot through the chest who developed shock and survived after 26 blood-lettings over the ensuing 15 days.

With the developments of surgery in the years 1880–90 it became apparent that shock was by then the chief cause of the high mortality. It was found that, in abdominal operations, rough handling of the viscera contributed to shock. In studies on dogs between 1895 and 1899, George Crile of Cleveland showed that tearing, stretching and crushing of tissues caused shock; whereas sharp dissection, meticulous control of bleeding and protecting exposed tissues with warm and moist coverings were most successful in avoiding it.

The First World War, with its huge numbers of ghastly injuries, brought the whole subject into the lime-light. Studies by physiologists and surgeons showed that a sudden and serious fall of blood-pressure was the predominant factor in shock, and two main schools of thought took shape. Firstly there was the toxic theory which explained shock as the result of some kind of poison, derived from damaged tissues, circulating in the blood. The second theory suggested that the fall in blood-pressure was the result of the escape of blood, especially plasma, from the general circulation into the wound. There is truth in both these ideas. The second theory is strongly supported by the fact that replacing the lost blood-volume by transfusion of blood or saline solution has now become accepted as the best way of preventing or treating surgical shock. This treatment has come to be used more and more as a supporting measure in all forms of operative surgery, as well as in other conditions such as road accidents and war wounds when shock is most to be feared. It is difficult to exaggerate the importance of this in modern surgery.

The conception of blood transfusion is not new, though its development as a safe and efficient means of saving life did not come about until well into the present century. Following William Harvey's discovery of the circulation of the blood in 1628, physicians began to contemplate the replacement of lost blood by injecting fluids into the blood-stream. Sir Christopher Wren began such experiments in 1659 and in 1667 Samuel Pepys described the

[1] Philadelphia, 1862.

transfusion (at the Royal Society's meetings at Gresham College) of twelve ounces of sheep's blood into a man, apparently without any ill effect. Later the patient claimed that 'he finds himself much better since, and as a new man', though Pepys goes on to say 'but he is cracked a little in his head'[1]. Although this particular patient suffered no harm, other transfusions during the next few years often ended in disaster, as might be expected in the light of modern knowledge.

Little more was heard of this subject for more than a hundred years. In 1818 James Blundell in London invented an apparatus for forcing blood along a tube into a patient's vein and he used this to transfuse human blood. In France and Germany such transfusions were done from time to time during the latter part of the nineteenth century, but the results were often fatal.

The invention of the hypodermic syringe, with its hollow pointed steel needle, made blood-transfusion a much easier procedure from a technical point of view. Alexander Wood invented this hollow needle in 1853 and in the same year Charles Gabriel Pravaz of Lyon made a similar syringe which quickly came into use everywhere under the name of the Pravaz syringe.

The technical problem of transfusion had now been solved, but physiological difficulties remained. The chief trouble was the incompatibility of animal blood with human. Leonard Landois of Griefswald, in his book on transfusion,[2] showed that the blood of one species of animal cannot be safely transfused into another species. Furthermore it began to emerge that even when human blood was used, it was often causing alarming and sometimes fatal results. In 1901 Karl Landsteiner, in Vienna, showed that the cause of incompatibility was the presence of substances in the blood of the recipient which brought about clumping of the red blood-corpuscles of the injected blood. This clumping (or agglutination) often caused the injected blood-corpuscles to break up altogether, releasing toxic products into the blood of the patient.

Much light was shed on this by Jan Janský of Prague, who showed that human beings could be classified into four groups according to the inherited properties of their blood. The classifica-

---

[1] *Diary*, November 21st and 30th, 1667.

[2] Landois, L., *Die Transfusion des Blutes*, Leipzig, 1875.

tions can be made by simple microscopical tests to find out whether the red blood cells of the prospective donor are agglutinated or not by the serum of the recipient. To avoid disaster it was important to use blood from a donor who was in the same blood-group as that of the patient. The simplest and safest method is to cross-match the actual blood of the donor and of the recipient directly against one another; though the formal classification of the patient into a definite blood-group is still of value and, indeed, is the routine procedure before any operation which is likely to require subsequent blood replacement.

In spite of the discovery of the blood-groups the actual process of transfusion remained technically difficult, mainly because blood was liable to clot quickly after it was withdrawn from the donor. In 1914 this difficulty was overcome by a new method, namely the addition of sodium citrate to the newly drawn blood. This is a comparatively harmless compound which prevents clotting entirely, by interfering with the chemical mechanism whereby clots are normally formed. Later it became usual to use blood plasma or serum rather than whole blood in the treatment of shock. (Plasma is the fluid part of the blood which has been prevented from clotting, whereas serum is the fluid that remains after clotting.) It was found that it was safe to give plasma or serum from a number of donors, mixed together, without having to ascertain the blood-group of the patient. Certainly the use of blood, plasma or serum has saved very many thousands of lives. Freeze-dried blood, subsequently 'reconstituted', has proved of immense value in combating shock under conditions of modern warfare.

Blood-transfusion is now universally accepted as a necessary service in all civilized countries. Stocks of blood are kept at convenient centres (often referred to as 'blood banks') throughout the country and blood of the right group is available to any hospital on demand. It should be added that this blood comes almost entirely from voluntary blood-donors among the general population. Though blood-transfusion began to be used in the First World War, it did not come into extensive and general use until the late nineteen-thirties. The conception of blood banks arose during the Spanish Civil War.

From 1927 onwards there were great advances in all the ancillary branches of medicine, without which surgery could not have progressed to its present high level of attainment. Indeed about this time it was widely thought that surgery had reached its limits and that nothing more could be hoped for except improvements in technique and operative skill. The more recent surgical advances relied upon improvement in X-ray techniques, anaesthesia and biochemistry and more recently still there have been startling innovations which have made heart surgery possible.

As we have seen, in the early part of the present century X-ray photographs, which at first had not been of much use except for fractures, began to be of the greatest assistance to the surgeon. Radio-opaque substances—now called 'contrast media'—were used to inject almost every hollow organ in the body. Sodium iodide was used to obtain X-ray pictures of the kidneys, lipiodol for the bronchial tubes and another iodine compound for the gall-bladder. Air was used to take pictures of the cavities of the brain (in this case visualization is due to the fact that air is *less* radio-opaque than the surrounding tissues.) Later blood-vessels of the brain could be photographed by the injection of a suitable contrast medium and this method was subsequently extended to all the arteries of the body, including those of the heart.

Progress in anaesthesia went far beyond the mere control of pain. New methods were introduced to extend the period during which a patient could be kept anaesthetized with safety. New anaesthetics came into use and techniques were changed. The use of cyclopropane allowed the operating-time to be much increased without risk. Among the most notable advances in technique was the introduction of the endotracheal catheter, that is to say a tube passed right down into the patient's windpipe, to provide a certain and ever-open airway. In this connexion the work of Ivan Magill was of outstanding importance as a contribution to modern anaesthesia.

Certain nerve-blocking drugs began to be used to produce muscular relaxation of the patient during major operations. The most interesting of these is curare, which had long been known as a powerful nerve-poison (Claude Bernard—1813–78—used it in many experiments on the nervous system). It was originally used by the South American Indians as an arrow-poison and was obtained from the plant *Strychnos toxifera*. All these improvements gave the anaesthetist almost complete control of the patient's respiratory system. This, with blood-transfusion during the operation, enabled the operating time to be extended indefinitely; it was now limited only by the physical endurance of the operator and his assistants. The new methods thus allowed the surgeon to embark on more intricate operations with far less damage to the patient's tissues, because the speed of operation was no longer the determining factor.

Among the most recent advances are the use of hypothermia and extra-corporeal circulation. Hypothermia simply means lowered temperature. The procedure is based on the work of W. G. Bigelow of Toronto. In 1950 he found that by lowering the temperature of an animal he could lessen the oxygen requirement of the body. (This is the way hibernating animals manage to survive.) For example, a dog with a temperature lowered to 20 degrees centigrade used 15 per cent less oxygen than a dog with a normal temperature. He went on to show that, because of the lessened oxygen consumption at 20 degrees centigrade, he could cut off the blood-flow through the heart for fifteen minutes without a fatal result. With lower temperatures the rhythm of the heart became interrupted; but he could restore this to normal by electrical stimulation. Here then was the key to successful cardiac surgery.

In effect, by reducing the human body temperature to about 30 degrees centigrade (86 degrees Fahrenheit), the whole blood circulation could be stopped for about ten minutes without any irreparable damage to the tissues of the body. The actual cooling was done in several ways. One was by drawing off the blood from an artery, passing it through a cooling-coil and then returning it into the veins of the patient. Another method was by immersing the whole body in cold water. This hypothermia enabled the heart to be excluded from the circulation for a short time and so made heart surgery possible. The first successful operation of this kind was done by Lewis and Taufic in 1953. They closed an atrial septal defect (the so-called 'hole-in-the-heart') with the body cooled to 30 degrees centigrade.

For more intricate operations ten minutes is not long enough.

A further development—profound hypothermia—bringing the temperature down to 20 degrees centigrade or even lower—enabled the heart to be stopped for about 45 minutes; though this method involved much more complicated techniques and expensive equipment than simple hypothermia.

The extra-corporeal circulation of the blood—technically known as perfusion—involves machines to keep the blood circulating and oxygenated outside the body, so that the heart may be kept free of blood while an operation is performed upon it. The use that can be made of these modern techniques is further considered in the section on thoracic surgery.

CHAPTER TWELVE

IMPORTANT ADVANCES IN SURGERY

IT is instructive to compare the number and kinds of surgical operations undertaken in the nineteenth century with those done, say thirty years ago and those of the present day. Let us take two examples, one from London and another from New York. In 1848 at St Bartholomew's Hospital there were 397 surgical beds, and the average number of operations per year (taken over a five-year period) was 370, of which 78 were amputations.[1] About sixty years later, when the beds were 390 in number, there were 3,561 operations of which only 25 were amputations. At the Presbyterian Hospital in New York in 1889 there were 130 beds. In that year 402 operations were done including 86 for incision of abscesses and 20 for amputation. Fifty years later, in in 1939, the total beds (including an additional wing) were 587. The number of operations in that year was 3,259, of which 60 were abscess incisions and 23 for amputation, while as many as 883 involved opening the abdominal cavity for appendicitis, gall-bladder disease, hernias and cancer of the stomach and bowel.[2] In 1889 the deaths directly due to operation had been 16·5 per cent; by 1939 it had been reduced to 2·1 per cent.

These figures show that the commonest operations of the older era—incisions of abscesses and amputations—had become, some fifty years later, a very small fraction of the surgeons' work. The enormous growth of surgery was chiefly due to new operations such as could not have been contemplated before the days of asepsis and anaesthetics. In the early decades of the twentieth century the surgeons had learned to attack almost every part of the body except the chest. The conquests of chest surgery will be described in a

[1] Godlee, R. J., *Lord Lister*, London, 1917.

[2] Haagensen, C. D., and Lloyd, W. E. B., *A Hundred Years of Medicine*, New York, 1943.

187

later chapter under the development of surgery in the last fifty years.[1] Here we may briefly touch on the history of six of the most frequent types of operation which formed the bulk of the general surgeon's work thirty years ago and which still loom large today.

I. APPENDICITIS

This is not a new disease, though the name dates from 1886. In the eighteenth century physicians made careful records of post-mortem examinations and among these appeared cases which we now recognize as undoubted appendicitis. Usually, by the time the bodies came to autopsy, the inflammation had proceeded to abscess formation and the abscess had burst into the abdomen and infected the whole peritioneal cavity (peritonitis). It was then no longer obvious that the disease had begun in the appendix and the condition was called perityphlitis, meaning inflammation round the caecum or blind gut. The early stages of appendicitis remained obscure for a long time, because surgeons dared not open the living abdomen to see what was going on. The result was that the various kinds of acute abdominal attacks with vomiting and pain were all hopelessly confused.

None the less there were certain acute observers who saw ahead of their time. In 1812, James Parkinson—whose name today is attached to the disease *paralysis agitans*—wrote a good account of fatal appendicitis in a boy of five. Post-mortem examination showed some impacted material in the appendix which had become inflamed, with obstruction, perforation and peritonitis. In 1827, François Melier, a young physician in Paris, wrote a paper on appendicitis. He saw that these abdominal infections resulted from acute inflammation of the appendix and even went so far as to suggest that, if a definite diagnosis could be made, it might even be possible to operate. This was a very bold assertion to make at the time.

It was many years before operation became usual. At first it was only attempted to relieve cases in which an abscess had already formed. Willard Parker, of New York, was a pioneer in this field. His first successful drainage of an appendicular abscess was in

[1] See below, p. 226.

188

1843 and by 1867 he had had three further successes. Moreover he had learned to diagnose appendicitis in its early stage; but he was reluctant to operate at this stage, for at that time abdominal surgery was held to be justifiable only as a last resort.

In 1886 Reginald Fitz of Boston published a masterly study of appendicitis, which cleared up much of the confusion which surrounded this and other forms of acute abdominal emergencies. It was he who named the condition appendicitis. He came to the conclusion that early operation was the best treatment. Charles McBurney carried on further extensive studies of appendicitis at Roosevelt Hospital. In 1889 he defined the anatomical position of the area which was found to be specially tender in many cases of the disease, and this has long been known to surgeons as 'McBurney's point'. He too stressed the necessity for early operation. This teaching was quickly accepted by most American surgeons, so that after 1890 appendicectomy became a common operation.

In England it became almost fashionable. The coronation of King Edward VII had been fixed for June 26th, 1902. On June 24th, amid general consternation, it was announced that the king was suffering from perityphlitis and an immediate operation was required. The coronation was postponed and the operation—conducted by Sir Frederick Treves—was highly successful and the king was pronounced out of danger within two weeks.

The principles of diagnosis and treatment have not changed much since then. As the public came to recognize that abdominal pain and vomiting may mean appendicitis and learned to call a doctor at once; and as surgeons realized that necessity of immediate operation, the mortality from appendicitis dropped steadily.

II. GALL-BLADDER DISEASE

As long ago as 1863, J. L. W. Thudicum, a London physician, wrote a book about gall-bladder disease, containing much of what we know today about the form and variety of gall-stones, the pathological changes resulting from them and the clinical signs of their presence. He knew that many people with gall-stones have no symptoms at all, that others have vague indigestion, while a few suffer the agonizing pains in the right upper part of the abdomen, which result when stones become lodged in the duct leading from the gall-bladder to the intestine. Thudicum knew of the fatal consequence of rupture of the gall-bladder and of obstruction of the duct by stones, which prevent the bile leaving the liver and so cause jaundice. As to treatment, he could only give opium or chloroform for the pain and then pack his patients—if and when convalescent—off to Vichy or Karlsbad for a 'cure'. At that time surgeons dared not open the vital upper part of the abdomen.

The first recorded incision and drainage of a distended gall-bladder was an accident, which took place in 1867 under the mistaken impression that the tumour was an ovarian cyst. Luckily the patient recovered, so that it became known that such a procedure was not necessarily fatal.

Eleven years later, in 1878, Marion Sims, an American gynaecologist, correctly diagnosed a distended gall-bladder and deliberately drained it. He called the operation cholecystostomy, and this treatment quickly became common. By 1885 the English surgeon Lawson Tait had done fifteen such operations.

The recurrence of symptoms proved to be the great disadvantage after these drainage operations. The symptoms persisted or recurred in nearly half the cases. Thus it was realized that some better treatment must be found.

Carl Langenbuch, chief surgeon at the Lazarus Hospital in Berlin, was the first to remove the gall-bladder together with its duct, so doing away with the focus of infection and stone-formation. This, the first cholecystectomy, was done in 1882 and the same operation was soon attempted by other European surgeons. By 1890 the Swiss surgeon, L. G. Courvoisier, working at Basel, was able to report on forty-seven cholecystomies in his important work on gall-bladder disease.[1]

The problem of removing stones from the common bile-duct was a more serious one, because surgical manipulations of this delicate structure are hazardous. Courvoisier was the first to cut open the duct and extract the stones successfully. Gradually it became the accepted practice to explore this duct as a routine in every gall-bladder operations, to make sure that no stones were left behind.

[1] Courvoisier, L. G., Casuistisch-statistische Beiträge zur *Pathologie und Chirurgie der Gallenwege, Leipzig,* 1890.

Important Advances in Surgery

III. HERNIA

Hernia (or rupture) is the protrusion of some structure in the abdomen through a weak point in the abdominal wall. A hernia is subject to unpleasant and sometimes disastrous complications, the main risk being that its blood-supply may be interrupted, when the contents of the hernia will die and fatal gangrene will ensue. Until about the 1870's the problem of how to treat hernia remained unsolved. The commonest type of hernia, the groin or inguinal hernia, incapacitated many men, and all the surgeon could do was to fit a truss which pressed on the opening in the abdominal wall and so kept the hernia from protruding.

When the era of abdominal surgery opened many surgeons attempted the cure of hernias. Several types of operation were devised. The simplest consisted in cutting down on the protrusion, tying it off and excising it after pushing back any gut that the hernia might contain, without any attempt at repairing the defect in the abdominal wall. Actual repair, by sewing the edges of the weakened opening together, was used by Vincenz Czerny at Freiburg in 1878. Gradually these methods became discredited, because up to forty per cent of the hernias recurred within four years; so the use of the truss once again became the accepted treatment.

This was the state of affairs in 1889 when Eduardo Bassini, professor of surgery at Padua, and William Halsted at Johns Hopkins Hospital, independently of each other, devised operations to effect the permanent cure of inguinal hernia. Their operations differed in detail but fundamentally they were the same, namely wide incision and exposure of the whole length of the weak place, dissection and excision of the protruding pouch of abdominal lining, and then carefully sewing up in layers the muscles and connective-tissues of the abdominal wall. These operations have proved very successful and recurrence of the hernia occurs in only a small proportion of cases. Certainly they have restored countless men to an active working life, who in earlier generations would have remained truss-bound invalids.

A Hundred Years of Medicine

IV. GOITRE

It was just a hundred and thirty years ago that T. W. King at Guy's Hospital described for the first time the elementary units of which the thyroid gland is composed—the follicles, filled with a gelatinous substance. After years of clinical studies it is now known that this gland supplies the body with an essential hormone.[1] This was identified as an iodine-containing compound in 1915 by an American chemist, E. C. Kendall, who called it thyroxine. It was subsequently synthesized in 1927 by two London chemists, C. R. Harrington and G. Barger. Our knowledge of the physiology and chemistry of the thyroid gland is intimately linked with the story of the surgeons' attempts to remove enlarged thyroids—or goitres.

There are certain parts of the world where these simple (i.e. non-toxic) goitres commonly occur. The incidence is highest in the mountains, but goitres also occur in the Great Lake district of the United States and Canada, the plains of Lombardy, some Swiss valleys and, in England, in Derbyshire (where it is known as 'Derbyshire neck'). One factor that all these districts have in common is a low iodine concentration in the soil and in the drinking-water. The medical aspect of goitre is discussed above in the section on hormones. Here we must confine ourselves to surgery.

Even after the advent of asepsis and anaesthesia, fear of uncontrollable haemorrhage deterred surgeons from operating on the thyroid gland, which is one of the most vascular organs in the body. None the less attempts were made. Between 1850 and 1877 about 190 operations were done, but the mortality was as high as 20 per cent.

Surgical success in the removal of goitre was largely due to Theodor Kocher, who was director of the surgical clinic at Berne from 1872 onwards. Kocher was a master-technician as well as an acute thinker. He devised new methods for obtaining satisfactory surgical exposure of the thyroid, for controlling haemorrhage and for avoiding damage to the nerves of the larynx (a grave danger in the early days and a disaster when it happened). In 1883 he was able to report on ten years of work, in which he had removed 101

---

[1] See above, p. 146, et seq.

goitres with 13 deaths. Unfortunately in 16 patients from whom he had removed the entire thyroid gland developed a new disease, characterized by lethargy, puffiness of the face and by dry skin. Kocher rightly concluded that this was due to complete lack of thyroid secretion and he named the condition *cachexia strumipriva*. He had in fact produced artificial myxoedema.[1]

Where there is a *toxic* goitre, i.e. one which is over-secreting thyroxine, the condition is referred to as hyperthyroidism. Surgical removal of part of the over-active gland became the best form of treatment. It was found by H. S. Plummer of the Mayo Clinic that great advantage was to be had by giving a pre-operative course of iodine treatment. The operation, originally developed by German and Swiss doctors, was taken up by American surgeons, notably William Halsted and C. H. Mayo. By 1908 the latter had operated upon 234 cases of hyperthyroidism with a mortality of 6 per cent.

As time has gone on, a better understanding of the abnormal physiology of this disease and refinements of operative technique have reduced the mortality to a small fraction of what it was. When the technical difficulties are considered these results must be seen as a noteworthy achievement of which surgeons may well be proud.

V. CANCER OF THE BREAST

This is the second commonest form of malignant tumour in women and, since the breast is easily removed, surgeons from time immemorial have tried to cure this disease by excision. It is unlikely that early crude attempts could ever have achieved success. John Aubrey, in his 'Brief Lives' tells of how William Harvey (1578–1657—the discoverer of the circulation of the blood) operated on 'my lady Howland, who had a cancer in her breast, which he did cutt-off and seared, but at last she dyed of it'.

Before Listerism the danger of sepsis became greater the larger the wound, so that surgeons did as limited an operation as possible. They removed only the part of the breast containing the tumour. The lymph glands in the armpit, to which cancer commonly spreads were left untouched, so that this kind of operation had but

[1] See above, p. 147.

little chance of success. The surgeons of the mid-nineteenth century were well aware of this. The two leading surgical textbooks of the day—that of Adolf Bardeleben[1] of Greifswald and that of Sir James Paget[2] of London—both stated that cancer of the breast could not be cured by surgery.

One school of thought held that cancer was a generalized disease from the beginning and that it was therefore useless to remove one focus, because others would inevitably appear. Two Germans, the surgeon Carl Thiersch and the anatomist Wilhelm Waldeyer were able to show by careful microscopical studies that this theory was quite wrong, and that cancer begins as a single primary lesion and that if this can be removed completely a permanent cure can be obtained. They showed that when cancer appeared at distant sites in the body, it did so from small groups of malignant cells which had broken away from the original lesion and spread through the lymphatics and blood-vessels. This discovery is of fundamental importance, for it is this knowledge that determines the management of every case of cancer today.

With this new knowledge surgeons began to operate again. Charles Moore of the Middlesex Hospital, in 1867, suggested removing the whole breast and axillary tissues in one piece, without cutting into the tumour. This idea received little recognition in England. Richard von Volkmann of Halle, who had introduced Listerism into Germany, devised and practised a similar operation in 1873. His operation became the standard one in German and Austrian clinics. For the first time cures were effected, though they were few. In Volkmann's own clinic, for example, out of a total of 200 operations in 1874-8, only 22 were alive and well three years later.

All these efforts fell short of the limits to which surgical removal could be carried out. In 1889 William Halsted took the next step by planning an operation which should remove all the tissues of the breast and axillary region, including a large area of skin, the subcutaneous connective tissues, the entire breast, both of the pectoral muscles and all of the lymphatic glands and connective tissue in the

[1] Bardeleben, A., *Lehrbuch der Chirurgie und Operationslehre,* 4th Edition, 1866, Vol. 3, p. 598.

[2] Paget, J., *Lectures on Surgical Pathology*, London, 1870, p. 651.

axilla. He covered the defect of the chest-wall with a skin-graft. This radical breast operation has not been improved upon and Halsted obtained results far surpassing those of his predecessors. The recurrence rate in his first 50 cases was 6 per cent, as opposed to Volkmann's 50 per cent.

It needed the development of the X-rays and their use in radiotherapy to lower the death-rate even further. By irradiating the surrounding tissues with a suitable dose of X-rays it became possible to kill any remaining cancer cells not removed by operation and so to reduce considerably the likelihood of any recurrence.

It has become increasingly clear that early diagnosis is the key to success. Every woman who detects a lump in her breast should seek immediate medical advice. There are many innocent breast tumours which require only local removal, whereas even the smallest cancer should be treated by the radical operation. In early cancer the miscroscopical appearance is the only reliable proof of the innocence or malignancy of a growth. In Halsted's time there was no method of microscopical diagnosis, so the surgeons had to rely on their own judgement of the naked eye appearance of the tumour; so that they sometimes made mistakes.

Biopsy is the term used to describe the removal of a small piece of tissue for microscopical examination as a preliminary to deciding on treatment. The idea came from Carl Ruge, a Berlin gynaecologist, in 1878, when he proved that many early cancers of the uterus could be diagnosed in this way, long before any signs or symptoms developed. The method was adopted and improved by German gynaecologists and in 1890 was introduced by Howard Kelly in his clinic at Johns Hopkins Hospital. At about this time the frozen section method was introduced both in Germany and the United States. A biopsy specimen is rapidly frozen by means of carbon dioxide and in the solid state it is comparatively easy to cut very thin slices. These can be mounted on glass slips and be ready for microscopical examination in a matter of minutes. Before this technique became available it took about a week to prepare a satisfactory microscopic slide.

This frozen section method was applied about 1905 to examine specimens of tumours. The practical importance of this in the control of breast cancer cannot be too strongly stressed, for it provides a way of diagnosing the early and curable case. It has now become standard practice to have microscopic examination made of every tumour of the breast, no matter how small and innocent it may appear.

VI. CANCER OF THE STOMACH AND INTESTINES

About one half of all cancer develops in the stomach or bowel. The chief difficulty in treating such tumours is that they rarely cause any signs or symptoms until the condition is well advanced. Moreover the abdomen is one of the more dangerous regions of the body from a surgical viewpoint, so that gastric and intestinal cancers present a far more formidable problem than breast cancer.

Resection (excision) of parts of the stomach or intestine could not be done until a satisfactory method of sewing together the cut ends of the digestive tube had been devised. It was only by animal experiments that this problem could be solved. It was found that such an artificial joining of the cut bowel was successful only when the outer layers of the bowel were properly united. All methods of joining up cut bowel (anastomosis) since contrived have been based on this principle. The method was first used in human beings in treating wounds of the intestine or excising strangulated hernias, because in those days surgeons never deliberately opened the abdomen.

About 1870, when German surgeons adopted Lister's teaching, the road became open to abdominal surgery and one of the first problems they took in hand was that of cancer of the stomach. In Vienna Theodor Billroth was the leading surgeon of his time and he saw that excision of the whole stomach was a possibility, and in 1881 he performed the first successful gastrectomy on a human being.

During the next few years many continental surgeons, mostly Germans and Austrians, removed cancers of the stomach but the results were very discouraging. In a total of 37 gastrectomies there had been 27 deaths from the operations. Of the ten survivors none lived for more than eighteen months. Thomas Welch, the American pathologist who produced these figures, drew the pessimistic, but very understandable conclusion that the disease was incurable.

Surgeons have since proved him wrong. Sixty years later gastrectomy was being done with increasing safety and a large number of patients were reported alive and well ten years after their operations. From this it must not be thought that the proportion of cures was at all satisfactory. Only about 2 per cent of those who developed stomach cancer were cured at that time mainly because four out of five patients had such advanced disease when first seen, that their condition was inoperable. For this reason two important aids to diagnosis were more than welcome. These were X-ray examination and gastroscopy; though of course even these cannot be applied until the patient develops symptoms which drive him to his doctor; and by then it is often too late.

The gastroscope, as devised by Miculicz in 1881, was an angled and rigid tube provided with mirrors. This rather clumsy device was superseded in 1932, when Rudolf Schindler of Munich perfected a complicated optical system which enabled him to make a flexible instrument, which was more easily introduced into the stomach.

If a patient has a stomach cancer which is early enough to be excised, then his chances of a cure are now quite considerable. It is a great tribute to surgical technique that the mortality following this difficult operation has fallen. It has been found that with this, as with other difficult surgical procedures, better results are obtained by specialists than by general surgeons.

Cancer rarely occurs in the small intestine, so that this need not detain us here; but it develops in the large intestine (colon) very often. The disease is more frequent at the lower end of the large bowel, that is, in the rectum. It often causes symptoms such as bleeding, constipation, diarrhoea or obstruction at a time when it is still early enough to be operable. X-ray examination and, for rectal cancer, local examination and the use of the proctoscope are indispensable diagnostic aids which can be relied upon to detect these tumours.

Operation for rectal cancer is one of the most extensive and serious. Generally it involves making an artificial outlet for the bowel through the abdominal wall—a so-called colostomy; together with total excision of the rectum. William Miles of London realized that an even more radical operation was necessary;

namely the removal of a wide zone of surrounding tissue, including the pelvic colon and the lymphatic glands in the neighbourhood— a truly formidable dissection. The operation had to be done in two parts, the first within the abdomen and the second from outside. This extensive operation necessarily carried with it some operative mortality (from 10 to 15 per cent at the time), but a very high proportion of the survivors were permanently cured.

CHAPTER THIRTEEN

SURGICAL SPECIALIZATION

DURING the present century our knowledge of disease and its treatment has grown at such a rate that it is impossible for one mind to encompass it all. This is particularly so in certain branches of surgery where accurate diagnosis depends not only upon extensive clinical experience but also on familiarity with a number of specialized instruments, such as the laryngoscope, the bronchoscope and the cystoscope. Moreover surgical procedures in treatment are now so varied that an adequate experience of them can be acquired only by the surgeons who limit their work to their own special fields. Thus specialization has become inevitable. Theoretically this may not be ideal, but in practice better results have been obtained by specialists than by general surgeons so far as the more difficult and intricate operations are concerned.

Thus a number of surgical specialities has come into being and they became universally recognized by leading medical schools and hospitals. The chief departments include obstetrics and gynae-cology (usually grouped together), genito-urinary surgery, nerve surgery, thoracic surgery and those branches of surgery which deal with the 'special senses'—the eyes, the ears and the nose. We shall deal in turn with the early history of each of these specialities.

I. OBSTETRICS AND GYNAECOLOGY

Obstetrics is the oldest surgical speciality, having developed before the nineteenth century, when the practice of midwifery began to pass from the hands of unqualified women into those of professional male obstetricians.

The most important advance in the early period was the inven-tion of the obstetric forceps, which for a hundred and twenty-five years remained the private and secret weapon of the remarkable family of English obstetricians, the Chamberlens. When the last Chamberlen, Hugh the younger, died in 1728, the secret had become known to many workers both in England and in France, and the forceps came into general use. The instrument consists of two fenestrated blades, curved to fit the child's head, and locking together at one end to form a handle. In a difficult labour the birth of the child can be assisted by the use of the forceps.

In the eighteenth century obstetrics began to be taught in medical schools. The first professorship was founded at Edinburgh in 1726 and other universities soon followed suit. Among the special hospitals founded in the United Kingdom during the last half of the eighteenth century were the Rotunda Hospital in Dublin (1745), the Lying-in wards of the Middlesex Hospital (1747), the City of London Lying-in Hospital (1750) and the General Lying-in Hospital—later Queen Charlotte's Hospital—(1752).

In Colonial America the transference of obstetric practice from midwives to trained physicians followed the British lead. Most of America's best doctors of that period had been largely trained in Britain and it was natural that they should bring home with them the new interest in obstetrics. The New York Lying-in Hospital was founded in 1791, the lying-in wards of the Pennsylvania Hospital were opened in 1803 and the Lying-in Hospital at Boston in 1832. The most famous American obstetrician of colonial times was Samuel Bard, who became professor of Obstetrics and Diseases of Women and Children at King's College, New York, in 1808.

Before the obstetricians could play their part in modern scientific medicine they had to solve the same two problems that held back the surgeons—pain and infection. They succeeded in conquering these and, curiously enough, they did so independently of the surgeons. The story of James Young Simpson has been told in an earlier chapter, but here let it be noted that Simpson was not a general surgeon, but the Professor of Midwifery at Edinburgh. His vigorous and successful fight for the use of chloroform in childbirth may be said to have achieved full recognition when Queen Victoria, in 1853, took chloroform herself for the birth of her eighth child. Simpson was created a baronet in 1866 and, when he died in 1870, he was given a public funeral; a bronze statue of him was erected in Edinburgh and a bust placed in Westminster Abbery.

The problem of anaesthesia in childbirth is rather different from that in general surgery. In uncomplicated deliveries the obstetrician wants a relatively light degree of anaesthesia, but sometimes over a long period. In America, when the dangers of chloroform became known, the most favoured form of anaesthesia in childbirth was a combination of several agents; the early part of labour being conducted under barbiturates or scopolamine, and the later stage, when the labour pains became more violent, under nitrous oxide ('gas'), supplemented if need be with ether. In England, about 1920, the use of scopolamine and morphine together came into vogue under the popular name of 'Twilight Sleep', a condition which was supposed to deprive labour of its terrors. It was said that the pains of labour were only dimly felt and, after parturition, only vaguely remembered.

The cause of infection contracted in childbirth—puerperal fever—was known to obstetricians long before the germs of sepsis had been discovered and long before Lister's antiseptic method for surgery was evolved. The discoveries of Gordon in Aberdeen (1795), O. W. Holmes in Boston (1843) and Semmelweiss in Vienna (1847) were all related to puerperal fever and not to general surgery. It was clearly demonstrated that the infection was conveyed from one woman to another by the doctors, nurses and students who attended them. Semmelweiss, by insisting on careful disinfection of the hands with soap and water, followed by rinsing in a solution of chloride of lime, reduced the mortality in the maternity wards of his hospital in Vienna from 18 per cent in April to 1 per cent in July of the same year.

In spite of these discoveries, it was not until Lister's methods had been taken up by continental surgeons that the same care was widely extended towards the prevention of puerperal sepsis. In 1870 A. S. Stadfeldt at Copenhagen began to use the carbolic acid technique for childbirth and was able to report ten years later that the mortality had been reduced from 1 in 14 to 1 in 116.

Antiseptic technique in childbirth developed in various ways in different countries. Bichloride of mercury soon became more popular than carbolic acid. The efficacy of this was well shown at the New York Maternity Hospital on Blackwell's Island. About one quarter of the women there had been dying of puerperal sepsis when, in 1883, J. H. Garrigues took charge and introduced sweeping changes. He instituted a strict antiseptic régime, using soap and water and a 1:2000 solution of bichloride of mercury to disinfect the beds, floors, the hands of the attendants and the genital passages of the patients. He forbade any contact with visitors or with attendants or students from the other wards or the mortuary. In three months the mortality-rate fell to zero.

Even after this and other convincing demonstrations, puerperal sepsis, though much less frequent, was not entirely eliminated. The sulphonamide drugs which became available in the thirties were a great help and penicillin in the forties made a magnificent contribution in safeguarding the health of women in childbirth.

In the latter part of the nineteenth century important advances in the technique of delivery were made. Etienne Tarnier, at the Maternity Hospital in Paris, produced a new type of forceps—the axis traction forceps—which was, mechanically speaking, a big improvement on the Chamberlen instrument.

Caesarian section, that is the opening of the uterus and delivery of the child through an abdominal incision, had been done occasionally as a last resort, but its mortality-rate had been frightening. In 1882, Max Saenger, a Prague obstetrician, made important improvements in the management of this operation, including the use of sutures to close the incision in the uterus. For the first time Caesarian section became safe enough to justify its use in special cases where the pelvic bones of the mother were so deformed that normal delivery was impossible.

The subject of maternal mortality is more fully discussed in the section on Health Organization.

Gynaecology is the branch of surgery dealing with female diseases other than those concerned with childbirth. It is a comparatively new speciality. Operations for ovarian tumours began to be widely done as early as 1840 in America, despite strong criticism. (The original ovariotomy by Ephraim McDowell in 1809 at Danville, Kentucky, was an isolated event, which, though successful, had little influence in promoting gynaecology.) In London

Spencer Wells became the great ovariotomist of his time, performing one thousand such operations between 1858 and 1880. These operations were done without antisepsis and about one-third of the patients died.

When antisepsis began to make abdominal operations relatively safe (from 1870 onwards) improved methods for removal of the diseased uterus were planned. The old technique of simply cutting a tumour out of the uterus and leaving the rest of the organ behind not only had a high mortality from haemorrhage and sepsis, but was quite useless in cancer of the uterus (which accounts for about one-quarter of all cancer in women). Removal of the entire uterus was necessary if a cure was to be effected. This had been tried in a few cases, but it had always ended in disaster.

In this operation—hysterectomy—the German surgeons led the way. Wilhelm A. Freund at Breslau was the first to devise a reasoned plan for complete removal of the uterus in cases of cancer. He carried it out successfully in 1878 under Lister's carbolic method, taking two hours over the operation. His patient was reported alive and well in 1904.

Unfortunately most uterine cancers develop in the neck—or cervix—of the uterus. It was soon found that even total hysterectomy, as carried out by Freund, was seldom successful in curing this form of the disease. About 1900 Ernst Wertheim, at Vienna, began to do the most radical operation possible, removing not only the entire uterus with its neighbouring structures and ligaments, but, also much of the tissues in the pelvis, which contained the lymph glands to which cervical cancer is so prone to spread. During the early years of the century Wertheim was chiefly responsible for popularizing this hazardous procedure among gynaecologists and for reducing the mortality to the low point of 15 per cent. The difficulty with this method is that it can be used only in a small proportion of patients, because in the others the disease is too far advanced when they first come for advice.

The next step in the fight against uterine cancer was the introduction of radium. A New York surgeon, Robert Abbe, was the first to use it in the treatment of cancer of the cervix. Before doing so he made a large number of experiments with germinating seeds, with ants, trout and mice, using the 150 milligrammes of radium chloride which he bought from the Curie Laboratory in Paris for 400 dollars in 1903. Two years later he reported his result in a case of cancer of the cervix, but although these pioneer attempts were interesting, Abbe failed to make any important contribution to the clinical development of radiotherapy.

The radiation treatment of cervical cancer developed mainly in French and German clinics between 1910 and 1915. Good results were reported from Freiburg, Berlin and Munich at the Congress of the German Gynaecological Society in Halle in 1913. They showed that large doses of the penetrating gamma rays from the filtered radiation of mesothorium produced some remarkable cures. After this systematic study of radiotherapy for uterine cancer began all over the world. Radiotherapy has developed into a speciality of its own. The use of very short-wave radiation—from X-rays, from radium or from man-made isotopes, often in conjunction with surgical removal of the cancerous organ—has certainly helped in many forms of cancer. Unfortunately the early hopes—engendered by a few impressive successes—that here was a cure for all forms of cancer have not been fulfilled.

II. GENITO-URINARY SURGERY

Since time immemorial there have been surgeons who specialized in 'cutting for stone', that is, removing calculi from the bladder by opening it, generally through the perineum. This kind of operation seems to have been practised by the Persians and may have been brought to Greece at the time of Alexander the Great. In medieval and renaissance times it was the second most frequently performed major operation (amputation taking the first place). Samuel Pepys, the diarist, underwent a successful operation for the stone in 1658 and he celebrated each anniversary of this important event of his life with thanksgiving.

In England the great exponent of this procedure in the first half of the eighteenth century was William Cheselden, surgeon to St Thomas's Hospital from 1719–38. He brought the operation to the highest pitch of perfection that could be attained in the days when there were neither anaesthetics nor antiseptics. His skill was such that he performed the operation in as little as 54 seconds. Even with this degree of dexterity, lithotomy, as the operation was called, carried with it a high mortality. Thus Morand, Cheselden's pupil, reported that among a total of 812 patients operated on at the Hôtel Dieu and the Charité at Paris, there were 255 deaths, and that many of the survivors were left with permanent urinary fistulae.

In 1822 Jean Civale, a young Parisian surgeon invented an ingenious instrument for crushing stones within the bladder. The lithotrite, as it was called, was inserted through the natural urinary passage, grasped the stone and then crushed it into fragments which could then be washed out of the bladder. This was a really important advance, for not only was it successful, but also, because it avoided any cutting into the tissues of the body, was almost without mortality. The lithotrite was much improved by Henry Bigelow of Boston in 1878.

This brings us to the modern or cystoscopic period of genito-urinary surgery. The cystoscope is an instrument for looking into the interior of the bladder. Before this instrument had been invented, diagnosis of disease of the urinary tract (that is, the urethra, bladder, ureters and kidneys) had to rest on clinical symptoms and external palpation. The surgeon was often not sure and dared not operate. The cystoscope, with all the information it could provide, made diagnosis more certain and so opened up whole new fields of treatment. An urgent need for such an instrument had long been felt. The problem was solved by Max Nitze, an ingenious Viennese surgeon. His first cystoscope was a tube with a system of lenses for viewing the lining of the bladder. It had a platinum wire loop on its tip, which provided illumination when heated white-hot by a galvanic current. Damage to the bladder by this hot wire was prevented by irrigation with cold water. When Edison invented the electric light in 1879, the Viennese cystoscope-makers quickly adapted it for their purpose.

Nitze himself and many other surgeons continued to improve the instrument, so that by the 1890's it was possible to inspect every part of the interior of the bladder. Minor operations inside could be done with small cutting, clamping and cauterizing instruments inserted through the tube of the cystoscope. Most important of all, it was found possible to catheterize the ureters. These are tubes which conduct the urine from the kidneys into the bladder, and each of the two ureters has a tiny opening into the base of the bladder. To examine the relative condition of two kidneys, it was necessary to insert a separate catheter into each of these openings. Alexander Brenner, also of Vienna, designed a special cystoscope for this purpose and he succeeded in catheterizing the ureters of a woman in 1888. For anatomical reasons the male ureters presented a far more difficult problem, but this was solved by James Brown at Johns Hopkins Hospital, Baltimore, in 1893 with a modification of Brenner's original instrument.

Now that samples of urine could be obtained from each kidney separately, various important microscopical and biochemical tests could be brought into play to determine the function of the individual kidney. Infection was detected by the presence of pus cells or leucocytes in the urine. Bacterial cultures could be made to discover the species of the organisms causing the infection. An ingenious test of kidney function was devised by a group of American workers, again at Johns Hopkins Hospital. The professor of chemistry, Ira Remsen, discovered a new purple dye, phenol-sulphone-pthalein in 1884. His colleague, the pharmacologist John J. Abel, found that it was passed by the kidneys into the urine, and in 1910 Leonard Rowntree and John Geraghty showed that the rate of excretion was lowered when the kidney was diseased and thus the amount of dye in the urine gave an accurate measure of the function of the kidney.

The new method of ureteric catheterization also provided a way of X-raying the ureters and the cavities in the hilum of the kidney. This could be done by injecting a radio-opaque liquid up the ureter. A colloidal solution of silver was first used for this purpose in Heidelberg in 1906. A few years later the method was improved by using sodium iodide solution in place of the silver.

With these new methods of examination the surgeon had information about the condition of the bladder, the ureter and the kidneys which he could not have had without cystoscopy. Armed with reliable data, he could decide upon treatment without recourse to exploratory surgery.

Kidney operations had in fact been done before the invention of the cystoscope. Gustav Simon, a Heidelberg surgeon, had removed diseased kidneys from 1869 onwards. With the improved cysto-scopic methods operations for many types of kidney disease began. In renal tuberculosis, for example, surgical removal of the diseased kidney gave the best chance of a cure. Stones could be removed from inside a kidney and its function restored, if it had not been too badly damaged.

Operations on the bladder became common from 1870 onwards, particularly for the removal of stones. Cancer of the bladder could also be successfully removed in cases where it had developed in the one portion of the bladder that could be safely excised. Unfor-tunately only about a quarter of such growths are so favourably situated.

In the early part of the twentieth century two new methods of treating tumours of the bladder were introduced. In 1908 Edward Beer of New York developed an electric-sparking technique for burning tumours away by means of an instrument passed through the cystoscope. Radium treatment was developed a few years later and radiotherapy by this and other means began to be widely used.

Enlargement of the prostrate gland is the commonest condition with which the genito-urinary surgeon has to deal. This gland surrounds the male urethra, just below the bladder. It often becomes enlarged in men after the age of fifty years and can cause varying degrees of urinary obstruction. If this becomes serious, the bladder cannot be completely emptied and the resulting back-pressure damages the kidneys to such an extent that, if the obstruc-tion is not relieved, death will ensue.

Until about 1880 sufferers from urinary obstruction of this kind could be relieved only by repeated catheterization or by a perma-nent fistula—miserable alternatives, because infection of the bladder inevitably ensued.

Operations for the relief of prostatic obstructions began as early as 1880, though at first they were incidental to the removal of stones from the bladder. Arthur McGill, of the Leeds Royal Infirmary, first realized the usefulness of prostatectomy in its own right. He did three such operations in 1887 and his success led to the widespread adoption of the operation in England, in Germany and in America.

Since that time the technique of the operation has become very much improved and the mortality-rate much reduced. The most important factor in making the operation safer was the careful study of kidney function before the operation and the provision, whenever necessary, of a preliminary period of bladder drainage to relieve the back-pressure on the kidneys and so allow them to recover before the major operation was done. Furthermore, with modern antibiotic treatment it is possible to clean up any infection before embarking on prostatectomy and to prevent reinfection afterwards. There is no doubt that, when successful, prostatectomy has given a new lease of life to thousands of men who without it would have lived and died in misery.

In a considerable proportion of men with prostatic obstruction this is due to cancer. Surgical excision of prostatic cancer was tried as early as 1867; but even the more radical resections subsequently carried out had little chance of success except with very early cancers; but for the most part the disease is far advanced when first detected. Radium and X-ray treatment were used in various forms, but with little success. The attack by means of synthetic hormones has been the outstanding discovery of recent times in connexion with prostatic cancer and this has been referred to elsewhere.[1]

III. ORTHOPAEDICS

The word orthopaedic was compounded in 1741 by Nicolas André, a Paris physician, from the Greek words *orthos*, meaning straight, and *paidion*, a little child. He used it in a work on bony deformities, which he attributed to faulty action of the muscles in childhood. The word has survived, though André's theory has long been discarded. Today orthopaedics means the branch of medicine dealing with bones and joints. It covers fractures and dislocations as well as diseases and deformities, both congenital and acquired.

Though the word orthopaedic did not become current in this country until the middle of the nineteenth century, the beginning of the speciality can be traced back to the eighteenth century when humanitarians began to be interested in crippled children. In 1828 Jacques Mathieu Delpech, professor of surgery at Montpellier,

[1] See above, p. 155.

published a work entitled *Orthomorphy*, on the subject of bone and joint deformities. He also planned and built a hospital for such cases in the country between Montpellier and Toulouse. About the same time Johann von Heine, an instrument and brace maker at Würzburg University, founded an institute in that city, which played a leading part in the development of orthopaedics in Germany. In England the first hospital of its kind was founded in Birmingham in 1817. William John Little, a surgeon who had club-foot himself, founded a similar hospital in London, which subsequently became the Royal National Orthopaedic Hospital, the leading British institution for the care of the crippled poor. In America two pioneer surgeons each established a special orthopaedic clinic in the same year, 1861. Lewis A. Sayre started his clinic at Bellvue Hospital, New York, while Buckminster Brown opened a private institution, the Samaritan Hospital, at Boston. In New York further special hospitals were opened, the Hospital for the Ruptured and Crippled in 1863 and the New York Orthopaedic Dispensary and Hospital in 1866.

These special hospitals and clinics enormously increased the knowledge of bone and joint diseases. As a result of new microscopical studies and clinical findings a number of new diseases of bones and joints were identified; but progress was mainly directed towards dealing with the well-known problems which crippling conditions already presented.

About this time experimental methods began to throw light upon the complex mechanism of bone growth and repair. There were two outstanding men. The first, Louis X. E. L. Ollier, was trained at Montpellier and Paris, and began experimenting on bones early in his career. He became professor of surgery at Lyon in 1859 and eleven years later published a two-volume work, *A Clinical and Experimental Treatise on the Regeneration of Bone and the Artificial Production of Osseous Tissue* which gave an excellent account of the process of bone growth and repair. Ollier believed that a bone grew chiefly from the periosteum, the fibrous envelope which is found round every bone.

In 1880 William MacEwen, at Glasgow University, was able to show that periosteum was not the sole source of new bone. He had as a patient a boy whose upper arm-bone had been almost entirely destroyed by osteomyelitis (infection of the interior of the bone) and he had been left with a limp and useless arm. Acting upon knowledge he had gained from animal experiments, MacEwen removed a series of bony wedges from the boy's shin-bone and embedded them in a row in the muscles of the arm. These separate pieces of bone lived and flourished and knit together to form a rigid and useful arm. This was the beginning of modern bone-grafting which is used so widely today.

The great advances in general surgery which began after 1870 were shared by orthopaedics. Surgeons were able to transplant muscles and tendons or could alter their lengths and their positions to correct deformities or overcome paralyses. The first tendon-transplantation was done in 1880 by Karl Nicoladoni at Innsbruck. He cut the tendons of the peronaeal muscles, which arise from the side of the lower leg, and sewed the ends to the cut end of the Achilles (heel) tendon. The patient was a boy of sixteen whose calf-muscles had been paralysed by poliomyelitis. In this way the peronaeal muscles were able to take the place of the calf-muscles and act upon the Achilles tendon to support the foot. Many ingenious modifications have been invented since then to improve the results of such tendon-transplantation. Nowadays even the small and slender tendons of the hands and fingers can be operated on with success.

Many operations on bones and joints were also devised in the new surgical era. In 1873 C. A. T. Billroth did the first operation for knock-knee, by chiselling part of the way through the tibia (or shin-bone), then deliberately breaking the bone at this point and so setting it in alignment with the thigh. Four years later MacEwen planned a much better operation by which the deformity was corrected by operating on the lower end of the femur instead of the upper end of the tibia. This procedure gained wide acceptance and the basic idea was applied to correct various other bony deformities.

Tuberculosis of the bones and joints had for long been an outstanding problem, because, if untreated, such cases almost always ended disastrously. The disease was commoner among children than adults, especially among those who lived under bad conditions of hygiene. Sixty years ago the outlook in such cases was tragic. If unchecked, the disease was progressive. It attacked the ligaments of the joints, softening them and often causing pathological dislocations. Effusions into the joints and abscess-formation were common. Tuberculosis could result in complete destruction of the joint, necrosis of the bone and secondary sepsis, and then amputation was the only course.

The treatment, as recently as twenty-five years ago, was something of an ordeal. A child with tuberculosis of the hip, knee or ankle could look forward to being put to bed for a matter of years, because absolute immobility in splints or plaster casts was essential. Surgical excision of the tuberculous joint had been carried out in a number of cases as early as 1820 by James Syme, the famous Edinburgh surgeon. Ollier much improved this operation towards the close of the nineteenth century and wrote a three-volume book on the subject.

Resection of a joint naturally abolished all movement. Surgeons attempted to prevent this fixation by a variety of procedures, usually by putting some of the patient's own tissues—fat or connective tissue, or even foreign materials like metal plates—between the cut ends of the bones. It was hoped that an artificial and movable joint could be obtained by this *arthroplasty*, as the new operation was called. The result was rarely so successful in curing the patient as the permanent and deliberate fixation of the joint, *arthrodesis*. This latter was introduced in 1878 by Edward Albert, professor of surgery at Vienna. It was, in effect, complete excision of the diseased joint. This did cure the tuberculosis by removing it. It is true the joint remained immovable thereafter; but a joint with active tuberculosis would have been unusable in the first place and would have caused endless trouble in the long run.

Russell Hibbs at the New York Orthopaedic Hospital applied the same principle to other diseased joints, notably those of the spine. This form of spinal fusion became the standard practice for tuberculosis of the spine. It will be appreciated that the whole picture has been changed—both as regards surgery and also prolonged rest—and the prognosis vastly improved in all forms of 'surgical tuberculosis' (as it was called) with the advent of streptomycin and the other anti-tuberculous drugs. In this country tuberculosis of bones and joints is far less common than it was, almost certainly because of better home conditions, better food and, above all, the provision of clean and safe milk.[1]

Fractures are one of the main concern of the orthopaedic surgeon. In earlier times broken limbs were fixed in crude wooden splints. Hugh Owen Thomas of Liverpool may be said to have started the modern treatment of fractures in the latter half of the nineteenth century. He was descended from a long line of Welsh bone-setters, but he himself had also obtained proper medical and surgical training at Edinburgh, London and Paris. He practised in Liverpool, first with his father and later by himself, near the docks where there was an abundance of surgical work of all kinds among the poor. Thomas was not only a well-trained doctor but a skilled mechanic as well. He planned many of the ingenious splints for which he became famous and he made them all himself. In place of the former clumsy wooden contraptions he made cleverly designed and well-fitting splints of iron (for strength) and padded with leather (for comfort). The basic principle he adopted was that the injured limb should be rested as much as possible. With some of his splints he was able to achieve just this, at the same time keeping the patient up and about; a very important advance in treatment. Thomas made it crystal clear that his basic ideas were what counted. 'A man who understands my principles,' he said, 'will do better with a bandage and a broomstick than another can do with an instrument-maker's arsenal.'[2] He was a man dedicated to the poor among whom and for whom he worked. It is said that he worked from dawn until late at night, seven days a week—every Sunday morning he held a free clinic for poor people—for years without a holiday and he died prematurely in 1891 at the age of fifty-seven.

Thomas's work was carried on by his famous nephew Robert Jones, whom he had thoroughly trained in his methods; but Jones had also had a sound hospital training, so he insisted on introducing the most scrupulous aseptic technique, surpassing that of any surgeon of his time. His progressive mind was quick to use any new knowledge that came his way. For example, hardly had he heard of Röntgen's discovery of X-ray in 1895, than he 'was off to Germany. He ordered and paid for an X-ray tube and he and

---

[1] See below, pp. 291 *et seq.*
[2] Watson, F., *The Life of Sir Robert Jones*, London, 1934.

Thurstan Holland, later to become an eminent radiologist, took what was almost certainly the first X-ray picture in England. It showed plainly a small bullet embedded in a boy's wrist. Jones saw at once that the new discovery was of immense value in bone surgery and especially in fractures; but at the same time he knew the dangers of short cuts to knowledge and did not allow himself to be carried away by the new invention. He acknowledged the X-ray machine as an invaluable adjunct, but he declined to let it take the place of accurate clinical diagnosis. He deplored the education of medical students who rarely bothered to acquire clinical skill in diagnosis but merely awaited the interpretation of an X-ray photograph. He wrote: 'While Roentgen's discovery has been to us of immense value, chiefly in the classification of our injuries, it has done little if anything to perfect or even alter our treatment of fractures.'[1]

In 1898 Robert Jones, much of whose work had been for crippled children, began planning for a children's hospital in the country, because he was convinced of the value of clean fresh air in the care and cure of his young patients. The hospital he envisaged was to have a resident doctor and regular weekly visits by a consultant surgeon from the nearest large town. The difficulties were many, but eventually the first hospital ward for the long-term treatment of crippled children was opened in 1899 at West Kirkby Convalescent Home for Children. Jones laid down the important principles that, in addition to surgeons of the highest skill, there should be abundance of fresh air and that the children should not be discharged from hospital until cured, however long it might take. Following this the foundation stone of the Royal Liverpool Country Hospital for Children, Heswall, was laid in 1900.

Agnes Hunt, descended from an old Shropshire family, completed her training as a nurse at the Salop Infirmary in 1890. Later she decided to start a small and entirely unconventional open-air hospital for children in need of country air and good food. In 1900 with a friend, Miss Greenford, she set up a ramshackle affair of crude sheds and outbuildings at Baschurch, a village near Oswestry. She regularly took such children as needed advice and possible surgical treatment into Liverpool; and there it was that she met

[1] Watson, F., op. cit., p. 80.

Robert Jones. He was immensely impressed by her intelligence and also by the obvious improvements in the health of the children in her make-shift open-air hospital. So it was that he became the consultant surgeon at Baschurch; and to this hospital came orthopaedic surgeons from all over the world, from the United States and Canada, from Europe, Australia and New Zealand, eager to meet Robert Jones and to watch and learn his methods. From these beginnings the Oswestry Orthopaedic Hospital (still affectionately known as 'Bobby Jones and Aggie Hunt') became famous throughout the world.

Early in the present century Robert Jones introduced the practice of setting fractures immediately under anaesthesia. In this way he could get a much neater result, with accurate alignment of the broken fragments of bone; furthermore it decreased the damage to the surrounding soft tissues, besides avoiding the terrible pain that setting without anaesthesia necessarily involved.

At the outbreak of war in 1914 Robert Jones was fifty-seven and had gained an international reputation. In the disastrous autumn of that year he foresaw, better than anyone else, how great a part orthopaedics would have to play in the war, if a huge total of hopeless cripples was to be avoided. A vast organization would be needed, but with the whole country, the Government and especially the War Office having but one thought uppermost—that of winning the war, whatever the cost—it would be futile to expect that this urgent problem would be tackled at headquarters.

Robert Jones had joined up as a captain, but was soon promoted to major and made a tour of inspection of military hospitals. He was aghast at what he found and sent a blistering report to the War Office. The main trouble was the policy of discharging soldiers as soon as possible from the hospitals, to make room for fresh casualties. The Army was not interested in a man who could not be made fit again for service, so he was discharged. This, Jones saw, would mean that half of the wounded men would be discharged from hospital at the most critical stage; that many of them would die and many of the survivors would be left with gross deformities and functional disabilities. Hospital accommodation must be provided for prolonged orthopaedic treatment to rehabilitate these men. Early in 1915 a hospital with two hundred and fifty beds—soon to be increased to five hundred and sixty—was opened at Alder Hey, Liverpool. This, together with the hospital at Shepherd's Bush, London, opened in 1916, was a great experiment, on the success of which depended the future of thousands of soldiers and indeed the future of orthopaedic surgery itself.

In the early months of the war the treatment of fractures was associated not only with much avoidable deformity, but also a high mortality. For example, in compound fractures of the femur, 80 per cent of the men died, mostly from sepsis. The clean bullet wound and the dry soil, of South Africa, which had given the Army surgeons such experience as they had, was a very different proposition from the lacerated wounds produced by shell-fire amid the well-manured mud of Flanders. Fortunately Robert Jones's outstanding ability as a surgeon was recognized. He was able to introduce important new methods of treating fractures on the battlefield. His chief concern was to splint the wounded men then and there, *before* moving them to the casualty clearing station. He advised the use of the Thomas hip splint for compound fractures of the thigh. Under his direction the mortality from this serious injury was reduced from 80 to fifteen per cent. His methods were copied enthusiastically by the Americans and as a result they found that their percentage of preventable deformities was less than any other armies could claim.

The need for doctors in the armed services was considered a top priority, but Robert Jones saw that the orthopaedic work at Alder Hey and Shepherd's Bush could not go on if the few specially trained surgeons were taken away. They were far too few as it was. Fortunately the Americans came to his help and a contingent of twenty carefully selected young orthopaedic surgeons arrived at Liverpool in May 1917: and to these young men much of the success of the orthopaedic centres was due.

The war had changed the whole outlook for the treatment of cripples and Sir Robert's name had become a household word throughout the land. It was clear that special orthopaedic clinics were needed to carry out reconstructive surgery of bones and joints in the severely injured, to correct their deformities and fit them for civil life. The lessons learned in the war were invaluable in treating not only old war injuries, but also deformities and injuries in civil life. Fracture clinics were set up in general hospitals where orthopaedic specialists could control the whole course of the patient's treatment and convalescence. The first of such fracture services were started at the Ancoats Hospital in Manchester in 1914 and at the Massachusetts General Hospital in 1917. Today most of the large hospitals have such special fracture clinics and the results obtained by these specialist services far excel those of the general hospitals of the past.

Long before this, treatment of fractures was improved by several new methods. The first of these was the use of plaster of Paris bandages. This idea was the invention of a Dutch Army medical officer, A. Mathijssen in 1852. Plaster of Paris is a fine white powder, consisting of calcium sulphate made anhydrous by calcining it. When wetted it swells and sets rapidly. It was originally prepared from the gypsums of Montmartre. This plaster had been used to make casts for many years. It was mixed with water into a thick paste and poured into a mould surrounding the limb. In this way a stiff case was made to support a broken arm or leg and keep the bony pieces in position; but the method was very messy and difficult to carry out. Mathijssen hit upon the idea of spreading the dry plaster on a roller bandage, wetting it and then bandaging the limb with it. The bandage itself then hardened into a perfect mould as the plaster of Paris set within the meshes of the cloth. This was one of the greatest surgical triumphs; simple, apparently obvious and thoroughly successful. It was now possible to prepare quickly and easily perfectly fitting light-weight splints for all fractures of limbs.

Plaster of Paris bandages soon came to be used in orthopaedic departments all over the world. Lewis Sayre, the New York surgeon, used such plaster bandages to make a well-fitting jacket for the whole trunk, applying the bandages while the patient was suspended by overhead cords supporting his head and shoulders. This manœuvre straightened and immobilized the spine. Today plaster casts are prepared in this way in a great number of orthopaedic conditions. They are an indispensable aid to this branch of surgery.

Another invaluable help to the orthopaedic surgeons was, of

course, the X-ray machine, which became available from 1895 onwards. The following year an American, an Austrian, and a German independently discovered how to take stereoscopic X-ray pictures. This was done by taking two separate pictures from different viewpoints, separated from one another by a distance equal to that between the two eyes of the observer. These pictures could be subsequently viewed by means of mirrors, so that each eye saw one picture only. The images fused in the brain, so that the picture appeared to be three-dimensional, the observer saw the broken fragments in perspective and found it much easier to establish their relative positions.

Another advance in treatment was that of the open reduction of fractures, that is to say the surgeon would cut down upon the bones and correct the position of the fragments very exactly. In pre-antiseptic days this involved a very grave risk, because, in effect, it converted a simple fracture into a compound one. None the less such operations were done to wire together ends of bones which had failed to unite. They had in fact been done with occasional success before Lister's day. He himself wired together a fractured kneecap, using his carbolic acid method, in 1877. A good many of these wiring operations were done in the next decade, but without much success. The first real advance came when metal screws were used to hold the bony fragments together. Early successes were achieved by Albin Lambotte of Antwerp in 1880 and William Arbuthnot Lane in London in 1894. Lane persisted in his efforts to fix difficult fractures by internal mechanical means and he eventually found the best way was to use long metal screws through the bones to fix metal plates in position. This method became widely used in all difficult fractures. The wires, bands and pegs used by Lane's predecessors were unsatisfactory because they worked loose and acted as irritant foreign bodies. The metal plates, on the other hand, held the whole bone together without movement; that was the secret of their success. Lane devised a specially rigorous aseptic technique for these open operations on bones, which required that all manipulations should be done with instruments. Infections can be disastrous in operations of this kind, because sepsis in bones is notoriously dangerous.

Later, screws and pins of various types began to be used in

treating fractures of the neck of the femur, which is a common accident in elderly people and often used to mark the beginning of the end. It was very difficult to get these fractures to unite. For one thing it was not desirable to immobilize old people in bed for any length of time, because they developed pneumonia and died. An operation was therefore devised in which a metal pin was driven through the shaft of the femur in its upper part, and through the broken neck into the head, thus uniting the femur mechanically.

These methods of inserting artificial materials into bones were always a little hazardous, because the body tends to react unfavourably to the presence of foreign bodies. If infection occurs the foreign body is almost always extruded by suppuration. Even with perfect asepsis trouble may occur. The secret of success seemed to lie in finding some substances completely without irritant action. This had to await industrial discoveries. Firstly, when stainless steel became generally available, it was found to cause very little irritation and so could be employed, using Lane's technique. Since the Second World War man-made substances, such as nylon, terylene and polyethylene have proved even more useful in that they seem to cause no irritation at all, and moreover these substances are extremely strong, which is of great consideration with any foreign material used in this kind of way.

Sometimes when a big joint, such as the hip, is badly damaged, say by osteo-arthritis, it has been found possible to replace the actual joint by some artificial contrivance. There were considerable difficulties. Firstly the artificial material must be completely non-irritant, as explained above. Secondly it must have great strength, because the actual forces exerted on a hip-joint are very large. Thirdly it has to be very resistant to wear and tear. The living joint of the hip is normally undergoing constant natural repair to the material of the joint surface, on which falls an enormous strain during such ordinary movements as walking and running. With an artificial hip-joint the wear and tear far exceed anything that an engineer would expect the moving parts of an engine to stand.

In 1938 the problem of material for artificial hip-joints was largely solved when Smith-Petersen found that the metal called vitallium was eminently suitable for this purpose. Many types of prostheses (as these artificial aids are called) have been tried, such as metal caps for joint surfaces, replacement of the whole head of the femur and, more bold than anything, a complete new artificial joint. This last involves screwing a metal cup into position in the pelvis to take the place of the acetabulum (the socket into which the thigh-bone fits). Such operations have been carried out and the patients have used their artificial joints for a number of years; but it is probably too early to be sure that the problem of wear and tear has been completely solved.

IV NEUROSURGERY

Surgery of the nervous system was born towards the end of the nineteenth century and it is singular in that it was largely the creation of two men, an Englishman and an American. Victor Horsley laid the foundations on which Harvey Cushing subsequently built an edifice of highly specialized technique. Neurosurgery deals with lesions inside the skull and the spinal cord. These lesions are injuries, tumours and certain kinds of inflammation. The subject also covers lesions of nerves outside the central nervous system, but these need not particularly concern us here.

Inside the brain and spinal cord and the membranes that surround them (the meninges) various types of tumours arise. Until neurosurgery became developed these growths were invariably fatal, for there was no treatment that offered any hope of a cure.

It was during his term as house surgeon at University College Hospital in 1880–1 that Victor Horsley began to think that the time was ripe for active surgical treatment in head cases; but, before anything of the sort could be attempted, it was essential to know how to localize brain or spinal lesions accurately so that the skull or spinal column could be opened at the right place. The first steps in this direction had been taken in Germany by Gustave Theodor Fritsch and Eduard Hitzig in 1870. They used a small electric current to explore the brain in animals. They found that local movements of limbs could be produced by stimulating definite small areas of the brain with a galvanic current, and that the precise site of the brain-stimulus determined the place and nature of the limb movements. Between 1872 and 1876 David Ferrier, a

London physiologist, developed this subject extensively with many experiments on the brains of birds, frogs, fishes and mammals, charting the various areas of brain-function, using a faradic in place of the galvanic current. From 1884 Horsley began working with Professor Edward Sharpey Schäfer at University College on the same methods of brain localization, but using monkeys. They employed both the method of faradic stimulation and that of removing tiny bits of the outer layer (cortex) of the brain to find out which bodily function was affected by each of the areas stimulated or removed. These animal experiments were done with rigorous anti-septic precautions and under anaesthesia, with chloroform or ether, supplemented by injections of morphia. These investigations, con-ducted over several years, added important knowledge to the physi-ology of the brain, besides enabling Horsley to evolve methods of opening the skull and the spinal column without undue risk.

In the same year 1884 enough information about brain-function was available in England to make possible the first clinical localiza-tion and removal of a tumour. The patient was a man of twenty-five who had developed twitchings and weakness of the left arm and leg, vomiting and headache. Alexander Hughes Bennett, a physician at the National Hospital for the Paralysed and Epileptic in Queen Square, London, diagnosed a tumour in a specific region of the brain cortex. He persuaded J. R. Godlee, a pupil of Lister's, to attempt to remove it surgically. Godlee opened the skull with a tre-phine at the point indicated by Bennett and found a tumour in the cortex of the brain. He removed it by blunt dissection. The patient survived the actual operation—the first of its kind—but the wound became infected and he died a month later of meningitis. This proved two points; firstly the possibility of cutting into the brain without immediate disaster, and secondly how essential rigorous asepsis was in any operation on the central nervous system.

In 1886 when Horsley was appointed surgeon to the National Hospital for the Paralysed and Epileptic, Queen Square, he was already well equipped. His early career was one of the best ex-amples in the history of medicine of the value of experimental work on animals as a preparation for clinical surgery. Horsley was the man the hospital meant to have and got. As to the hospital itself, Queen Square was not the only institution of its kind in London, but it was 'the oldest, the largest, the richest and the best; and it was known far and wide for its work and teaching'.[1]

Before this time it is no exaggeration to say that the methods of treating head injuries were no more advanced than those taught by Ambroise Paré, the famous French surgeon, in the sixteenth century. Horsley put forward six cardinal points to be observed in brain surgery; firstly rigorous asepsis; secondly, complete familiarity with the action of anaesthetics on the brain; thirdly, a long curved incision of the scalp to give adequate access to the brain; fourthly the use of a miniature circular saw to open the skull, fifthly never to use a galvanic cautery and lastly his own invention of stopping bleeding from the cut edges of bone by the use of antiseptic wax.

Horsley's first brain operation was done in May 1886. The patient was a Scot of twenty-two, who had been run over at the age of seven, with extensive brain damage. When admitted to Queen Square he had sluggish mentality, partial paralysis of one arm and one leg and frequent fits—2,870 of them in his first thirteen days in hospital. Horsley succeeded in removing the scar tissue from the brain, 'the wound healed well, the mental condition improved and the fits ceased'.

Later the same year Horsley removed a tumour from the brain of a man who was completely paralysed on the left side, was having fits and had been half-comatose for ten days before the operation. He correctly diagnosed a brain growth and specified its situation. At operation he removed a tumour (a glioma—a growth originating from the nervous cells of the brain) of $4\frac{1}{2}$ ounces in weight. The patient regained full consciousness, the fits stopped and the paralyses improved. Unfortunately this kind of tumour is prone to recur and the patient died of a recurrence about six months later. By the end of his first year at Queen Square Horsley had done ten brain operations with only one operative death, an accomplishment hardly imagined up to that time.

In the following year, 1887, he achieved the first successful removal of a tumour from the spinal cord. The patient was an army officer who was having excruciating pains, with partial paralysis of the bladder and complete paralysis of the legs. Horsley

[1] Paget, S., *Sir Victor Horsley*, London, 1919, p. 116.

was able to undertake this extensive and difficult operation because he had already done such an operation in the course of his animal experiments. He removed the tumour. The wound healed well, the pain and the paralyses vanished and the patient returned to work, lived in the best of health and died twenty years later of some unrelated cause.

In the same year Horsley showed that, in cases where a brain tumour was not removable by surgery (because of its situation in a dangerous area), free trephining of the skull—decompression, as Harvey Cushing called it later—gave very great relief, though, of course, it was a palliative measure only and in no sense a cure.

In the meantime Frederick Bramwell, a physician and pathologist in Edinburgh, had been studying the clinical and pathological aspects of brain tumours. In 1888 he published a monograph[1] which was the first comprehensive work on the subject. His descriptions of the symptoms; headaches, vomiting, eye-signs and paralyses caused by these growths, were so accurate and clear that his book can still be read with profit today.

In 1893 Horsley developed a method of treating paraplegia (paralysis of the lower limbs and part or whole of the trunk) resulting from tuberculosis of the spine. In this disease the vertebrae are attacked and one or more of them may collapse, causing pressure on the spinal cord, with paralysis of all muscles supplied by nerves originating from the spinal cord below the site of the lesion. In this condition Horsley advised early resort to operation to relieve the compression. It should be noted that his work for surgery of the spine was just as important as his more spectacular operations on the brain.

By 1899 Horsley had done forty-four brain operations with only ten deaths, and nineteen on the spinal cord with only one death. Although this was an unparalleled feat, his London colleagues remained unimpressed and even went so far as to suggest that Horsley was prepared to operate for the sake of operating. Nothing could have been further from the truth. He was always at great pains to assess each case on its merits. His critics may have had the impression that he operated unnecessarily just because he saw the importance of *early* operation on brain tumours, without waiting

[1] Bramwell, F., *Intracranial Tumours*, Edinburgh, 1888.

for the progressive symptoms of compression—neuritis of the optic nerve, vomiting and headache.

Incidentally, Horsley had many other interests and threw himself enthusiastically into medical politics and into the fight for women's suffrage and for complete abstention from alcohol. He gave evidence about venereal disease before the Committee on Physical Deterioration,[1] and also before the 2nd Royal Commission on Animal Experiments. To the latter body he insisted on the importance of animal experiments, because of the need for teaching students how to operate and how to administer anaesthetics, as well as the need for working out new methods in surgery.

In the First World War he volunteered for military duties. In the course of these he was sent first to France, then to Egypt, to India and finally to Mesopotamia where, in 1916, at Amarah he died of heat-stroke in his sixtieth year.

After Horsley's work, surgeons elsewhere began to attempt occasional brain operations. At first it was found difficult to secure adequate exposure of the brain by the early methods of drilling one or two holes in the skull and enlarging them with a chisel. In 1891 a French surgeon, J. Toison of Lille, suggested the modern method of cutting a bone-flap. He bored a series of primary holes and then cut the intervening bone with a chain saw, cutting from within outwards. In 1896 an Italian, Leonardo Gigli, introduced his flexible wire saw into surgery and four years later he used it for cutting a bone-flap from the skull. With these improvements opening the skull became a less hazardous procedure.

Nevertheless neurosurgery made little progress. Its status at the turn of the century was well summed up by Harvey Cushing, the man responsible for the great advances which have since been made. He reviewed the records of Johns Hopkins Hospital and found that the diagnosis of brain tumour had been made only 32 times in the 36,000 patients admitted in the last ten years. Thirteen of these 32 had been transferred to the surgical wards, where two of them had been operated on, both with fatal results.

At the time when he reviewed this depressing record, Cushing was a well-trained surgeon of thirty-one, just returned to Baltimore

[1] See below, p. 274.

from a year's work in a physiological laboratory in Switzerland, where he had studied the problems of intracranial pressures and the experimental pathology of the nervous system, and he resolved to devote himself to neurosurgery. At Johns Hopkins, during the ensuing twelve years, he developed the method of precise localizing technique for operating on the brain. To this he brought the general principles of surgery that he had learned from his great chief, Halsted. These included meticulous control of bleeding, great care and gentleness in the handling of living tissues and the use of layers of separate sutures in closing wounds.

Cushing applied these principles to brain surgery with great skill. He controlled bleeding from the scalp by putting a tourniquet round it. For tumours at the back and lower part of the brain he devised the so-called cross-bow incision, which has been the standard one ever since. When he had the tumour exposed, he would shell it out of its bed by the gentle use of cotton-wool pledgets, instead of plunging his fingers into the substance of the brain and digging it out as his predecessors had done. It was through such crude methods that the majority of their patients had died from haemorrhage. Cushing not only reduced bleeding by gentleness in manipulation, but devised new methods for checking it. These included small pieces of fresh muscle which he placed over oozing surfaces, tiny silver wire clips with which small blood-vessels were clamped and the electric coagulation of bleeding-points.

All these methods were designed to combat surgical shock, and thus he was able to carry out extensive operations in one stage, instead of several stages as had been the custom before. He introduced the practice of keeping a running record of the patient's blood-pressure throughout the operation so as to have early warning of the onset of shock, a practice which has since been adopted in all types of surgery.

In 1912 Cushing went to Harvard as Mosley professor of surgery and surgeon-in-chief to the Peter Bent Brigham Hospital. There his clinic for neurosurgery became world famous. He perfected his methods in detail, collected a huge mass of data about brain tumours, and trained a succession of young men who carried his teachings abroad and established neurosurgery as a speciality in the chief centres of medical education everywhere.

Cushing's contribution to neurosurgery did more than anything else at that time to establish this as a special branch of surgery, for he proved so strikingly the dividend it paid in improved results. He was a strong influence in raising the standards of surgical teaching. As an essayist and medical historian, he won wide recognition, his life of Sir William Osler having become one of the best known medical biographies of our time. He died in 1939 at the age of seventy, honoured all over the world.

In the last two decades neurosurgery has been successfully applied to the treatment of Parkinson's disease, or paralysis agitans. This is a progressive disease of insidious onset, generally starting in middle-age and usually in men. It is characterized by involuntary rhythmic tremors of the hands, an anxious, mournful and change-less facial expression ('Parkinson's mask') and a hurried, shuffling gait. The disease was quite incurable and practically untreatable and, after a varying number of years, led to complete helplessness, ending in death from pneumonia or some other intercurrent cause. The very nature of the symptoms suggested that they had their origin in some definite area of the brain; and this has proved to be so.

At the beginning of this century Robert Clarke invented an apparatus, which he patented, for performing operations inside the skull. It enabled a probe to reach with great accuracy any prede-termined point inside the brain through a very small hole, thus avoiding extensive opening of the skull. Victor Horsley and Clarke together used this new machine in a number of animal experiments, but it was not used on human beings until 1950. In that year E. A. Spiegel and H. T. Wycis used a modified Clarke's machine to treat involuntary movements of the limbs in 'spastics'. By electro-coagulation of small areas of the brain, they succeeded in abolishing the involuntary movements altogether. Later they applied the same principle to improve tremor and rigidity in Parkinson's disease, by destroying specific areas of the brain tissue, where the symptoms had their origin. Many patients with this disease now have a fair chance of amelioration of their symptoms, provided the disease is not too far advanced. The probe is passed through a 'silent' area of the brain cortex (i.e. one which, when stimulated or destroyed, gives rise to no observable changes in the body) and the modified Clarke's machine can ensure that the point reaches the selected spot to an accuracy of one millimetre. Most sufferers from Parkinsonism have bilateral disease, so that two operations are necessary, one on each side of the brain. It is usual to leave an interval of some months between the first and second operations. It would appear that age is no contra-indication to operation, provided the patient's general condition is satisfactory. For example L. Oliver[1] recorded a number of patients over seventy who had been treated with success. It should be added that this treatment, though it can give great relief, is purely palliative and in no way stops the degeneration in the central nervous system, the cause of which remains unknown.

V. THORACIC SURGERY

Chest surgery is the newest of the major surgical specialities, and it is only within the last twenty years or so that it began its most spectacular achievements. Seventy years ago Stephen Paget, son of the eminent Victorian surgeon Sir James Paget, published a scholarly work, *The Surgery of the Chest*,[2] and it is fair to regard this as marking the opening of the new speciality, though Paget himself thought that chest surgery by then was nearing its zenith. He wrote that 'surgery of the heart has probably reached the limits set by nature to surgery, no new method, and no new discovery can overcome the natural difficulties that attend a wound of the heart ... There are signs that we have reached a stage in this portion of our art beyond which, on our present lines, we cannot advance much further'.[3] He did well to include the clause 'on our present lines,' because fresh discoveries were just round the corner—discoveries which were to alter the whole situation most profoundly. In Paget's time there was no blood-transfusion, no kind of anaesthesia suitable for open chest work, no hypothermia, no kind of

---

[1] Oliver, L., *Parkinson's Disease*, London, 1967.
[2] London, 1896.
[3] Cited by R. H. Meade, *A History of Thoracic Surgery*, Springfield, Illinois, 1961, preface.

heart–lung machine and indeed X-rays had been discovered only the year before Paget wrote those words.

Up to the time of the Second World War chest surgery was pretty well limited to treating empyema, bronchiectasis, lung cancer (occasionally) and tuberculosis and these developments all depended on adequate antiseptic methods.

Empyema is an accumulation of pus in the pleural space, which is formed by the thin envelope of tissue which surrounds the lung and lines the inside of the chest wall. Empyema is generally the result of pneumonia. Unless the condition is treated, the volume of pus increases and compresses the lung more and more and leads to complications which are eventually fatal. Until about 1880 surgeons dared not open the pleura to provide free drainage. The only treatment was to draw off the pus with a syringe, using a wide-bore needle, and repeating this again and again—usually to no purpose. Thus, out of a series of 48 patients with empyema, Paget was able to report only six that were cured in this way.

With the adoption of Listerism, surgeons in Germany found that wide incision through the chest-wall, preferably with excision of a portion of a rib to provide better drainage, gave much better results than the old aspiration method. In 1891 Franz Koenig of Göttingen reported 66 cures in a series of 76 cases so treated. This method was adopted in France and England and Paget himself made use of it. Gradually it became the standard method of treating empyema all over the world. None the less the disease continued to be one of the most dangerous conditions confronting the surgeon. In most hospitals the mortality ranged between 20 and 30 per cent.

The next advance in the treatment of empyema came with the First World War, when the great influenza pandemic of 1918 swept through the armies of Europe. Enormous numbers of empyemata followed. Most of them were of a special type, the infecting organism being a streptococcus rather than the usual pneumococcus. In these streptococcal infections massive pleural effusions often occurred. It soon became clear that the standard method of prompt open drainage gave disastrous results. In some American camps the mortality was over 70 per cent.

At this time Evarts A. Graham at Washington University School of Medicine at St Louis made an experimental study of empyema in dogs. He was able to induce streptococcal empyema experimentally. He then treated one series of animals by the standard open-drainage method, while in a second series no operation was done. Most of the first series died, whereas most of the second survived. Graham showed that most of the deaths were due to air entering the pleural space on the operation side, in such quantity as to push the central partition of the chest (the mediastinum) across to the other side, so compressing the sound lung and causing fatal interference with breathing.

Applying these findings to human beings, Graham advised against early open drainage, and dramatic results ensued. At Camp Lee, Virginia, where the Empyema Commission worked, the new treatment reduced the mortality in this disease from 48 per cent to 4·3 per cent. When necessary, drainage could be done later in the course of the disease, when the mediastinum had become stiffened by inflammation, and so not readily pushed across to the other side. This drainage at a later stage was found to be far less hazardous; but the wound generally took a long time to heal and it was necessary to wash out the empyema cavity repeatedly with Dakin's solution (sodium hypochlorite).

Later on the method of 'closed drainage' was adopted in order to avoid the pressure on the lungs. This consisted in making an airtight connexion between the drainage-tube and the chest-wall, and putting the lower end of the tube beneath the surface of some water in a large bottle, well below the level of the chest. In this way the water acted as a simple one-way valve, allowing discharge from the wound, but permitting no air to get up into the chest. This method became generally adopted and is still in use today.

Another disease of the lungs, bronchiectasis, became amenable to surgical treatment in the 1920's and 1930's. In this disease the innermost parts of the air tubes of the lung, because of infection or congenital defects, become dilated and filled with pus. The condition generally involves the lower lobes of the lungs, which suggested to the surgeons at the turn of the century that local removal of the diseased part of the lung might effect a cure. Encouraged by some successful removal of one lung in animals, surgeons did in fact attempt removing the affected lobe in bronchiectasis. Lothar

Heidenhein of Worms has been widely credited with the first successful lobectomy; but this has been questioned. Meade[1] stated that Heidenhain's case was in effect the opening and draining of a multiple lung-abscess, followed much later by piecemeal removal of the major part of the damaged lung, first with a knife and later a cautery. He said that it was in no sense resection of a lobe, such as is practised today. A few daring surgeons in Germany and in America attempted this operation, but it proved to be so dangerous, with a mortality of more than one half, that only the most desperately ill would consent to it; and of course their poor general condition constituted an added risk.

Howard Lilienthal did his first resection in 1914 on a three-year-old child who had become bronchiectatic as a result of having inhaled a nut some time before. This patient recovered. By 1925 he had operated on 34 patients, but with the alarming mortality of over 60 per cent.

After 1920 further advances were made. Bronchoscopic and X-ray examinations simplified and made certain the diagnosis of bronchiectasis and provided a larger number of cases for study. In 1923 Graham devised a method of destroying the diseased lung in stages with a cautery; but the risk was great and surgeons were reluctant to undertake such procedure. In 1929 Harold Brunn, professor of Surgery in the University of California, reported six cases of lobectomy with only one death. The first of these operations was in 1918 and they were all done as one-stage operations, followed by drainage and with a suction apparatus connected to the tube to produce a negative pressure and so help the remaining lung to expand.

Norman Shenstone and Robert James, of Toronto, improved on the method by using a snare type of tourniquet. In 1932 they reported on 15 lobectomies. All the patients had previously had one phrenic nerve deliberately paralysed shortly before the main operation, so as to stop the movement of the diaphragm on the affected side. Further improvements in anaesthesia—local nerve blocks and spinal anaesthetics—enabled the operators to avoid the added hazards of inhalation anaesthesia.

Abscess of the lung was another serious condition which had a

[1] Meade, R. H., op. cit., p. 49.

very high mortality until quite recently. Many lung abscesses were due to inhalation of infected material from the mouth, or they followed the accidental inhalation of a foreign body—generally in infancy or childhood—or a portion of tooth during dental extractions under gas. Operation to remove the contents of such abscesses and to bring about free ventilation of the affected lung (to discourage the growth of anaerobic bacteria) was frequently undertaken. This operation was not always successful; for example, in a high proportion of the adult cases there was a cancer underlying and causing the lung abscess. The introduction of antibiotics in the 1940's greatly improved the outlook in non-malignant cases.

The surgical attack on pulmonary tuberculosis has already been described.[1] Artificial pneumothorax, section of pleural adhesions, artificial paralysis of the diaphragm, thoracoplasty, resection and pneumonectomy all come under this heading. Though of great historical importance and interest, surgery for pulmonary tuberculosis is but rarely used now, the standard treatment of today being the use of antituberculous drugs.

One of the most serious problems the thoracic surgeon has to face is that of lung cancer. Fifty years ago the disease was held to be without hope of cure. Yet today many people are alive and well years after surgical removal of cancer of the lung.

This disease is distressingly common and both the number of new cases and the number of deaths is mounting year by year. Its presence should always be suspected where there is persistent cough, pain in the chest and, above all, where there are traces of blood in the sputum. The disease can often be accurately diagnosed and located by X-ray examinations and bronchoscopy; but unfortunately it cannot always be excluded with absolute certainty even by the most painstaking investigations.

As with other forms of cancer, if surgical excision is to have any chance of success, it must be radical. Since most cancers arise in the central part of the lung, removal of the entire lung is generally required. This formidable operation was first done successfully by Rudolf Nissen in Berlin. The patient was a twelve-year-old girl with advanced bronchiectasis. The first success with lung cancer was announced by Evarts Graham in 1933. He had done a total

[1] See above, p. 138 *et seq.*

pneumonectomy on a physician, and subsequent microscopical examination of the tumour proved that it was unquestionably cancer. After removing the lung with an electric cautery, he further cauterized the lining of the bronchus and put in some radon seeds for good measure. He then had to decide what to do about the large empty space in the chest, which he feared would become infected if he left it as it was. He decided to do a thoracoplasty to obliterate this space. The patient was alive and living an active life twenty-five years later.

Since then many pneumonectomies for cancer have been successfully carried out and a great number of these patients have survived. At first only a few lived much longer than a year. The main reason for the lack of success was that the disease was too far advanced when the patient was first seen by the surgeon. Early diagnosis was (and still is) the key to success; but unfortunately many cancers develop without giving rise to any symptoms until it is too late. Furthermore many patients are deterred by fear from seeking early medical advice. Once a diagnosis has been made, the case has to be fully investigated by bronchoscopy to confirm the diagnosis and to decide whether the case is likely to prove operable. Breathing tests have also to be done to measure lung function, to be quite sure that the patient will have enough breath left to lead a reasonable life if the whole of one lung is removed.

X-rays, radium and other forms of gamma radiation are valuable in post-operative treatment to kill off any malignant cells that may have been left behind. Radiotherapy is also used in cases where operation is impossible; but the results for the most part have been depressing.

Before the Second World War very little heart surgery had been done. Repair of injuries, such as stab wounds had on occasions been attended with success. H. Souttar, of the London Hospital, had done an operation on the mitral valve of the heart as long ago as 1925. A few operations on the pericardium—the membranous sac which encloses the heart—had also been carried out. But, in general, surgeons were very reluctant to operate on the heart. Later on a number of new discoveries were made which ensured pretty complete control of the opened chest, and so made thoracotomy a comparatively safe procedure. Among these new inventions we may mention in particular the notable advances in anaesthesia; the introduction of cardiac catheterization, which made X-ray assessment of the heart and blood-vessels a possibility, as well as measurement of blood flow, blood-pressures and blood-gases inside the heart.

The invention of cardiac catheterization was the result of an act of supreme courage on the part of one man. In 1929 a German, Werner Forssmann, was considering means of getting drugs quickly into the heart in certain emergencies. He thought it might be possible to pass a catheter up a vein in the arm into the interior of the right side of the heart. He found that he could do this quite simply in a dead body. He then proposed to try it on himself. He asked a doctor to put a wide-bore needle into one of his (Forssmann's) arm veins and he then pushed a catheter through this needle a distance of 35 centimetres up his arm. At this point his colleagues persuaded him to stop; for who could foretell what would happen if a tube were passed into the living, pulsating heart?

A week later Forssmann tried again, this time all by himself. Under local anaesthesia he passed a radio-opaque ureteric catheter up an arm vein a distance of 65 centimetres, which he calculated as the length required for the tip of the tube to enter his heart. He then walked to the X-ray room and with the aid of a nurse he was able to view his own chest on the fluorescent screen, reflecting the image in a mirror; and, sure enough, the tip of the tube was in the right auricle of his heart. Surprisingly he experienced absolutely no symptoms following this courageous experiment.

Further advances (referred to in Chapter XI) included anti-coagulation techniques which made blood-transfusion practical; hypothermia and perfusion methods, which gave the surgeon all the time he needed and a blood-free heart to operate upon. It will be seen from all this that successful surgery of the heart required well-organized team-work. It was no longer the surgeon alone that counted; he needed diagnosticians, biochemists, physiologists, blood-donors and blood-transfusion experts, radiologists and highly skilled anaesthetists, besides a great deal of very expensive equipment, with well-trained engineers and nurses to look after it. The result of all this was (and is) that heart surgery can only be carried out where all these doctors, nurses, technicians and machinery can be concentrated at centres which have accommodation enough for them to work and money enough to afford the enormous expense.

The heart conditions now amenable to surgery are very many and we cannot enter into details about them here. They include putting electrical pace-makers into the body to regulate the rhythm of the heart-beat in some forms of disease and machines to re-start hearts that have stopped under hypothermia or for other reasons, besides repair of heart valves. Surgeons have also been able to replace damaged heart valves with completely artificial contrivances which have worked satisfactorily for years.

In short it may be said that cardiac surgery is still advancing with rapid strides, though the complicated organization described above must of necessity make all these procedures extremely expensive. None the less as Sir Thomas Holmes Sellors has succinctly put it: 'The risks are small and the results are good.'[1]

ADDENDUM. Since this Chapter was written, the first successful transplant of a living heart from one man to another has been carried out, early in 1968, by Christian Barnard in South Africa.

[1] *British Medical Journal*, 1967, I, p. 385, 'The Genesis of Heart Surgery'.

PART III

Health Organization

Having reviewed some of the most important scientific discoveries which have contributed to the prevention and cure of disease we must turn our attention to the administrative and legislative aspects of medicine. Before considering the rise of the Public Health services and the State Medicine it will be convenient to give some brief account of the reform of the hospitals which play so large a part in the cure of sickness today. The latter began almost entirely through voluntary effort and is consequently better described separately from the sanitary services which had their origin largely through the law of the land.

CHAPTER ONE

THE REFORM OF THE HOSPITALS

WE have seen what dirty and disorderly places the hospitals were in the past. To write of the early stages in their reform must be to give a very brief outline of the work of Florence Nightingale. The story is only too well known, but it is of fundamental importance. From her came the main inspiration and it is the direct result of her influence that the hospitals are managed in the efficient way in which they mostly are today. To be really effective the reform needed the combination of good nursing and organization with the new Antiseptic Method of Lister: but the campaign for reform began before either the germ-theory or the antiseptic principle had been announced.

Florence Nightingale began her career in 1832, when she went for three months to Kaiserswerth in Germany to the Institute for Deaconesses, where there was a school for infants and a hospital where some sort of training in nursing was given. How little this was may be judged from her own words: 'The nursing there was *nil*. The hygiene horrible. The hospital was certainly the worst part of Kaiserswerth. I took all the training there was to be had— there was none to be had in England—but Kaiserswerth was far from having trained me.'[1]

Shortly after her return she became Superintendent of the *Establishment for Gentlewomen during Illness* in Harley Street; but she left this for a while to help to nurse the patients at the Middlesex Hospital during the cholera outbreak of 1854. In the same year England and France declared war on Russia. Thus it came about that the Crimean War gave her the opportunity to try her mettle. Her experiences in Harley Street and the Middlesex hospital had prepared her for the ordeal that was to come. It was her work at

[1] Cook, E., *The Life of Florence Nightingale*, revised by R. Nash, London, 1925, p. 45.

237

Scutari and the magnificent results that she obtained that were to be the guiding lights towards hospital reform.

The situation in the war area was horrible indeed. The old army pensioners who had been sent out to nurse the sick and wounded proved quite useless and in fact spent much of their time nursing one another. The shortage of medical supplies was scandalous. 'Not only are there not sufficient surgeons—that, it might be urged, was unavoidable: not only are there no dressers and nurses —that might be a defect of system for which no one is to blame: but what will be said when it is known that there is not even linen to make bandages for the wounded?'[1]

It was through Sidney Herbert, who was Secretary at War, that Miss Nightingale both volunteered and was asked (the letters crossed in the post) to undertake the formidable task of organizing the nursing at Scutari. She rapidly collected a body of thirty-eight women who were to be her staff. She had to choose these with care from the volunteers who applied for service; for she was very well aware that the women she needed must not only be able-bodied and tender-hearted but must also be persons of prudence and capacity and have as much previous experience and training as was possible. Thus the great experiment (for such it was) began.

It must not be supposed that this was absolutely the first experiment in female attendance on sick soldiers. The French had their Sisters of Charity, while, through the influence of the Grand Duchess Helena Pavlovna, the great Russian surgeon Pirogov introduced female nurses to tend the wounded in the Crimea.[2]

The state of affairs at Scutari could hardly have been worse when Florence Nightingale arrived. There were more than seventeen hundred patients in the military hospital and among them raged cholera, dysentery, erysipelas, fever and gangrene. Amputations were carried out in the very wards so that the soldiers watched their companions dying under the surgeon's knife. To add to this, hundreds were dying of inanition simply because they were unable to digest the only available diet of boiled beef.

There was a complete breakdown of all medical organization.

[1] *The Times*, October 12th, 1854 (cited by E. Cook).
[2] Garrison, op cit., p. 498.

There was dirt, confusion and neglect. The floors were rotten and the walls encrusted with filth. The beds were both insufficient in their number and overcrowded in their arrangement. Vermin and lack of ventilation helped to make the place a stinking inferno. There were not only no medical supplies, but there was no ordinary bedroom furniture. Basins, soap, towels, mops, knives, forks and plates—all were wanting. There was no laundry and often not even enough fuel.

That the new matron was undaunted by the task set before her was surprising enough; but she had also to fight against fierce opposition not only from the military authorities, but even from the medical men themselves who resented her interference. We find her complaining to Sidney Herbert that Dr Hall was trying to root her out. An accusation that she was 'spoiling the brutes' was all the encouragement she got for providing reading-rooms 'to avoid the convalescents coming in *dead* drunk (they *die* of it)'.

The success of Florence Nightingale's great campaign is well enough known. It is necessary to give but a few examples of her figures. 'In the first seven months of the war the mortality among the troops had been at the rate of 60 per cent per annum—from *disease alone*—a rate of mortality which exceeds that of the great plague of London.'[1] After she had been at Scutari for six months she was able to report that of the 1,100 patients left in the Barrack Hospital only 100 were in bed and the death-rate had fallen from 42 per cent to 22 per mille.

By what means did she accomplish this extraordinary result? By methodical and unremitting hard work and by discipline. To aid her in her work she had with great foresight armed herself with medical and household supplies in huge amounts—in spite of the assurance she had received before she set out from Dr Andrew Smith, the head of the Army Medical Department, that nothing was wanting at Scutari. Furthermore she had money, both her own Fund and that collected by *The Times*. She had also the loyal support not only of the Government through the influence of Sidney Herbert but also of public opinion at home.

Besides her battle with officialdom and etiquette she had to fight

[1] Cook, E., op. cit., p. 173.

mainly against dirt and chaos. She procured and made use of soap and water. She provided a new laundry where the washing was done by the soldiers' wives. She produced socks, boots, shirts, trousers and dressing-gowns. She reorganized the kitchen and the cooking. She provided stores of all sorts and routed out much of the Government supplies which were hidden away under the munitions in the transport ships and in the labyrinths of the Turkish customs house. She even engaged workmen to make fresh quarters fit for the reception of new consignments of sick and wounded. In fact, far from being simply the matron of a hospital, she became practically 'mistress of a barrack and indeed assistant purveyor to the British Army'.[1]

It was while this organizing was in progress that Miss Nightingale developed her idea of what a nursing service should be. Nurses were not to be an entirely separate service of domestics; much less were they to interfere with the work of the doctors. They were to be 'a subordinate branch of the medical service under the doctor's orders as to matters of treatment while under their own superintendent as to matters of discipline'.

Florence Nightingale also introduced uniforms to promote cleanliness and to give the nurses a smart and sober appearance and to 'disarm criticism and belie the untoward reputation of nurses'; for the nursing profession was one of the most disreputable and it says much for her courage that she ever embarked on a career which carried with it so grave a stigma. Indeed it was just this sordid reputation which was at the root of the bitter opposition which her family and her friends put up in their efforts to stop Florence from doing any nursing at all.

Her work at Scutari was an outstanding success and her contention was proved that soap and fresh air meant health and that good hospital hygiene could make all the difference between a death-trap and a house of recovery. Furthermore she had overcome the prejudices against female nurses. She was about to create an entirely new profession for her sex. But the strain, physical and mental had been tremendous. The news came that Miss Nightingale was down with Crimean fever; but she refused to leave her mission and remained at Scutari until the last invalid soldiers had

[1] Cook, E., op. cit., p. 77.

gone. It was extremely fortunate that she did not die at this time, for her magnificent achievements were only a preliminary to a life-long fight for reform in nursing and hospital organization. But her health was broken and only her indomitable will enabled this per-petual invalid to carry on her great work.

Florence Nightingale returned home a heroine. She was ill, but she could not and would not rest so long as the old methods of organization existed in the Army Medical Service. Another war might easily see a repetition of the Crimean disaster. She set about to collect statistics. She found that the state of affairs in the Army at home was deplorable. 'We had, during the last six months of the war, a mortality among our *sick* not much more than among our *healthy* Guards at home, and a mortality among our troops, in the last five months, two-thirds only of what it is among our troops at home.'[1] Here were some figures for contemplation. Further she showed that 'even among the Guards, men of picked physique, the death-rate was nearly double what it was in civil life'.

Armed with such figures as these with which she could, and would if necessary, have caused the gravest public scandal, she was able to browbeat the Government into appointing a Royal Com-mission to inquire into the whole matter. The mortality could only come from the grossest mismanagement and it was high time that something should be done; but what? In her *Notes on the British Army* Florence Nightingale gave the answer which contained 'not only the scheme of all Sidney Herbert's subsequent reforms, but the germ and often the details of further reforms in the same kind'. She was the adviser to the Commissioners and the power and the knowledge behind the scenes.

Many of these recommendations were carried out in Army barracks and hospitals. Buildings were ventilated and warmed; water supplies were improved, while drainage was introduced or reconstructed; kitchens were remodelled and reorganized; gas-lighting was provided and many buildings were entirely recon-structed and others condemned. More than this, in 1860 was founded the Army Medical School to furnish proper training. This developed later into the present Royal Army Medical Corps.

The results of all this began to be evident almost at once. The

[1] Cook, E., op. cit., p. 174.

death-rate during the years 1859 to 1861 was just halved; in fact it was brought down to that of the civil population. Immense improvements were also seen when the Army was on field service in the China expedition, where the mortality, including that of the wounded, was little more than 3 per cent per annum.

During the same time Miss Nightingale also applied her ideas to the reform of hospitals and nursing in civil life. This she was enabled to do by making use of the Fund that had been raised for her to establish a Nightingale School of Nursing. This was to be an experiment in the proper training of nurses. In June 1860 the first probationers were admitted for a year's training at St Thomas's Hospital. The previous year she had published her *Notes on Nursing* in which she had defined nursing as signifying 'the proper use of fresh air, light, warmth, cleanliness, quiet and the proper choosing and giving of the diet—all at the least expense of vital power to the patient'. She added that it ought to include 'nursing the well' or domestic hygiene. This outlook might almost pass for commonplace today, but at the time of publication the *Notes* contained much that was new. The book was a startling success, for 15,000 copies at five shillings each were sold within the first month.

We cannot follow Florence Nightingale's career at further length, but her work was far from completed. She took an active part in the reform of the workhouses, which may be said to have begun in 1867 under the Metropolitan Poor Act. She was also in the forefront of the bitter controversy which raged over the attempt to control venereal disease by legislation, as we shall see in good time.[1] From her bedroom in South Street she also reformed the Army in India. She had even conducted a vigorous but unsuccessful fight to reform the War Office itself. It was in this battle that she literally worked poor Sidney Herbert to death.

There was plenty of room for improvement in English hospitals, for the so-called hospital diseases were still very prevalent. Lister's antiseptic campaign began in 1865, but at first it made but slow progress in this country. Until the surgeons adopted this system there was very little chance that these septic diseases could ever be banished from the surgical wards. Miss Nightingale herself

[1] See below, p. 297.

smiled at the germ-theory, but much of her soap, water and fresh air was certainly instrumental in removing the bacteria of sepsis. The striking results of the application of the work of Pasteur and Lister to hospital practice may be seen by taking just one example, this time from Germany, which was one of the earliest countries to adopt the new methods. In 1875 in the hospital at Munich no less than 80 per cent of the wounds, whether surgical or accidental, became gangrenous. Everything had been tried, wrote Professor von Nussbaum, when 'in a single week, with great energy and industry we applied to all our patients the newest antiseptic method now in many respects improved by Lister, and did all the operations according to his directions, we experienced one surprise after another . . . not a single case of gangrene occurred'.[1] Today these methods are universal and gangrene in an operation wound is a rarity and is rightly considered a disgrace.

Towards the middle of the nineteenth century special hospitals began to appear. Before that there were no hospitals for special diseases, with the few exceptions mentioned in our introductory chapter. Knowledge was rapidly growing and it became apparent to the younger men that specialization was imminent. The whole field of medicine was becoming too wide for any single individual to cover. First of all special departments were set up in the general hospitals; but it was so easy for the older practitioners who disapproved of specialization to refrain from sending their patients to these departments. In this way grew the conception of having special hospitals for particular diseases.

Specialist departments are a valuable asset to any large general hospital, but there is room for doubt about whether special institutions for particular complaints are a desirable feature of modern hospital service. At the present time there are specialized hospitals for cancer, tuberculosis, ears, nose and throat diseases, skin disease, venereal disease, women's ailments, for sick children and many other purposes. All of these do excellent work, but probably no better than could be done in general hospitals. In certain circumstances the existence of special hospitals can be completely justified. This is particularly so in the case of fever hospitals (which, as will be seen, came mostly under Local Authorities)

[1] Godlee, R. J., *Lord Lister*, London, 1917, p. 340.

where isolation is of the first importance. Special hospitals for
tuberculosis are also justifiable, for this, too, is a contagious disease.
Institutions for children flourished especially by reason of the
sentimental appeal they made to their supporting public. In
general, however, it may be said that the multiplicity of special
hospitals was uneconomic and increased the difficulties of co-
operation between specialists in different subjects.

One of the most striking changes in hospital practice was the
rapid rise of the municipal and county rate-paid institutions. These
were built and maintained by Boroughs or Urban and Rural
Districts under powers given them by the Public Health Act of
1875.[1] County Councils also acquired similar powers under the
Local Government Act of 1929,[2] although they could build hospitals for infectious disease under the earlier Isolation Hospitals
Acts.

There was always much discussion about the relative merits and
demerits of the voluntary and the rate-paid hospitals. In general
the advantages of the voluntary system may be summed up as
follows. They lived by competition and efficiency so that only the
best could survive. There was no charge on the rates and the
voluntary hospitals offered better facilities for teaching and research
than did their rate-aided rivals. Their senior staffs were unpaid and
worked under the constant criticism of their juniors and of the
students, circumstances which must have kept them up to a high
pitch of efficiency. Against the voluntary system it was urged that
the various institutions were often too jealous or too self-centred to
co-operate effectively with one another or with outsiders. Furthermore they were often situated far nearer the homes of the honorary
staff than those of the patients they were designed to serve. In
the rate-paid hospitals on the other hand, it was thought that there
was grave danger that lack of publicity, criticism and competition
might have allowed them to fall into an uninspired level of medi-
ocrity.

The reform of the hospitals was a very slow process, so much so
that in 1871 a Commission was appointed under Sir William

[1] Section 131.
[2] Section 14.
[3] 1893 and 1901.

Fergusson to inquire into hospital abuses. Soon after this the worst features began to disappear. None the less Sir D'Arcy Power, one of the senior surgeons at St Bartholomew's Hospital in the City of London, told of the far from satisfactory conditions which prevailed in the out-patient department as recently as 1898. The huge crowd of patients assembled in Smithfield in all weathers to await the opening of the doors at nine o'clock in the morning, including 'the man who sold bottles and ointment pots to those who had forgotten to bring them and the woman who was reputed to buy confection of senna and linctus for her open jam tarts, and the cod-liver oil for use in her neighbours' lamps'.[1] The hall was small and overcrowded and the atmosphere poisonous. There were so many patients that it was impossible for the best-intentioned doctor to give a proper examination to each one. The Poet Laureate, Dr Robert Bridges, stated that 'he saw and prescribed for 7,735 persons during this year of office [as house physician at St Bartholomew's] in 1897 and that 5,330 of these were new patients. The average time spent on each case was 1·28 of a minute and he congratulated himself on having given a separate audience to the troubles of 150 talkative women in $3\frac{1}{2}$ hours'. An amusing tale is told of the wholesale methods of one apothecary at the same hospital. When the crowd was assembled in the hall, he would say 'All those with a cough stand up!' and he gave them each a ticket for a bottle of physic to be obtained at the dispensary. Then he would continue, 'All those with the belly-ache, stand up! . . .' and so forth.

The available accommodation both in voluntary and rate-paid hospitals increased very rapidly in the decades before the Second World War; but the former were outstripped by the latter. In the first instance voluntary hospitals were supported entirely by endowments, subscriptions and contributions from the public, and no charges at all were exacted from the patients; but later, owing to the ever-increasing cost of modern treatment, it became necessary to ask the patients to contribute according to their means. The money so obtained made an appreciable contribution to the immense and ever-mounting cost of running the hospitals.

[1] *Lancet*, 1932, I, p. 1000.

In Great Britain the distinction between voluntary and publicly-supported hospitals disappeared with the advent of the Welfare State. This latest phase in the history of the hospitals resulted from the passing of the National Health Service Act of 1946. This will be discussed later when we consider the socialization of medicine which has occurred in the last twenty years.

CHAPTER TWO

MEDICINE AND THE STATE

1. SANITARY LEGISLATION IN THE NINETEENTH CENTURY[1]

IN the first half of the nineteenth century the knowledge of the principles of health was surely and steadily growing, but the ignorance of the masses was abysmal and there was hardly a vestige of interest taken by the public in the health of the community as a whole. It was becoming more and more clear that many of the diseases which inflicted so much hardship and so many fatalities on the people were the result of demonstrable causes and, what was of the greatest importance, that these causes were largely removable.

Thinking men began to see that action by the State was imperative if anything was to be done to mitigate preventable disease. The knowledge was there, but legislation was needed to apply it and to give shape to an organization which might be capable of enforcing the fundamental principles of health.

Such laws as there were for safeguarding the public health were for the most part valueless, incomplete or fallen into disuse. In early times common law right was the only means of redress from sanitary nuisance. As early as 1388, we find the first Sanitary Law which prohibited, under penalty of £20, the casting of animal filth and refuse into rivers and ditches in urban areas.[2] Certain restrictions were undoubtedly in force in many parts of the country in the sixteenth century. It is interesting to note, for example, that Shakespeare's father was fined on two occasions at Stratford-on-Avon for insanitary behaviour.[3] From time to time legislation was

[1] A fuller account is given in Sir John Simon's *English Sanitary Institutions*, London, 1890.

[2] Second Report of the Royal Sanitary Commission, London, 1871,

[3] ibid.

enacted against extraordinary pestilences—against the plague, for instance, in the reign of James I. It will be remembered, too, that early in the eighteenth century Richard Mead had published his very sound recommendations for the prevention of the spread of contagious disease.[1] These excellent suggestions were put on the Statute Book,[2] but unfortunately the most important clauses were repealed the following year—as Mead alleged, through political acrimony.

As early at least as the reign of George II individual towns began to ask for special legislation to enable them to improve their sanitary condition, but there was no compulsory Act for the redress of the state of the country as a whole.

On the other hand there were very encouraging aspects in the views held by some of those in authority. Jenner's discovery of vaccination had been taken up by the Government which had made an annual monetary grant to the National Vaccine Board for the upkeep of the supply of lymph for vaccination. The grant itself was beggarly; but it was a beginning. The first Vaccination Acts were passed in 1840 and 1841. The first of these prohibited the highly dangerous practice of attempting to immunize people by deliberately inoculating them with true smallpox. The 1841 Act provided that the expenses of public vaccination should come out of the Poor Rate. By these Acts the Poor Law Guardians and overseers were empowered to contract for the vaccination of all persons resident in their unions and parishes respectively.

The various sicknesses, acute and chronic, which were constantly taking their toll among the people were not likely to arouse men to the consciousness of the necessity for action. These diseases were always with them and, being 'natural', they were taken as a matter of course. A sudden and violent visitation of an unknown or unusual pestilence was far more likely to arouse alarm and a clamour for protection. The Asiatic cholera, therefore, played a large part in moulding public opinion in matters of public health.

The Great Reform Bill of 1832 may be fairly called the beginning of public health legislation, despite the fact that it contained no

[1] See above, p. 24.
[2] 7th Geo. I; Cap. 3.

provisions which were directly concerned with preventive medicine. Nevertheless, as a direct result of this Bill's becoming law, there followed in 1833, 1834 and 1835 respectively the Factory Act, the Poor Law Amendment and the Municipal Corporations Acts. The first of these aimed at limiting the working hours of children; the second had its importance in the formation of the Poor Law Commission which, as will be seen later, was to be the beginning of a *central* Public Health Authority; while the third began the system of elected local authorities which are still today in control of the local administration of preventive medicine, besides wielding many of the powers that were formerly in the hands of the magistrates.

It was in 1834 that Edwin Chadwick was appointed secretary to the Poor Law Commissioners, and Chadwick was to be the leading spirit in the demand for sanitary reform. He saw clearly that those diseases which abounded wherever there was filth could and should be prevented by the removal of that filth. It was the needy and squalid that took the diseases. Disease itself produced poverty and squalor. It was a vicious circle that must be broken.

That such disease could be checked was the accepted medical opinion. Had not John Howard, the Bedfordshire squire, shown what could be done in the prisons of England? Through his work, conducted in a spirit that was both philanthropic and scientifically methodical, the gaols offered the prisoners such hygienic conditions few of them could have experienced outside. The prisons need no longer have been incubators of typhus fever.

It was shown that disease-prevention was not only a possibility but also sound economy. Good health would diminish pauperism and small expenditure for prevention would avoid greater outlay for the care of the sick and the burial of the dead. Prevention was not only better, it was cheaper than cure.

The Poor Law Commissioners made a very extensive inquiry into the state of towns and the health of the labouring classes. The results of this were made public in Chadwick's historic report.[1] As we have seen in the introductory chapter, the discoveries were appalling and revealed the vilest conditions of physical and moral decay. None the less it seems certain that in some ways, or in some

[1] *General Report on the Sanitary Condition of the Labouring Population of Great Britain*, 1842.

areas, conditions were improving, because during the eighteenth century the death-rate had been falling. Chadwick made urgent recommendations for the removal of all filth and the provision of adequate drainage. He stressed the importance of liberal supplies of water without which it would be impossible to maintain any thorough system of sewage-removal. He also insisted on the important principle that waterworks, sewage-disposal and land-drainage should always be controlled by one authority.

It was to be expected that there would be opposition to any attempted legislation, especially any endeavour to coerce reluctant local authorities. There were also the vested interests of the landlords and of the speculative builders and of the water companies. But in addition to these there was the public itself. People fear sickness and want to be protected, but they also hate interference. It was essential, if real sanitary improvements were to be made, that there should be active interference with insanitary persons as well as with property. Other objections were raised on the score of wasteful expenditure by those who were short-sighted enough not to see that ultimate advantages would well outweigh the unpleasantness of increased rates.

Bills were introduced in Parliament by Lord Normanby and later by Lord Lincoln, but both these reformers met with very great opposition and both had their projects wrecked by the fall of the respective ministries. But while legislators were wrangling much good work in educating public opinion was being done by certain voluntary societies. The Health of Towns Association, on which sat such distinguished men as Anthony Ashley Cooper (later Lord Shaftesbury), Benjamin Disraeli and a doctor, Southwood Smith, was founded in 1839 and was active in its agitation for reform. The Association for promoting Cleanliness Among the Poor took more concrete steps by founding bathing establishments and wash-houses in the East End of London. There were other societies which set to work to provide decent lodging-houses and improvements in the houses of the labourers. Much, too, was done from this time onwards by the generosity of philanthropists. The American, George Peabody, for example, gave half a million pounds sterling towards the building of dwelling-houses for artisans. Indignation had been aroused and an example set.

The first of a series of Acts for the removal of nuisances (defined as 'the filthy or unwholesome condition of any dwelling-house or other building, or any accumulation of any offensive matter, dung, etc., or the existence of any foul drain, privy or cesspool') was eventually passed in 1846. Two years later, after a great fight and with many alterations, a Bill, introduced by Lord Morpeth, was made law as the Public Health Act of 1848. This is the ground work of all sanitary legislation. Its provisions were, for the most part, adoptive and not compulsory except when enforced by the Board of Health on evidence of exceptional mortality.

The main effects of this legislation were to enable local authorities to obtain by a simple means powers which previously had demanded a special local Act of Parliament. They could have powers to construct and manage sewers and drains, wells, pumps, waterworks and gasworks; to control deposits of refuse, water-closets, slaughter-houses and offensive trades; to remove nuisances; to pave streets and regulate dwellings, common lodging-houses, cellars, etc.; to provide burial and recreation grounds and to supply public baths with water. For the first time local authorities could easily obtain these very comprehensive powers for the public good.

The 1848 Act furthermore set up the famous General Board of Health as a central Health Authority. It had three members, one *ex officio* being the Commissioner of Works, while the other two were to be appointed by the Queen. These two were Anthony Ashley Cooper and Edwin Chadwick. The new Board rapidly acquired unparalleled odium, mainly because of Chadwick; for he was widely hated as the indefatigable busybody who had brought to light so many abuses. As Poor Law Secretary, led on by zeal for reform, he had made himself execrated by both rich and poor through his complete inability to make allowances for the personal feelings of others. Chadwick, too, had been the great exponent of the Poor Law principle which has been well summed up as giving 'the paupers exactly what they don't want and then they get tired of coming'. The Board, then, started at a disadvantage. Its chief function was to act as a Central Authority from which local Boards of Health could acquire powers voluntarily and cheaply for sanitary improvements. There was also, as we have seen, a provision that in districts where there was an abnormally high death-rate the General Board could thrust powers on to any authority which might prove recalcitrant. Unfortunately the Board had no power to see that its instructions were carried out and consequently could be, and was, defied with impunity. Nevertheless many towns made use of the Act to secure improvements.

The principle of the setting up of the General Board should be noted, for it is on this model that the Public Health system of this country has been based. This principle is that the actual sanitary work should be done by each district for itself, but that there should be a Central Authority, with limited powers, which could advise, direct, inspect and, if need be, compel.

The General Board of Health made many useful investigations; for example, that on the water supply of London: but its chief claim to fame, as Sir John Simon pointed out,[1] was that it awoke in the whole country 'a conscience against filth'. None the less the Board was openly accused of ignorance, incompetence, intolerance and aggression and was dubbed a hopeless failure in matters of both theory and practice. Although most of the accusations levelled against the 'bashaws of Somerset House', as the Board was nick-named, were conspicuously unjust, its unpopularity led, in 1854, to the overthrow of the Government which attempted to continue its existence. The Board was reformed on a changed plan and continued in office for another four years, when its functions were taken over by the Privy Council.

The Year of the Public Health Act was marked by another important event, the appointment of John Simon as Medical Officer of Health to the City of London. It was largely to this man's immense energy and extreme ability in directing the methods by which the structure of sanitary practice was built up, that is due the excellent system of hygiene that we enjoy today. This was an entirely new experiment in State service which was started in England and which Simon directed towards the success which it ultimately achieved.

Simon was not the first medical officer of health in this country. Before this towns had been able to obtain private Acts to give them powers for improvement. Two years before Simon's appointment

[1] Simon, J., *English Sanitary Institutions*, London, 1890, p. 224.

Liverpool had availed itself of this and had its own Act for street improvement and to provide proper sewers and drains. The following year the same town appointed W. H. Duncan as its Officer of Health. Duncan's was the first of these appointments in the country and with commendable zeal he managed to rid the town of many of the most noxious infamies.

Simon was quick to perceive that if good was to be done, it was essential to collect far more knowledge than was then available. It was statistics that he needed. There were no good statistics that went back far into the past. There were the old Bills of Mortality, weekly returns of the deaths in the various parishes in his London district, which had been published with varying accuracy for more than two hundred years. These were of little use for medical purposes until 1728, when the *ages* of the dead were first given. Really reliable figures began under the Births and Deaths Registration Act in 1836. Returns of illness, as opposed to death, were not to be had.

What Simon required was not grand totals of the deaths in the City from various causes, but detailed figures for each district so that he could see at once where the dangerous areas lay and could exercise prompt inquiry and act. He was fortunate in securing the willing co-operation of the Registrar-General and of eleven Poor Law medical officers of the City, and thus was able to obtain weekly information of all new cases of fever arising in each separate area.

He was quick to use the information thus obtained. He instituted weekly inspections, secured orders for removing every nuisance and, what was of the utmost importance, he planned subsequent visits to see that those orders had been carried out. The results demonstrated to all who cared to see what could be done by a really able and energetic man. Within the seven years in which Simon held this office, he had carried out almost all the necessary improvements which had been advised by Chadwick. There was a new drainage system, good water supply, strict street and house cleaning, the mitigation of all nuisances and 'at a time when cesspools were still almost universal in the metropolis and while, in the mansions of the West End, they were regarded as equally sacred with the wine-cellars, they had been abolished for rich and poor throughout all the square mile of the City'.

This sterling example seems to have been well appreciated, for when in 1855 the Government proposed to appoint a Central Medical Officer to the reconstituted Board of Health this position was given to John Simon. His duties, as far as any details were concerned, were of the most nebulous kind, but again he set himself to the diligent collection of facts and figures. During his term of office he initiated systematic scientific inquiries throughout the whole country and on a wide range of subjects. In addition to reports on the direct sanitary condition of the country he published a number of very valuable studies of different individual diseases among which were tuberculosis, bronchitis, ague, diarrhoea, industrial poisoning and the diseases which different industries seemed to produce.

In one of his reports he bitterly laments the lack of facts. How could one organize an efficient public health system without knowing exactly where there was lack of health and in what this lack consisted? This time Dr Edward Greenhow came to his assistance. The Registrar-General's office contained much of the needed information, but the published returns gave only general death-rates. Greenhow, using the accumulated mass of papers in the Registrar's office, with great labour produced some very informative and particular statistics for the seven years 1848–54. Now, for the first time, could be discovered the numbers, the sexes, the diseases and the districts of the dead. The importance of this was immediately clear to Simon. The figures demonstrated that the incidence of disease varied tremendously in different parts of the country. This could have been expected, but it was vital to know the particular areas in which each disease was most prevalent, so that the cause could be sought. If there were several districts in which the same disease carried off above the average number of victims, there must surely be a common cause in these districts. In this way Simon was able to show that there were removable causes of disease, differing in different areas. The value of such arithmetical methods in public health work began to be understood. Shortly after this the task of producing the required figures was undertaken by the Registrar-General. Today the returns of the Registrar-General are one of the most important of all medical periodicals.

It was not long before the results of Simon's work began to be convincing. The Ninth Report of the Central Medical Officer (1866) showed encouraging figures of the decline of certain diseases in definite districts where considerable improvements had been carried out. In Cardiff, to name the town where the greatest effect was observed, the general death-rate had fallen by almost one-third, from 332 per ten thousand population in the years 1847–54 down to 226 per ten thousand in the years 1859–66. In the particular instance of typhoid fever the death-rate had been reduced from $17\frac{1}{2}$ to $10\frac{1}{2}$ and of diarrhoea (other than Cholera) from $17\frac{1}{4}$ to $4\frac{1}{2}$. Such figures as these could not fail to impress even the most sceptical. It was unfortunate that in a few places improvements in sanitation did not produce the expected results. Chelmsford, for example, showed a rise in the death-rate from each of the diseases classified in the tables. None the less the general improvement was very striking.

It was a relief to the sanitarians as it was a lesson to the country that the efforts to improve the public health had not been in vain. In these results lay the justification for attempting further advance. There were many abuses yet to be abolished. Power was often lacking to bring the offenders to heel. A water company which might be poisoning thousands could be fined no more than £200. This was hopelessly inadequate, especially if we are to believe that the spread of cholera in the outbreak of 1866 could be justly ascribed to the guilty mismanagement of the East London Water Company.

Up to this time nearly all the sanitary legislation had been adoptive: that is to say there were at hand means for hygienic action which any district could adopt at its pleasure. But now, under pressure from the growing volume of intelligent opinion, the great Sanitary Act of 1866 made sanitation the duty and no longer the whim of local authorities. Compulsion was found necessary and penalties were enacted against sins of omission. Overcrowded houses and workshops were brought into the category of nuisances, which before had been confined to filth alone. Here again it was the fresh outbreak of cholera that helped to sway public opinion on the need for action.

Following this important step came a number of other Acts dealing with merchant shipping, drugs, vaccination and a variety of other subjects. Before following the history of sanitary legislation any further, it will be convenient to mention one other Government measure that has had an important influence for the good of the medical profession and of the public. This was the Medical Act of 1858 which set up the General Medical Council. This consisted of twenty-three members, of which seventeen were appointed by the various bodies (universities, the Royal Colleges of Physicians and Surgeons) which at that time granted their own degrees or licences to practise, while six were appointed by the Crown. Later the total number was increased to twenty-nine, including three who were elected by the medical profession as direct representatives. The General Medical Council was charged with important duties which it still fulfils today. Firstly, it compiles and keeps up to date the Medical Register, which is the official list of all medical practitioners who have followed certain approved courses in medicine, surgery and midwifery[1] and have passed certain examinations. This list at once provides a means for the general public to distinguish between a properly trained doctor and a quack. No one whose name is not on the register may pretend that he is a qualified doctor, but there is nothing whatever to prevent his practising 'medicine' on any members of the public who may care to submit to his treatment. An unregistered practitioner, however, works under certain disabilities in that he may not sign a death certificate, procure dangerous drugs or sue for his fees. The importance of the Register in protecting the public will at once be obvious.

There is no one statutory course of training (as there is in some countries) which must be followed to obtain admission to the register. Today there are in fact many different bodies, including colleges, societies and universities which are empowered to issue licences to practise medicine and, as the number of medical schools, attached to the ever-growing number of universities, becomes greater, doubtless the number of ports of entry will correspondingly increase. In 1964 there were 18 universities in Great Britain and the Republic of Ireland granting degrees in medicine and surgery. Thus there is no uniformity in the training required, but

[1] This last was added by the Medical Act of 1886.

[2] The registration of women is permitted by the Medical Act of 1876.

each licensing body must satisfy the Council that its standards do not fall below some reasonable standard of excellence.

The Council is also concerned with keeping up the respectability of the profession by removing from the Register the name of anyone found guilty of felony or infamous conduct in a professional respect. Here again it will be noticed that the Council exists mainly to protect the public, not the profession.

The second duty of the General Medical Council is that of compiling an official list of drugs and medicaments, the *British Pharmocopoeia*. This book gives also standards of purity below which the *materia medica* must not be sold. It lists the official strengths and doses of the various drugs.

Soon after these events it became very clear that the hygienic machinery constructed by legislation in instalments and *ad hoc* amendments could not run smoothly. Progress could only have been made step by step as the enemies gave way, the result of which was a piecemeal body of enactments and amendments which often resulted in anomalies and sometimes in confusion. Two separate authorities might find themselves severally responsible for the same duties, while each authority might be under more than one central control. The Boards of Guardians were responsible for the removal of nuisances, yet the sewers were under the vestries of the parishes. Where there was a Medical Officer of Health he did not co-operate with the Registrar of Births and Deaths. Unless some attempt was made to weld the whole sanitary system into one unified organization, there was danger that the people would never receive those benefits which it was the object of the law to confer.

A Sanitary Commission was appointed and its reports[1] advised that 'the administration of the law should be made uniform, universal and imperative throughout the Kingdom'. A direct result of this was the Act of 1871 which set up the Local Government Board which acted as the central health authority up to the time when its functions were taken over by the Ministry of Health in 1919. The new Board was to have powers advisory, permissive and mandatory to achieve the acceleration of sanitary progress. It was also to be a stimulus towards new legislation and the prevention of such diseases as were on all hands admitted to be preventable. It was to

[1] 1869–71.

257

exercise medical and legal supervision over local authorities. It was to concern itself with the administration of the existing law and to promote fresh legislation to achieve the recommendations of the Sanitary Commission. Yet all was not plain sailing, for the Board was greatly troubled by refractory local authorities. For example, an attempt to force the universal appointment of medical officers of health led to appointment of nominal officials with beggarly stipends, while two authorities often appointed the same man, who consequently exercised his duties over an unmanageably large district. Furthermore there was nothing to ensure that the officers appointed had any skill or experience in sanitary matters or even had leisure enough from their practices to undertake any of the work at all.

The Board took steps to concentrate the whole administration of Public Health and Poor Relief into one bureau.

The Commission had advised that a complete system of medical officers and nuisance inspectors should be created, and half of the cost of this was to be borne by the Government where the appointments were considered satisfactory. The aim of the legislation was to secure just this, namely for every district a medical officer with special knowledge, with special powers and duties to supervise and advise in matters of the health of his own particular district. The Act of 1872 permitted the compelling of authorities to appoint medical officers, but the enforcement of satisfactory obedience was another matter.

A later Act, the Public Health Act of 1875, became the groundwork of the modern public health system in England and Wales. It formed a comprehensive code of sanitary law containing more than 300 sections. It gave local authorities control over sewers, empowered them to construct new ones and ordered them to keep them in repair. It provided that sewage must be purified before it was discharged into any stream, watercourse, canal, pond or lake. It gave wide powers to construct and maintain waterworks. Nuisances were to be dealt with summarily. For the first time insanitary houses could be dealt with because, included in the list of nuisances were 'any premises in such a state as to be injurious to health' as well as overcrowded houses. Other nuisances were named; including accumulations of filth, animals improperly kept and any chimney (other than those of private houses) sending forth black smoke in such a quantity as to be a nuisance. There were also extensive powers for the prevention and treatment of infectious diseases. The Act also allowed any sanitary authority to build hospitals, though it allowed the authority to recover the cost of treatment and maintenance from any patient who was not a pauper. It is from this important Act that the modern public health machinery has come. In spite of the wide powers it gave, it was in one way an unhappy event, because it followed at once that preventive medicine became permanently separated from everyday medical practice.

Housing was a subject that came much to the fore in the latter half of the nineteenth century. Considerable improvements had been made by the private enterprise of enlightened landlords as well as by voluntary charities and philanthropists. In this connexion mention must be made of the great work of Octavia Hill and of John Ruskin, not only in bringing the facts to the attention of the public, but also in their highly practical schemes for improving the housing conditions of the poor. On the other hand, so far as the law was concerned, it was not until the Public Health Act of 1875 that local authorities had any statutory powers to abolish slums. The clause about nuisances specifically mentioned 'any premises in such a state as to be injurious to health' and this definition should have been wide enough to cover all forms of bad housing; but unfortunately there were no effective provisions for bringing pressure to bear on refractory landlords, so that it soon became clear that the housing problem had not been solved.

In 1884 a Royal Commission was appointed to report on the Housing of the Working Classes. The evidence showed that there was gross overcrowding in all the big cities and especially in London. The difficulties in trying to solve this problem together with the abolition of slums were enormous. For one thing, any scheme of slum clearance aggravated the housing shortage and so led to further overcrowding. The number of sanitary inspectors was woefully inadequate and many of them were hopelessly inefficient. Furthermore, as John Simon alleged, the law had to a great extent been inefficiently, not to say at times corruptly, administered and the Royal Commission was of the opinion that this was the work of councillors who sought election with the deliberate object of protecting their property from the law. Following the report of the Commissioners came the Housing of the Working Classes Acts of 1885 and 1890. The second of these Acts made it the duty of Medical Officers of health to seek out and report on bad housing and it gave ample powers to local authorities to build houses for the working classes. Here was the germ of the 'council house' which is so prominent a feature of every town today; but it must be made clear that most of the houses built by the local authorities at that time were in huge blocks or tenement houses, rather than the cottage-type building which the words 'council house' bring to mind today. Unfortunately at the time the vested interests of private property combined with the unhelpful attitude of the magistrates to ensure that comparatively few houses were in fact built by local authorities. There seems little doubt that private builders, including co-operative societies, did much more towards improving the standard of living, though it cannot be claimed that the new houses were always of satisfactory quality. Big improvements there certainly were, but they could not keep pace with the expanding population, so that overcrowding continued well into the present century.

II. SANITARY LEGISLATION IN THE TWENTIETH CENTURY

At the turn of the century, in spite of the great discoveries in bacteriology and the growing knowledge of how infectious diseases spread, there remained many problems which could only be solved by extensive alterations in the law. The huge volume of *preventable* illness was becoming obvious to all thinking people and there was an awakening of the public consciousness to evils which had for so long been taken for granted. The agitation and enthusiasm for reform were mainly aroused by the frightening facts that were brought to light by many social workers. Among these stand out Charles Booth and B. Seebohm Rowntree. Booth's volumes on the *Life and Labour of the People in London* in 1889–97 and Rowntree's findings in the city of York[1] had shown that the root cause of much

[1] B. Seebohm Rowntree. *Poverty; A Study of Town Life*, London, 1901.

sickness was simply poverty. Rowntree clearly proved, by a most painstaking investigation, that the total earnings of 4·2 per cent of the working population of York fell short of the 'sum required to provide *food alone*, without taking into consideration other necessary expenditure such as that on clothes and fuel'. With totally inadequate food and the lack of facilities for personal hygiene, good health was quite out of reach for an appreciable proportion of the town workers.

Gradually the public became alive to the need for action in matters of public health. It was evident that the local authorities could do much to help by assuming new responsibilities. Over the first twenty years of this century a whole series of new Acts of Parliament thrust more and more duties on to the local councils which became responsible for education, school meals, maternity and child welfare, the school medical service, and the local health authorities were required to provide facilities for the prevention, diagnosis and treatment of infectious diseases, in particular tuberculosis and venereal disease.

Perhaps the most far-reaching of all the reforms at that time was the National Health Insurance Act for manual workers, which reached the Statute Book in England in 1911. Such insurance did not begin in this country. Germany had instituted such a scheme more than a quarter of a century before and it was mainly on this that the new Bill was modelled. Health Insurance was one part of the measure brought in by Lloyd George as Chancellor of the Exchequer in the Liberal Government. This was not a preventive measure, but was designed to provide for medical treatment of disease.

The main idea was that all persons between sixteen and seventy years of age who were under contract of service (with certain exceptions) should be compulsorily insured, the premiums being paid partly by the workers and partly by their employers, totalling ninepence per week per person. For this payment the workers were to secure free medical treatment at home, payment during sickness of ten shillings for men and seven shillings and sixpence a week for women up to twenty-six weeks, disability payments and a maternity bonus for women. Furthermore, sanatorium treatment for tuberculosis was to be provided. These benefits were to be obtained through 'approved societies', that is to say the trade unions, Friendly societies, etc., or, for those who did not, could not or would not belong to such societies, through the Post Office.

This was clearly an important social measure; but there was much opposition on a variety of grounds from the working classes, including domestic servants, and from employers. Here we must confine our attention to the objections raised by the medical profession. It was to be the duty of the local authorities to arrange with the local practitioners for the medical treatment of the insured at the rate of payment of six shillings per head per annum. The British Medical Association, which could justly claim to represent the view of the general practitioner, was fully decided that the payment must be larger than this. The Government increased its offer to nine shillings, but this too was thought too small, and more than twenty-seven thousand doctors signed an undertaking to support the British Medical Association in its determination to fight the Government by withholding their services.

An offer was made to treat the insured for a minimum of eight shillings and sixpence a head, or a fee of two shillings and sixpence per visit, under some arrangement to be made between representatives of the doctors and of the patients, with the express proviso that a free choice of doctor should lie with the individual insured person. The Government, however, meant that there should be control of the public moneys by the insurance committees of the local authorities and the Central Insurance Authority and it could not let the matter pass purely into the hands of the doctors and the approved societies. The Government therefore decided to rely on those doctors who would repudiate their pledges and flout the opinions of the British Medical Association. Lloyd George carried the day and gradually the 'strike' was broken, so that by 1913 the Association was compelled, by large-scale secessions from its ranks, to release members from their promises.

None the less the doctors had protested to some purpose, for their more reasonable demands, such as the free choice of doctor and the increase in the capitation fee, had been granted. The Act came into force and gradually its unpopularity faded until National Insurance became accepted as a necessary part of the social system.

Before the advent of the Welfare State more than fifteen thousand general practitioners were working under this scheme which provided for about one-third of the population. Any doctor might become a 'panel' doctor and the central authority (later the Minister of Health) alone could remove him from the panel and only for some very good reason. The patient had complete freedom of choice of doctor, being limited only by geographical distances; but no one doctor could take more than 2,500 panel patients on his practice. On the whole the system worked smoothly, in spite of occasional outcries that the panel patient got perfunctory treatment, that the doctors gave disability certificates too easily, or that over-prescribing constituted an unnecessary expenditure to the State.

There is little doubt that the good work done by the National Health Insurance scheme far more than compensated for any minor flaws or irregularities which critics were only too anxious to expose. Any tendency towards neglect or slackness on the part of the doctors was obviated by the right which every patient had to change his doctor at will.

In 1919 legislation was enacted to bring under one authority all the various matters affecting public health. Such legislation became the more urgent because of the growing unpopularity of the Local Government Board which had become apathetic, if not obstructionist, particularly in its attitude towards local medical officers of health. The new Act set up the Ministry of Health under a Minister who, as a member of the House of Commons, should be responsible to Parliament. There was to be a Chief Medical Officer to advise on reforms and other public health matters, but it was the Minister who was to be answerable to Parliament. Dr Addison was the first Minister of Health, though, as appeared thereafter, the Minister is not necessarily a medical man. Sir George Newman was appointed the first Chief Medical Officer.

The Minister was put in charge of duties previously performed by other bodies, notably the Local Government Board (which disappeared unlamented) and the Insurance Commissioners. He also took over the work of the Board of Education concerning the health of mothers and children of pre-school age and to some extent those connected with the school medical services. Other powers—those dealing with disabled soldiers and sailors—were to be taken over at some time to be determined later. The Minister was also charged with taking measures for the prevention and cure of disease, the initiation of research, collecting statistics, publishing information and training persons for the health services. He was also to appoint Consultative Councils of persons (including women) with good experience of various subjects, such as National Health Insurance and Local Health Administration. In this way the Ministry became the central supervising authority in England and Wales. In Scotland the Secretary for Scotland became Minister of the Scottish Board of Health, with four Consultative Councils, three of which functioned like the English Councils, whilst the fourth dealt with the public health of the Highlands and Islands.

The next stage in the unification of the health services came with the Local Government Act of 1929, an extensive measure of which only a part is concerned with matters of health. The most important provision in this respect was the transfer of the functions of the Poor Law Authorities to the County and County Borough Councils, each of which was forced to appoint a Public Assistance Committee (some members of which had to be women) to carry out its new duties. In this way the councils were to provide all assistance, including medical help, that was legally possible to any person without his being classed as a pauper. The Act also gave powers to the County Councils to provide hospitals and this marks the beginning of the municipal rate-paid hospitals. The Act further stressed the importance of appointing whole-time medical officers of health who were to be restricted from private practice.

It was during the Second World War that plans began to take shape for the Welfare State. In 1941 Sir William Beveridge (with an appropriate committee) was asked to undertake a comprehensive examination of the national insurance and all the other social services and in 1942 the famous Beveridge report was launched. The recommendations made in this historic paper formed the basis of our socialized medicine. Beveridge recommended the widest possible health service which was to include prevention, cure and rehabilitation for every member of the community. Family Allowances were brought in in 1945 and the following year the much-disputed National Health Service Act was passed. The Government scheme, as outlined in the White Paper of 1944, advised that the new medical services should be run almost entirely by the local authorities. This scheme was hotly contested by the British Medical Association which rejected any proposal that the doctors should be controlled by local councillors and by the Society of Medical Officers of Health which, though it agreed in principle to control by local authorities, insisted that these should be thoroughly overhauled and reformed before they could be considered fit to act as controlling health authorities. While the Coalition Government and the medical profession continued to wrangle and confer, the Labour Party was returned to power and Aneurin Bevan produced a completely different plan which he proceeded to force through against a good deal of bitter opposition.

The National Health Service Act of 1946 came into force in July 1948. In brief it created the fourteen Regional Hospital Boards, under which all specialist services and all hospitals (except the teaching ones) were to be administered. Each regional board was to place its hospitals in local groups under Hospital Management Committees. The general practitioners, on the other hand, were to be controlled by executive councils, each covering the district controlled by a County or a County Borough Council. Each of these authorities was to appoint a health committee, which was to run the public health services, including domiciliary care. The Minister himself, on whom the responsibility to Parliament rested, was to be advised by a central council. This is the briefest outline of the scheme which, with a few exceptions, has continued as originally planned.

The 1946 Act has certainly done much to unify the health services throughout the country. It brought all the hospitals, including general hospitals, specialist hospitals, sanatoria, fever hospitals and those for the chronic sick under one authority. In this way it was able to ensure that every hospital had its share of attention from consultant medical and surgical specialists. The public health services, that is to say the preventive side of medicine, in particular the maternity and child welfare, the Health Visitors, District Nurses, Home Helps, immunization procedures and the care of mental health were all embraced in this unifying Act.

The chief merit of the new scheme was that it offered medical care, preventive as well as curative, to every member of the community. The advantage of this must be obvious to all, though the whole scheme has been widely criticized, sometimes fairly and often unfairly. The chief objection seems to be that, so far from being all-embracing, the Act left out the one thing necessary for completeness, namely welfare itself, which continued under the National Assistance Act until quite recently, when it was transferred to the new Ministry of Social Security.

The most serious criticisms of the National Health Service are three in number. Firstly the Health Service has not stressed the importance of *prevention* of ill-health in the way that was intended (for example the hospitals, that is the curative side of medicine, absorb the lion's share of the available cash). Secondly, so far from being under one controlling authority, the Act left the Health Service under three different bodies—the specialist and hospitals under the Regional Boards, the general practitioners under the executive councils, while the preventive services were for the most part left with the local authorities to be paid for out of the rates. Thirdly, from a financial point of view, the Government of the day had underwritten an unlimited liability for a service whose cost has continually mounted and will clearly continue to do so in the foreseeable future.

Having now reached the point where the public health services, the welfare service and the medical and surgical treatment services are all available to every individual in the community, we must turn back to survey some of the more specific services in greater detail.

III. FOOD ADULTERATION

About the middle of the nineteenth century the increasing scandal of food adulteration began to receive a long-deserved publicity. It must have been clear to almost every consumer that certain foodstuffs were of very unpredictable quality and that unscrupulous purveyors were obviously swindling their customers by mixing cheaper ingredients with the more expensive foods. If such food had been diluted merely with inert substances, no more harm would have befallen the consumer than a small financial loss or perhaps some degree of malnutrition. It began to appear, however, that many common articles of food contained substances that were definitely injurious to health.

In 1851 the *Lancet* began to publish analyses made by an Analytical Sanitary Commission. Various articles were dealt with in turn. The microscope and the test-tube revealed a disgraceful state of affairs. Out of thirty-four samples of coffee, thirty-one were adulterated with chicory, and corn was found in twelve. Every single sample of bread out of two dozen contained alum, which was used not only to 'improve' the colour and taste, but also to give additional weight. Milk was often found to be 'sophisticated', generally with the comparatively harmless liquid tap-water, but it frequently contained as well thickening agents like flour and chalk in order to mask the thinness caused by the addition of up to 45 per cent of water. Sugar, cocoa, arrowroot, pepper, mustard and vinegar were all subjected to analysis. Chicory used to dilute coffee was itself diluted with other cheaper substances, while vinegar was often diluted with water and then brought up to strength with powerful mineral acids.

The *Lancet* gave public notice that three months after it began to publish these results it would mention in full the names and addresses of all tradesmen found to be selling adulterated food—and the names were duly printed as well as those of the few firms who were selling pure foods and so got free but well-earned publicity.

This public exposure of such fraudulent practices led to agitation which grew greater when it was discovered that poisonous preservatives were often added to perishable food, deodorants were being used to mask the smell and taste of articles of questionable freshness, while boiled sweetmeats were being coloured with red lead, vermilion (mercuric sulphide), arsenic, copper and chromium compounds—all poisonous in varying degrees.

Revelations such as these produced legislation in 1860 to stop the adulteration of food and drink. This was the beginning of an outcrop of preventive laws which were consolidated by the Food and Drugs (Adulteration) Act of 1928. Under this and earlier Acts the Ministry of Health (set up in 1919) makes regulations to prevent danger to the public health from the importation, preparation, storage and distribution of food and drink.

At the present time every local authority, through its Medical Officer of Health and his Sanitary Inspectors, is required to exercise a careful watch over the purity of food sold or exposed for sale in its district. The inspector purchases samples of foodstuffs and has them analysed. Should they be found not to be genuine, prosecutions occur and heavy fines, and even imprisonment for subsequent offences, may be meted out to offenders. It is this constant supervision which ensures that our foods are not polluted with chemicals, so that it is no longer true that: 'Chalk and alum and plaster are sold to the poor for bread.'[1]

As a result of the very extensive legislation between 1875 and 1928, the position with regard to preservatives was this. Most, including boric acid, formalin and salicylic acid were forbidden altogether. The permitted substances, benzoic acid and sulphur dioxide, were only to be used in specified foods and drinks and in strictly limited quantities. Certain articles of food, if they contained preservatives, were to be clearly labelled to that effect and the amount of the preservative plainly stated.

It should be made clear that many of the forbidden substances are not particularly harmful if present only in the minimal amounts necessary to achieve their object; but there is considerable risk that anyone eating a number of different foods, all of which contain the same preservative, may easily receive an injurious dose. The term 'preservative' is not held to include such agents in common use, such as salt, saltpetre, sugar, vinegar, alcohol and spices.

Certain colouring matters were forbidden under regulations made by the Minister of Health (1925–7). These included firstly compounds of the poisonous metals, antimony, arsenic, cadmium, chromium, copper, mercury, lead and zinc; secondly the vegetable gamboge which, besides being a strong yellow dye, is also a drastic purgative; and lastly certain specified coal-tar colours, Picric Acid, Victoria Yellow, Manchester Yellow, Aurantia and Aurine.

Owing to the importance of milk as a food, particularly for infants and young children, a whole body of legislation has been introduced to deal with this one article. The law concerning milk deals with every aspect of the attempt to secure a clean and

[1] Tennyson, *Maud*, I, i, 39.

wholesome supply, but owing to the large number of Acts and Order lack of space makes it impossible to consider them in detail.

A strict watch has also to be kept in order to ensure that certain poisons do not find their way into food and drink apart from any deliberate action of the manufacturers or purveyors. Poisoning from the metals used in tinning processes or from metal cooking utensils has been recorded. In 1900 several thousand beer drinkers in the North-West of England were taken severely ill, and some seventy died from arsenic poisoning. The cause was eventually traced to the impure sulphuric acid which was used in the preparation of the 'invert sugar' added to the wort during the manufacture. Outbreaks of poisoning have occurred from the use of cheap enamel utensils, glazed with antimony, for the preparation of fruit drinks. These few examples will show how important is the watchful eye of the Medical Officer of Health.

IV. MOTHERS AND CHILDREN

During the nineteenth century one of the gravest features of the mortality statistics was the immense number of children who died in the first few years of life. A huge total of infants in arms was carried off by epidemic summer diarrhoea, which is undoubtedly a disease of dirt abetted by malnutrition. Measles and whooping-cough accounted for many under five years of age, while rickets handicapped so many others that they died of some intercurrent disease. These are some of the direct causes of mortality among children. Indirectly the two chief factors were undoubtedly poverty and ignorance. Florence Nightingale in her *Notes on Nursing* showed that she was very well aware of this.

Infant mortality is, by definition, the number of deaths of children under one year per 1,000 live births. As late as the five years from 1896 to 1900 the figure was as high as 156 per 1,000 live births, which means that out of every hundred babies at least fifteen were dead before their first birthdays.

The spectacular decline in the mortality rate of children under five years dates from the beginning of the present century and, be it noted, it began before any specific action had been taken by the

State to reduce the appalling number of deaths. However, long before this medical men like Simon and Farr had written extensively on this very subject. They had foreseen that improved hygiene was bound to produce remarkable results. Most of the deaths were certainly due to faulty environment, in which must be included not only bad housing but also absence of sunlight and fresh air, dirt, poisonous food, lack of breast-feeding and a hundred other details in the lives of the children. The cause of the decline in the death-rate must therefore be sought in those factors which improved the general status of the people, and in particular that of the poorest sections of the community. It was these general improvements rather than any measures expressly directed against child deaths that began to take effect.

Besides the building of more and better houses, the sanitary conditions inside the homes of the poor were immensely improved towards the end of the nineteenth century and these improvements have continued ever since. It is probable that much of the advance in hygiene can be fairly attributed to the effects of elementary education which became compulsory after the passing of the Education Act in 1870. Everyone was taught to read and by this means information could reach the homes in a way that was not possible before. Today, of course, information pours into every household in ever-increasing volume through the media of the press, the radio and television; but long before this the teaching of elementary cleanliness and personal hygiene in the schools must have had considerable influence for good, though these benefits could not have any immediate effect upon the infant mortality rate. Time was needed for the new generation to grow up. It is significant that, thirty years from the introduction of compulsory education, when the girls born after the year 1870 were in the prime of life and becoming mothers, the decline in the death-rate among the children began.

In the first half of the present century more specific legal measures were enacted to protect the lives and healths of mothers and children. The most effective of these schemes of preventive medicine are the Midwifery, the Maternity and Child Welfare and School Medical Services, each of which must be briefly described.

Medicine and the State

(a) Midwifery

We have already seen that it was as late as 1886[1] that a knowledge of midwifery became compulsory for any student taking a medical degree. There was no control at all over the midwives themselves. They conducted large numbers of labours, often without medical direction and often in a most slatternly way, so that the damage to life and health must have been considerable. The discoveries of Semmelweiss and Lister could hardly have been put to any effective use by the ignorant 'bodies' who, by attending labour after labour, could spread puerperal sepsis far and wide.

In 1902 legislation was enacted to ensure that practising midwives should have proper scientific training. The Act set up the Central Midwives Board, which was to exercise control over the midwives in some respects similar to the control of the medical profession by the General Medical Council. The Board was to frame rules for the training of midwives, to appoint examiners and arrange for the examination of candidates and to publish annually an official roll of certified midwives. The Board was also to remove from the roll the name of anyone found guilty of disobeying its rules or of misconduct. Lastly the Board was to make regulations concerning the proper conduct of midwives in the exercise of their profession.

The rules of the Central Midwives Board are exceedingly strict. A midwife must visit the mother before the birth of the child, check that the lie of the baby is normal, test the urine and in some districts arrange for various blood tests, in particular the Wassermann reaction or some equivalent. The midwife is required to keep written notes about each patient. She must make all the necessary arrangements, personal and general, for the impending confinement. Scrupulous personal cleanliness is enjoined and the necessary medical equipment to be provided is described in detail. The exact duties both to the mother and the child are defined and a list given of the conditions in which medical help must be sought without delay. No operative procedure is permitted except in grave emergencies. The midwife must notify the Medical Officer of Health of certain well-defined circumstances; in particular of any

[1] See above, p. 256.

still-birth when no doctor has been in attendance; any contact of the mother with infectious disease; the death of a mother or a child and she must also inform the Medical Officer of Health if she herself has helped in the laying-out of a dead body.

The rules decide the conditions under which a midwife may be temporarily suspended from practice to prevent the spread of infection, as well as those under which her name may be removed from the roll altogether. Any woman thinking herself aggrieved by having her name struck off may appeal to the High Court of Justice. In this respect she had at the time an advantage over a medical practitioner, for whom a decision of the General Medical Council was final.[1]

The Midwives Act took the further and important step of prohibiting uncertified women from practising, although it made provision for the certification of those untrained women who were actually in practice when the Act came into force. Unfortunately it was necessary to certify a very large number of these and so it came about that more than half the midwives were in fact unqualified and this state of affairs came to an end only gradually, as the untrained midwives died out in the course of nature and only fully qualified women were enrolled thereafter. No woman may pretend to be a midwife unless certified. No one uncertified may attend a 'woman in childbirth otherwise than under the direction and personal supervision of a duly qualified medical practitioner', except in a case of sudden or urgent necessity. The Act, subsequently amended in some details in 1918, 1926, and again in 1951, also makes it the duty of every County Council and County Borough Council to exercise a strict supervision over all midwives practising in their districts, to investigate charges of malpractice, negligence and misconduct and 'if a *prima facie* case be established, to report the same to the Central Midwives Board'. A midwife must notify the local supervising authority every year of her intention to practise in her area.

Under the Nursing Homes Registration Act of 1927 Nursing Homes (including Maternity Homes) could be strictly supervised and penalties were enacted for conducting such institutions if they

[1] In 1950 right of appeal to the Judicial Committee of the Privy Council was created.

were unregistered. Local authorities could refuse to register an improperly conducted home or if it was considered that the situation, construction, accommodation, staffing or equipment was unfit. The homes must be open to inspection at all reasonable times.

It should be noted that the Midwives Acts, like the Medical Acts, are designed more to protect the public than the profession.

(b) Maternity and Child Welfare

This service, the name of which is self-explanatory, developed mainly in the twentieth century when publicity was being given to the wretched condition of the health of the poorer children. Alarm was raised about the ever-decreasing birth-rate and people began to see the national importance of preserving in good health the diminishing numbers of the newly born.

The germ of the service may be traced back into the last decade of the previous century. In 1892 Florence Nightingale began a campaign for home visits by trained visitors. She started with the villages in Buckinghamshire in the neighbourhood of Claydon House,[1] the historic seat of the Verney family, which she had made her second home, through the kindness of her brother-in-law Sir Harry Verney. Florence Nightingale may be said to have invented the profession of Health Visitor in her entirely new scheme for home visits by Lady Health Visitors, who were to be trained to teach the village mothers the first principles of home hygiene. She insisted that the work should be personal; the Health Missioners were 'not to lecture the village women, but to work *with* them'.[2] Similar schemes were started in a small way in other areas; in Warwickshire and Worcestershire.

In the same year 1892 Pierre Budin at the Hôpital de la Charité in Paris developed the idea of the infant welfare centre. This notion spread to England almost at once and was quickly developed all over the country. Again everything was done by voluntary effort at the start. First of all free additional food was provided for

---

[1] This house now belongs to the National Trust and is open to the public. It contains the Florence Nightingale museum.

[2] Woodham-Smith, C., *Florence Nightingale*, 1950, p. 583.

mothers, then free instruction in the proper methods of nursing young children. Later Parliament was to show its appreciation of this kind of work by allowing monetary grants towards the expense of providing doctors, midwives, health visitors and welfare centres. In the meantime it had become increasingly clear from the 1904 Report of the Committee on Physical Deterioration that some more effective scheme must be devised. Many of the excellent suggestions made by this Committee have subsequently been accepted and universally applied. In particular the report advised the creation of the School Medical Service, a nation-wide service of Health Visitors and it stressed the pressing need for whole-time Medical Officers of Health.

The State control over the care of mothers and children was greatly helped by the Notification of Births Act of 1907. This was something quite different from the 1836 Registration of Births; for this latter was used only for statistical purposes. The new Act, which was adoptive, required the father of the child *and* any person attendant on the mother at the time of or within six hours of the birth to notify the fact in writing within thirty-six hours to the Medical Officer of Health for the district concerned. The importance of this will be seen at once, for it enabled the Medical Officer to make immediate arrangements to see that everything possible was done for the mother and the newborn child. Before this new law was passed the child might be dead long before the local Medical Officer even knew of its existence.

Eight years later another Act made notification compulsory in all districts and also allowed local authorities to exercise their powers as Sanitary Authorities to look after the health of expectant and nursing mothers and young children. This power was extended under the Maternity and Child Welfare Act in 1918 to include children up to the age of five. Before this local authorities had had no special powers over children between the time when they ceased to be infants in arms and the time when they reached the usual school age and so came under the control of the Education Authority.

Under the 1918 Act it was ordered that local authorities should establish Maternity and Child Welfare Committees. One-third of the members need not be members of the council (i.e. they could be co-opted) but must be persons qualified by training or experience in subjects relating to health and maternity. At least two of the committee must be women. A parliamentary grant was made towards the expense. In this way the elected councils became the special guardians of the health of women and infants, just as before they had been made the protectors of the public as a whole against nuisance and disease.

It must be noted that at this time a general domiciliary service by medical practitioners was not authorized.

From these beginnings a complete system of health supervision arose, including the Maternity or Antenatal Centre and the Infant Welfare Centre. The first of these institutions was designed to advise expectant mothers about their own health and thus it was both educational and preventive. The staff of such a centre was to include a doctor (who was generally a woman) and a certified midwife, who might be one of the Health Visitors of the district. The main functions were these. The doctor gave consultations which were followed by a domiciliary visit by the midwife. Educational classes were given in the special hygiene of pregnancy, in 'mothercraft' and in sewing. Special dinners or milk could be provided when necessary. Dental treatment could also be included, since septic teeth constitute a grave risk to the mother. Special attention was provided in separate institutions to any women suffering from venereal disease; for this is one of the most potent causes of congenital illness and deformity of children.

The Infant Welfare Centre was mainly intended for teaching mothers the best method of caring for the health of her offspring and was consequently a preventive institution rather than one for treating the ailing child.

Soon after the midwife has paid her final visit to the mother's home the Health Visitor makes her appearance on the scene and, besides giving good advice, she encourages the mother to bring her children regularly to the welfare centre and not to wait until the babies fall ill. Classes are held both in hygiene and in such highly important matters as cooking and sewing. Information is further disseminated by home-visiting. Treatment of minor ailments may also be given at such a centre, but it is most undesirable that the centre should become a clinic for sick children or a kind of out-patient hospital. Any sickness but the most trivial should be reported to the family doctor and if need be treated at a children's hospital. The Welfare Centre should be for the maintenance of health, not for the treatment of disease.

Since the socialization of medicine in the United Kingdom, from 1948 onwards, local authorities have added to the Maternity and Child Welfare a number of new services. These include Home Nursing in pregnancy and infancy and Home Helps for mothers delivered at home. Another important function of the Service is the vaccination and immunization of infants against diphtheria, poliomyelitis, smallpox, tetanus and whooping-cough (B.C.G. vaccination against tuberculosis is normally given at ten years and upwards and is offered through the School Medical Service).

Until the incidence of tuberculosis fell so spectacularly in the last fifteen years, the prevention of tuberculosis and the rehabilitation of the tuberculous was one of the main pre-occupations of the local authorities and occupied a very large share of the Health Visitors' time; but this will be discussed more fully in a later section.

Under the Maternity Service special arrangements are made for the large numbers of unmarried mothers which is such a conspicuous feature of our present-day society. Particular measures are necessary, not only for obvious social reasons, but also because such cases carry with them a higher maternal mortality and infant mortality than normal.

(c) The School Medical Service

From the age of five years the child is normally at school and comes under the control of the Education Authority, which is a County Council or County Borough Council. The service in the elementary schools was established in 1907, so that the School Medical Service has in fact been in existence some years longer than the Maternity and Child Welfare Service.

At the beginning of the present century much concern was felt about the deplorable physical conditions of the young men of England. This was largely brought to light by the statistics of recruiting for the Boer War, which showed how many men of military age were physically unfit. Even before this it had been found necessary to provide special educational facilities for the very large number of children who were blind, deaf, mentally defective or epileptic. It was time to investigate the whole question. of the health of the children in the elementary schools.

In 1903 a Royal Commission on Physical Training in Scotland pointed out the unventilated condition of many of the school buildings and the dirty and under-nourished appearance of the children. In England the work of the 1904 Committee on Physical Deterioration has already been mentioned. The facts, where they were available, were more than disconcerting and the Board of Education was goaded into action.

The first legislation was concerned with providing meals for necessitous children, but shortly afterwards much wider powers were obtained. The Education (Administrative Provisions) Act of 1907 gave power to the Education Authorities to open vacation schools and classes, to make arrangements for the health of the children and, what was most important, to provide for medical inspection of the children, both on their first admission to school and as often afterwards as the Board might see fit. It was doubtful whether it was legal to compel the children to undergo inspection and indeed a subsequent Act expressly states that there is nothing that can force the parents to submit their children to examination or treatment. Tact and persuasion were—and still are—better weapons than force, and at the present time the parents who refuse the inspection are only a very small minority. The 1921 Act also empowered the local authorities to provide school meals, and to recover the cost from the parents, except when any of the children were held to be unable to take full advantage of the education on account of lack of food. Especial attention to the nutrition of the children was one of the main features of the scheme and today the School Meals Service provides a dinner at a subsidized price to about two-thirds of all the children in council schools. This school dinner is designed, on scientific lines, to be highly nutritious, with a high protein content. It should contain about one-third of the total calories needed daily and in this way it provides the main meal of the day. It should be noted that this Act expressly exempted teachers from duties in relation to the feeding of the children.

The first inspections showed only too well how much needed they were. Between 20 and 40 per cent of the children had bad teeth and one-tenth had serious defects of vision. One in every hundred had tuberculosis.

There was no power before this time to provide the treatment which was clearly necessary. Suggestions could be made to parents and inquiries made to discover whether they had acted on the proffered advice. The new Act provided for the medical treatment of the children, but at that time the parents were to contribute towards the cost. Later, grants were made towards the expense and later still the Education Authorities were made responsible for seeing that treatment was provided if the parents failed in their duties. This provision of treatment through the School Medical Service was of enormous importance to the children at this time, because they could get treatment from the family doctor only by paying for it. Under the Lloyd George National Insurance scheme it was only the worker himself that was insured—not his family.

The School Medical Service has been closely co-ordinated with the National Health Service since 1948, but it has continued its independent existence under the local authorities. Today all the medical and dental services provided through this service are free.

At the present time every child in every publicly-maintained school throughout the country is regularly inspected by the school doctor. The first inspection takes place shortly after the admission of the child to school. Parents are encouraged to attend, particularly with the school entrants. The last inspection is done at school-leaving age, and there are at least two other intermediate inspections during the child's stay at school. Full medical and dental records are kept and these follow a child who moves into another area or school.

Minor ailments can be dealt with by the school nurses under the direction of the school doctor. More serious disabilities, requiring further investigation, are referred to local clinics and to specialists, normally through the National Health Service.

In addition to the general medical inspections and treatment, Child Guidance clinics, for the treatment of maladjusted children are provided by most local authorities. Each of these is staffed by a psychiatrist, an educational psychologist and one or more psychiatric social workers. Health Education is often given in senior schools including hygiene and such subjects as the problems of adolescence and the dangers of cigarette-smoking. This educational service is of great importance and is growing fast.

(d) Results

The consequences of these schemes for watching over the children are very striking and the number of lives that have been saved is very large indeed. It will be recalled that in the five-year-period 1896–1900 the infantile mortality rate was 156 per 1,000 live births. In each succeeding quinquennium the figure decreased. By 1931 it was 65 per 1,000; that is to say that in the first thirty years of this century it had decreased by more than half. In 1965 it fell to a new low figure of 19·0. The still-birth rate also dropped to the record low figure of 15·7 per 1,000 total births. The very big drop that has occurred in infantile mortality in the last twenty-five years is certainly due to the introduction of chemotherapy and antibiotics particularly penicillin, in controlling infections of the gastro-intestinal and respiratory tracts.

Before 1948, the year the National Health Service came into operation, when a child left school he ceased to be under the medical care of any authority until he reached the age of sixteen when, if employed, he came under the compulsory health insurance scheme. It was extremely unfortunate that there should have been this unprotected gap of two years at this unimportant period in the life of the adolescent. This gap in the protective wall which the State had built round each individual has now been closed both by the raising of the school-leaving age and by the all-embracing National Health Service.

In tragic contrast to the lowered mortality among the children was the complete failure of all the efforts made to reduce the maternal mortality right up to about twenty years ago. At the beginning of the present century the mortality of women in or associated with childbirth was 5·56 for every thousand children born alive. From that time onwards, in spite of the new midwifery and maternity services, the figure hardly altered until quite recently. In 1931 the maternal mortality rate was still as large as 5·55 per thousand; and this did not include the deaths resulting from illegal interference with pregnancy, namely criminal abortion, suicide and murder.

The direct causes of these deaths were, in order of numerical importance, puerperal sepsis, toxaemias of pregnancy, haemorrhage, accidents of pregnancy and certain causes of sudden death (e.g. pulmonary embolism). It was strange that the discoveries of Semmelweiss and Lister had failed to eliminate sepsis. Many reasons were given to explain away the deaths. It seemed clear that either the whole conduct of midwifery was wrong or else that it was inefficiently performed. Bad treatment, lack of facilities for obtaining treatment, bad conditions of confinement and neglect of proffered medical advice all played their part in keeping up the number of deaths. It was pointed out that the mortality rate from sepsis in Holland was just about half of that in this country.[1] Furthermore certain institutions had records which were conspicuously favourable compared with those of the country as a whole. There was little doubt therefore that sepsis was preventable. Such measures as the compulsory notification of puerperal fever and compensation for midwives who had been suspended from practice owing to contact with septic cases, were designed to prevent the spread of sepsis, but somehow the expected results did not occur.

There was much concern among responsible bodies over this urgent problem. The final Report of the Committee of the British Medical Association on the Causation of Maternal Mortality was published in 1928. It affirmed that, though the committee did not doubt the existence of a minority of inefficient practitioners and midwives, yet on the whole conscientious use was being made of all the available knowledge and facilities. The report advised increased co-operation between doctors, midwives and maternity homes, the absolute minimum interference with labour, intelligent anticipation and treatment of complications, more facilities for antenatal supervision, more midwifery beds and an intensive

[1] Jellet, H., *The Cause and Prevention of Maternal Mortality*, London, 1929

educational campaign among members of the general public. Dame Janet Campbell, the Senior Medical Officer of the Maternity and Child Welfare at the Ministry of Health, roundly stated that the training of students and midwives was by no means satisfactory.[1]

Things began to take a turn for the better after the Second World War and some at least of the improvement can be attributed to the use of antibiotics. In 1964 the maternal mortality rate was only two-fifths of what it had been ten years before. Since 1957 the Ministry of Health has conducted four Confidential Inquiries into Maternal Deaths in England and Wales. The last report, covering the years 1961–3, appeared in 1966[2]. It showed that since the first period, 1952–4, the maternal death-rate had been more than halved. The causes of 876 deaths were examined and it was found that the four main causes of death were abortion, pulmonary embolism, toxaemia and haemorrhage. No less than 55·4 per cent of the cases of abortion were illegally procured. The report stressed that altogether there were avoidable factors in 262 out of 692 deaths analysed. This is clearly much too high. Most of the deaths occurred in the antenatal period and could have been avoided by proper foresight. It would seem that both mothers and doctors, in some instances at least, are tempted to take a quite unnecessary risk.

V. OCCUPATIONAL DISEASES

Under this head will be described the diseases which occur almost exclusively among industrial workers and which are caused by the particular conditions under which they work. Certain ailments have long been known by names which indicate their occupational origin. Housemaid's knee and tennis elbow are two with which everyone is familiar. In the industrial world we find such names as grinders' rot, potters' asthma, chimney-sweeps' cancer and wool-sorters' disease.

[1] Campbell, J., *Protection of Motherhood*, Ministry of Health, No. 48, London, 1927.

[2] Ministry of Health Reports, No. 115. Report on Confidential Inquiries into Maternal Deaths in England and Wales 1961–3, 1966, H.M.S.O.

The earliest comprehensive study of such maladies seems to be that of Bernardino Ramazzini, Professor of Physic at Padua, who published his *De Morbis Artificum Diatriba* at the beginning of the eighteenth century. This work[1] contains forty-three chapters dealing with as many different vocations from the lowest to the highest, from *Diseases of the Cleansers of the Jakes (de morbis Foricariorum)* to those arising from the sedentary pursuits of *Learned Men*. It includes detailed descriptions of the effects of many industrial poisons. For example, Ramazzini tells of the dismal plagues inflicted by quicksilver upon goldsmiths. At that time gilding and the silvering of mirrors were done by dissolving gold or silver in mercury, applying the solution to the appropriate article and finally driving off the mercury by heat. With the greatest precautions it was impossible to avoid inhaling considerable quantities of the poisonous mercurial vapours so that workmen 'do quickly become Asthmatick, Paralytick and liable to Vertigos; and their Complexion assumes a dangerous Ghostly Aspect . . . Their Neck and Hands tremble, their Teeth fall out, their Legs are weak and maul'd with the Scurvy'.[2] The modern processes of electrical plating and silvering of mirrors by the use of ammoniacal solutions of silver nitrate have relieved these particular craftsmen from the dangers of mercurial poisoning, but casualties may still occur among the manufacturers of thermometers, barometers, mercury-vapour lamps, mercurial explosives and other products.

A valuable study of occupational disease was made in Leeds by C. T. Thackrah over a hundred and thirty years ago. His book on *The Effects of the Principal Arts, Trades and Professions*[3] described many of the diseases which continued to trouble industry for a long time after. He wrote of the dangers of dusty employments and of the injury to the lungs from vapours. He called attention to skin diseases among grocers and bakers, to chimney-sweeps' cancer, to lead-poisoning among potters, house-painters, plumbers and braziers, and he insisted that wet and cold do not produce all the disorders so commonly attributed to them.

[1] Editio Secunda, Utrecht, 1703.
[2] Ramazzini, B., op. cit., translation, *Diseases of Tradesmen*, London, 1705, p. 15.
[3] London, 1831.

At the time of publication of Thackrah's book attention was being drawn to the deplorable effects of industrial fatigue in the mills, especially among the young children who were employed there for twelve hours a day during six days a week. Factory legislation began in 1833 with an Act that forbade the employment of children under nine years of age in the spinning and weaving trades. This was the beginning of the limitation of ages and hours which has continued ever since. Four Factory Inspectors were appointed to see that the provisions of the Act were carried out. Eleven years later the Inspectors were given powers to appoint Certifying Factory Surgeons who were to give certificates of age for the children and also to inquire into the nature of accidents in the factories. The employment of children in factories continued until much later and they did not get full protection until the Children's Act of 1889 and an amending Act of 1904. Factory legislation, none the less, was considerably extended throughout the nineteenth century to include many different aspects of the problem of securing safeguards for the health of the workers. Most of the provisions governing this are to be found in the Factory and Workshops Act of 1901. This contains ten parts and more than a gross of sections dealing with health, safety, conditions of employment, education of children, homework and various specified trades which are known to be particularly unhealthy. We cannot detail the numerous sections which deal with the general health of the workers, although it must be noticed that these are the provisions which are the most effective in preventing disease. Here we must turn to some of the so-called dangerous trades which have a more particular medical interest.

In the latter half of the nineteenth century attention was especially directed towards certain trades which were injurious to health apart from any general considerations of fatigue, age or bad hygiene. As a preliminary the Act of 1895 specified certain maladies which were made compulsorily notifiable to the Chief Inspector of Factories. These were poisoning due to lead, phosphorus, or arsenic as well as the disease anthrax. The notification was the duty of any medical practitioner called in to attend any patient whom he believed to be suffering from any of these conditions. By later legislation poisonings from mercury, carbon disulphide, aniline and benzene were included among the notifiable conditions, as well as ulceration due to chromium compounds, cancers of the skin and toxic jaundice.

We have already referred to anthrax, the deadly disease of animals against which Pasteur had discovered a means of preventive inoculation with attenuated cultures of the anthrax bacillus. Certain classes of workers were, and still are to a lesser extent, very liable to infection with anthrax. In man the disease may begin either in the skin as an inflammatory swelling or in the lungs, when it is known as wool-sorters' disease, from the circumstance of its having been comparatively common in the woollen industry at Bradford. Cutaneous anthrax is extremely dangerous to life, whereas the pulmonary kind is almost invariably fatal.

The skin of workers may become infected through contact with the hides, fleeces or skins of animals which have died of anthrax. Dust from such material may contain myriads of the highly resistant spores of the bacillus and may remain infective for years. When such dust finds its way into cracks or cuts on the human skin, the spores quickly germinate into anthrax bacilli, a swelling appears at the site of the infection and after a short interval the whole body becomes invaded by the bacteria. In a similar way those who came into contact with infected wool or horsehair may inhale the spore-laden dust and so develop pulmonary anthrax.

The ideal method of prevention would be to prevent animals from becoming infected. In this country Acts have been passed to make certain diseases of animals notifiable. Under the Anthrax Order, 1928, animal anthrax was made notifiable and stringent regulations were laid down for the disposal of any infected carcass and for the disinfection of premises. However, since most of the bacilli responsible for industrial anthrax are imported, these measures cannot be wholly effective. A second line of defence lies in disinfecting hides or wools. Unfortunately wool becomes useless for many industrial purposes if it is heated for too long. A reliable method has been found and is now used to disinfect the more dangerous kinds of material. The best preventive measure is that adopted in this and certain other countries, namely the attempt to prevent any infected hides or wool from reaching the market; but since so many countries, particularly in Asia and

Africa, are liable to produce diseased animal products, the problem is exceedingly difficult. Further preventive measures have been introduced to stop the workers becoming infected by any spores which may be present in the materials they handle. Of these, exhaust ventilation in places where the dust is likely to arise is probably the most effective, but so long as infected stuffs are used, then there is always danger.

Once the disease has been contracted, prompt treatment is of the utmost importance. A highly effective anti-anthrax serum was first prepared by Professor Sclavo of Siena in 1895. This treatment reduced the mortality from cutaneous anthrax from 48·3 per cent to 4 per cent. To ensure prompt treatment it is important to warn employees of the danger so that they can seek early advice. Excellent coloured plates showing typical anthrax pustules are used for warning notices.

Lead poisoning is liable to occur in a number of different trades— for example, in metal-smelting, the preparation of red lead, white lead and paints, coach-painting, house-painting, enamelling, pottery, plumbing, the making of electric accumulators and in the manufacture of tetra-ethyl lead (used as an 'additive' to petrol). Stringent precautions were enforced on every industry in which lead-poisoning occurred. Exhaust ventilation in the work-rooms did much to avoid the inhalation of the vapour and dusty compounds of lead. Factory hygiene, including the provision of protective clothing and washing facilities, and the prohibition of eating in the workshops greatly reduced the quantities of lead which the workers consumed. The use of wet rubbing for removing old paint lessened the risk for painters. Water is also very effective for laying the lead-containing clouds of dust which would otherwise fill the rooms where accumulators were made. During certain operations in this process it was necessary for the operators to wear gas-masks. In some industries it was found possible to substitute harmless materials for the poisonous lead substances. For example, it was discovered that in the preparation of glazes for pottery, the solubility of the glaze, and consequently its toxicity, could be much reduced by using lead mixed with silica instead of the highly poisonous red or white leads. In painting it was often possible to use zinc oxide in place of white lead. More recently satisfactory paints which do not contain lead at all have been widely used.

An important factor in controlling this form of poisoning is the weekly medical examination by the Certifying Surgeon which every employee in the lead-using factories was required to undergo. Lead is a slow and cumulative poison so that the inspection is especially valuable for the detection of early signs, of which an alteration in the microscopical appearance of the blood is one of the most characteristic.

In the manufacture of lucifer matches it was customary to use white phosphorus, an insidious poison which attacked the workers, giving rise to inflammation of the gums with eventual necrosis (death) of parts of the jawbone—a condition known as phossy jaw. Poisoning from this cause was very prevalent wherever matches were made and considerable public agitation followed. The discovery that phosphorus sesquisulphide is equally effective for matches and also quite innocuous provided an easy way of prevention. Under the International Conference at Berne in 1906 all civilized countries undertook to prohibit the use of white phosphorus for matches. This undertaking was carried out in England by the White Phosphorus Prohibition Act of 1908. The remedy was immediately effective and fresh cases of phossy jaw are now unknown.

Arsenical poisoning in industry occurs either from the salts of arsenic or from breathing in the highly dangerous gas 'arsenurietted hydrogen'. The salts cause local irritant action on the skin, whereas arsenurietted hydrogen is a potent blood-poison. Poisoning from the salts has occurred in the manufacture of certain chemicals—sheep-dips, paints, preservatives for the use of taxidermists and others. The symptoms include intense local irritation leading to eruptions and ulceration with general ill-health and cramps. Poisoning from the gas is rare, but has occurred in chemical works.

The methods of prevention are similar to those used against lead. The actual incidence of poisoning from arsenic is very small and this is undoubtedly due to the stringent precautions that are enforced.

Besides all these powerful chemical poisons there are certain substances which, though not particularly poisonous in themselves, have a highly deleterious effect when inhaled in finely powdered form into the lungs. The 'dusty' trades are responsible for a very large amount of occupational illness among many different kinds of workmen. The substance silica, which occurs abundantly in every part of the world, is the chief cause of the damage. The diamond miners of South Africa, the tin miners of Cornwall, the workers in the rock upon which New York is built, stonemasons, potters, the manufacturers of scouring powders and coal miners in certain districts are all liable to suffer from the effects of constantly inhaling air containing silica over long periods of time.

It used to be thought that silica caused damage to the lungs simply from the mechanical irritation due to the fineness, sharpness and hardness of the particles inhaled. More recently it has been supposed that the effect is mainly a chemical one due to the gradual solution of the particles in the secretions of the lungs. Whatever the mechanism of the process, the damage is undoubted. Firstly a chronic inflammation is set up and this leads to the formation of increasing masses of fibrous tissue throughout the lungs, until ultimately the function of the lungs is so badly damaged that the sufferer is breathless on the smallest exertion, or even when at rest. Before the advent of modern anti-tuberculous chemotherapy the gravest danger was that tuberculosis so often supervened on top of the silicosis. This is not now the fatal complication that it used to be.

The prevention of silicosis, as the disease is called, presents a difficult problem. Water to allay the dust, exhaust ventilation at points where the dust is first raised, masks and dust-traps have all been used with varying success. In some trades harmless substances have been substituted for silica. For example, in the processes of sand-blasting the use of steel grit has given good results. If the workers are examined regularly, those that show signs of early silicosis can be removed to other employment and may recover, though in some trades the proportion of those that can do so is very small.

Even more dangerous than silica is the dust of asbestos which is a compound of silica and magnesium. Asbestosis is at least twice as swift in killing as silicosis. The recognition of asbestosis was a specific disease, though it was suspected early in the present century, was delayed by the current view that silica was only dangerous in the free (chemically uncombined) state. In the late twenties W. E. Cooke and others were able to demonstrate peculiar nodules in the lungs of dead asbestos workers and in the centre of each nodule were found spicules of asbestos. Since that time the insidious course of the disease has been studied from the gradual onset of shortness of breath until, after a few years, the fatal bronchitis or pneumonia terminates the scene. Here, too, before the discovery of streptomycin, tuberculosis was frequently the cause of death.

In the last few years the danger of asbestosis has been much in the news, particularly when it was discovered that it often gave rise to malignant changes in the lungs or pleura.

These discoveries led to the strict rules which have controlled the industry in the last thirty-five years. Besides the segregation of the dangerous processes in special rooms, exhaust ventilation and humidity, special gas-masks, overalls and head-protectors are required. It was hoped that with all these precautions the incidence of asbestosis would become negligible. Unfortunately there has been growing evidence to show that asbestos is even more dangerous than was thought, because it has been found to affect people not actually working with asbestos but living in the neighbourhood of the places where it has been used. Probably the best way of dealing with this particular menace would be to employ other materials whenever possible. For example in the past asbestos was often used as a heat-insulating material (for lagging hot pipes) in spite of the fact that it is not specially notable for its non-conducting properties (its one claim to usefulness is that it is fireproof). It should always be possible to use some other material, say fibre-glass, for heat insulation.

Finally, among dust diseases, farmer's lung is a condition which has recently come to the fore. In 1965 it became officially recognized as one of the diseases caused by industrial injuries and sufferers are now entitled to compensation. The condition was originally described over thirty years ago. It is a lung disease caused by the inhalation of the dust from mouldy hay and it gives rise to acute respiratory distress. The symptoms generally subside if the patient can keep away from mouldy hay: but repeated attacks can produce chronic lung disease, with progressive breathlessness, ending in secondary heart failure. Farmers who are subject to recurrent attacks have to be advised to change their farming methods or even to give up farming altogether.

Farmer's lung is not uncommon, but it varies very much in different parts of the country. It is found particularly in Cumberland, Devon, Wales and Northern Ireland, being much less frequent in the drier areas of East Anglia. It is widely thought that a high rainfall at harvest-time is an important contributory cause. The disease is almost certainly an allergic response: that is to say the individual sufferer has become unduly sensitive to certain specific moulds. At present there is no known cure. Severe attacks can often be suppressed immediately by cortico-steroid hormones: but relapses generally follow further exposure to mouldy hay.

6. TUBERCULOSIS

The medical and surgical treatment of tuberculosis has been described in some detail in an earlier section of this book. None the less the outstandingly successful result of the anti-tuberculosis campaign could hardly have been achieved without the active intervention of the State and it is this aspect of the matter that we must now examine.

Now that the infectious nature of the disease had been proved, public opinion was aroused to the necessity of urgent action. Voluntary efforts began the movement for new facilities for the effective treatment of consumptives. Sanatoria were opened at Frimley and Midhurst. In 1887 the first voluntary tuberculosis dispensary was opened at Edinburgh. It was dispensaries such as this that were to form the central clearing-houses in the huge anti-tuberculosis schemes that developed in the first two decades of the present century. In England the first dispensaries were opened at Paddington and St Marylebone in 1909 and 1910 respectively.

Since tuberculosis was infectious the desirability of making it notifiable followed at once. Certain towns in England had schemes of voluntary notification as early as 1899, but it was not until four years later that notification was first made compulsory in Sheffield by means of a private Bill. In 1908 the Local Government Board used its powers under the Public Health Acts to make regulations providing for the compulsory notification of all cases of consumption which came under the Poor Law Medical Officers and three years later further regulations required the universal notification of all cases. Armed with this information the appropriate local authority could at once take steps not only to provide advice and treatment to the sufferer, but also to protect his family and neighbours from the worst risks of becoming infected.

The National Insurance Act of 1911 provided, among other benefits, for the domiciliary treatment of consumptives by their panel doctors, for the building of sanatoria and hospitals and for research into tuberculosis. Such advantages unfortunately were only available to persons who were insured under the Act. It therefore became increasingly clear that, if any scheme for the eradication of tuberculosis was to be effective, it must be all-embracing and available to the whole community. The Astor Committee on tuberculosis recommended that the organization of a complete anti-tuberculosis scheme should be put into the hands of each local authority. Accordingly in 1912 the Local Government Board invited each County Council and County Borough Council to prepare its own scheme. Such plans as were approved were to be financed by the State to the extent of four-fifths of the cost of dispensaries and three-fifths of the cost of sanatoria and hospitals. The annual cost of the schemes were to be paid by the local authorities, but they were to be reimbursed partly by payments from Insurance Committees and half the remaining deficit was to be provided by the Local Government Board. All responsibility for sanatoria and dispensaries was subsequently transferred to the Country and County Borough Councils by the Tuberculosis Act of 1921.

The anti-tuberculosis campaign was thus launched on a most ambitious scale. Its declared object was that no single case of tuberculosis should be uncared-for and that all services should be free and available to everyone. This was a great advance on any benefits which could be had under the National Insurance Act. Schemes developed in every area, consisting of several co-operating units, the tuberculosis dispensary forming the main link between the individual units and between the public, the outside doctors and these units.

General practitioners sent their suspected cases to the dispensary where they were examined by the tuberculosis officer—a physician with special experience in the diagnosis and treatment of tuberculosis. Besides being merely a centre for diagnosis, the dispensary was also to be a centre for the observation of the progress that the patients made, for the treatment of those not in institutions, for the examination of persons living in close contact with the tuberculous and for the 'after care' of those discharged as cured. The ideal was that no patient who was definitely tuberculous should cease to be under observation until he was cured or dead. The dispensary was also to be an office for the dissemination of antituberculous propaganda.

The dispensary would normally send its tuberculosis patients to a sanatorium. Through its care committee it kept in touch with employers and social welfare centres, and it co-operated with the Maternity and Child Welfare Centres and the School Medical Service in caring for the needs of children. Special 'tuberculosis visitors' attended the dispensaries and it was their duty to visit the homes of the patients. Here they obtained information about the home life of the patient and those in close contact with him, and gave advice as to the best methods of improving the hygiene of the home. The visitors could also engage in the actual nursing of sick patients in their homes under medical supervision.

The above paragraphs give only a rough outline of the particular measures designed to prevent the spread of infection and to provide treatment for the sick. In addition to such a scheme more general measures were to be taken towards the general health of the community as a whole. This was to be interpreted on the widest scale. For example, it included the teaching of hygiene in schools, the provision of fresh air, open spaces and recreation grounds in towns, the provision of an ample and varied diet for every child and, exceedingly important, a supply of clean and uninfected milk.

In considering the importance of pure milk, it must be said that there was considerable controversy, not only over the best means of assuring such a supply, but even over the desirability of such a thing. As soon as it became known that tuberculosis was infectious, it became obvious that there was need to inquire into the possibility of people becoming infected through meat and drink. It was suggested that all meat found to be tuberculous should be seized and destroyed; and in some places this was done. Unfortunately Koch confused the issue by asserting in 1901 that the tuberculosis of cattle was not transmissible to human beings and he said that the risk of contracting the disease from milk or meat was so small that he considered precautions unnecessary. None the less it was subsequently shown that an appreciable proportion of human tuberculosis was of bovine origin.

Accordingly action was taken to improve the standard of the milk supply. A bewildering number of Acts, Orders and Regulations followed over the ensuing fifty years. All milk-producers must be registered. Cows may be inspected and milk samples taken. Cowsheds and milking-sheds must be adequately lighted, ventilated and equipped with a supply of water. Tuberculous persons were prohibited from handling milk.

In addition to these precautions a number of special designations of milk were laid down. There were Certified Milk, Grade A tuberculin-tested, Grade A Pasteurized and simply Pasteurized milks. Certified milk was the product of special herds of cows, every animal of which had to be examined and tuberculin-tested every six months. Any animal reacting positively to the test had to be removed at once. Every individual cow of such a herd had to be marked and registered. Milk from such a herd could not contain tubercle bacilli, but there could be no guarantee that it was bacteriologically safe in other respects. Pasteurised milk was safer, as it had been heated to 145 degrees Fahrenheit for half an hour, then cooled and bottled at once. Such a procedure killed almost all bacteria and in particular *M. tuberculosis*. Pasteurized milk could be sold at the same price as untreated milk because it kept longer. (Unkind critics alleged that the big distributing companies were more interested in prolonging the life of the milk than that of the customer.)

After the Second World War special areas in the country were designated, in which no milk could be sold unless it came from tuberculin-tested herds and by now nearly all the milk in this country comes from such safe sources.

Medicine and the State

The campaign for pure milk brought about the almost total disappearance of tuberculosis of the neck glands in children, which used to be so common in this country some twenty years ago.

The campaign against pulmonary tuberculosis in the United Kingdom—and even more so in Europe—met with a major setback as a result of the First World War and both the number of new cases and of deaths showed a notable increase. Between the wars the campaign was resumed on the same basis as before, because the experience gained between the inception of the scheme in 1909 and the outbreak of war had shown most encouraging results. The number of sanatorium beds, dispensaries and tuberculosis officers was increased, but the provision of beds never really caught up with the need, so that effective isolation of infectious (sputum-positive) cases could not be universal.

The Second World War precipitated a further disaster. On the outbreak of hostilities a large number of sanatoria were almost completely emptied by Government order, to provide beds for the emergency medical service. Mass bombing of towns was universally expected and these beds were to be used for the reception of the expected casualties. The result was that every tuberculous patient who could stand on his feet was sent home, so that hundreds of infectious cases were returned to their families. Thus whole new crops of cases arose. Furthermore the sanatorium beds were kept empty for many months, and still the expected bombing did not occur; so that by the time the beds were made available again, waiting-lists had piled up. The lost months could never be recovered and in most areas there was a waiting list of between three and six months, before a patient could be treated. The results of this were extremely disheartening to the tuberculosis officers who by then had patients dying on the waiting-list. The situation was aggravated by the food shortages, though the Government was able to help in this respect by making extra rations, particularly of milk and fats, available to tuberculous patients.

After the war energetic efforts were made to wipe out the waiting-lists by opening other tuberculosis beds in different institutions, such as fever hospitals and by providing convalescent homes where patients from sanatoria could complete their treatment and so make sanatorium beds available to those awaiting admission.

About 1943 it was realized that financial conditions often made it difficult or impossible for a wage-earner to accept treatment, involving, as it did, many months in hospital. For a breadwinner the diagnosis of pulmonary tuberculosis meant disaster to himself and his family. To help such cases the Government brought in special maintenance allowances (under Memorandum 266 T) which were to be paid to patients who agreed to stop work to undergo treatment. These quite substantial weekly sums were to be paid in addition to National Health Insurance benefits and they could be paid to a patient still on the waiting-list, provided he was resting at home. The allowances were also available after the patient left hospital, so long as he was off work under medical instructions. There is no doubt that this measure induced many patients to undergo treatment which they would otherwise have refused.

In the same year, 1943, mass miniature radiography began to be available to the general public. It had been introduced earlier in this country by the Royal Navy under the name of the pulmograph. It had been highly successful in bringing to light many cases of pulmonary tuberculosis, particularly among middle-aged men who, though not seriously ill in themselves, were infecting their younger and more susceptible shipmates. The number of mass radiography units available to the public was gradually increased until today there are over a hundred mobile and static units operating under the regional hospital boards in co-operation with the local public health authorities. The mass miniature radiography service did very valuable work in bringing to light thousands of completely unknown cases of tuberculosis. When the campaign began, even in the healthier areas it was found that more than one in every thousand persons X-rayed for the first time had active tuberculosis. In the industrial areas things were much worse. As time went on the percentage of newly discovered cases became smaller and smaller, so that it was found desirable to switch the units away from the general surveys they had been doing. Today they are concentrating on special areas where there are bad records of tuberculosis and on specially susceptible sections of the people.

That the law of diminishing returns governed the pick-up of new cases by the mass radiography service came as no surprise, but, though it was to be expected, it should furnish no good reason for complacency. A simple calculation, based on the total number of persons known to have been X-rayed,[1] the percentage of tuberculosis found and the total population figures (as recorded by the most recent census) shows quite clearly that there must still be many thousands of unknown and actively infectious cases at large among the general population.

There was always difficulty in getting patients back to work after treatment, partly because they were not always fit to resume their former occupation, especially when it involved heavy physical exertion, and partly because employers were reluctant to take on workers who were known to have had tuberculosis. To help to overcome this difficulty the Disabled Persons Employment Act of 1944 provided that employers of more than twenty persons must take at least three per cent of their staff from those whose names were on the Disabled Persons register. It was open to anyone with tuberculosis to have his name put on the register and so improve his chance of getting employment.

In 1948 the National Health Service Act transferred all the sanatoria, dispensaries, tuberculosis officers and Mass radiography services to the various regional hospital boards. In this way most of the tuberculosis services became unified under single bodies, with the exception of the prevention and after-care which was left in the hands of the local authorities. The dispensaries were renamed chest clinics and the tuberculosis officers became chest physicians, signifying that the service was now to include not only tuberculosis, but all forms of lung disease.

It was not until 1950 that the campaign for mass immunization with B.C.G. began in this country, although, as we have seen, the vaccine had been used in France more than twenty years earlier.[2] Indeed by 1948 the total number of vaccinated persons in other countries (excluding Japan) had risen to about ten million. In the United Kingdom the scheme began in a modest way with the vaccination of those known to be at risk (i.e. the contacts). At first the B.C.G. had to be imported in liquid form from Denmark. This

---

[1] In 1965 the total number of such examinations in England and Wales was 3,263,670.

[2] Vide Supra, p. 127 *et seq.*

type of vaccine had the grave disadvantage that it would keep for only two weeks, so that it was not always easy to arrange clinics to coincide with the arrival of the supply of vaccine. B.C.G. is now made in this country and distributed free of charge to chest clinics and school clinics. It is supplied as a freeze-dried powder which will keep for a full year without losing its immunizing power. This form of protection is now offered to all schoolchildren of ten years and upwards, as well as to those particularly exposed to risk, such as medical and nursing students. There is no doubt that this widespread immunization has been a decisive factor in the enormous reduction of tuberculosis in the young adult population of today.

A further measure for the protection of children has been introduced since the end of the Second World War. This is the compulsory X-ray examination of all adults working in contact with children. In particular, all new teachers are required to have their chests X-rayed before taking up their appointments.

The antituberculous campaign has been one of the most successful public health measures ever attempted. Thirty years ago the sanatorium wards were full of sick and dying adolescents and young adults. Today the picture is quite different. The tuberculosis wards are far fewer in number and the beds are filled for the most part by elderly men; and of the few fatalities that occur, the average age at death is rapidly approaching that of man's allotted span. The actual mortality rate in this country is now about one-thirtieth part of what it was at the beginning of the century. However, the disease is far from having been conquered, because it is still a major scourge in many parts of the world, particularly in over-populated countries such as India and Pakistan, where the actual numbers of the population and consequent overcrowding makes tuberculosis particularly difficult to control.

VII. VENEREAL DISEASE

The problem of State interference in the matter of venereal disease has always been a thorny one. The whole subject has been inevitably mixed up with sex and tabu and these, added to the general hatred of any kind of interference with personal liberty, have made the task of improving the health of the people in this respect an exceedingly thankless one. Nevertheless the ravages of syphilis and gonorrhoea in the middle of the nineteenth century were of such dimensions that it was thought essential to try some sort of experimental legislation.

Before the causal organisms had been found and before there was any worthwhile treatment, it was difficult to know what action would be effective. In France and other continental countries there was legal machinery for licensing brothels and registering prostitutes; so when the prevalence of syphilis in the British Army came to be considered by the Medical Department of the War Office, it was just this continental system which caught their fancy. It was actually proposed to have licensed prostitutes, who were to be medically examined at regular intervals and, when necessary, forced to submit to treatment.

Needless to say Victorian morality was outraged by this suggestion. Florence Nightingale was up in arms. She averred that the continental system was 'morally disgusting, unworkable in practice and unsuccessful in results'.[1] She was sure that the root causes of vice in the Army were physical rather than moral and she listed them as the filthy overcrowded conditions of living, drink and boredom; and she was convinced that the proper remedy lay in improving the living conditions of the soldiers and providing proper accommodation for their wives. She was not content with mere assertions; she actually produced statistics to prove that compulsory licensing and inspection of prostitutes did not in fact decrease the incidence of venereal disease.

The Army Medical Department still bore Miss Nightingale a grudge because of her exposure of their system (or lack of it) during the Crimean War and her opposition to their scheme still further infuriated them. The result was that, in spite of all the facts which the opposition put forward, the venereal disease Bill— euphemistically styled the Contagious Diseases Bill—was passed in 1864. (Miss Nightingale said the War Office deserved the V.C. for their cool intrepidity in the face of facts.)[2]

The Contagious Diseases Prevention Act applied only to some

[1] Woodham-Smith, C., *Florence Nightingale*, London, 1950, p. 400.

[2] Woodham-Smith, C., op. cit., p. 402.

eighteen naval and military stations where it was thought it would be comparatively easy to enforce the provisions of the Act and ascertain whether any benefit accrued. The Act provided, on the continental model, for the compulsory examination of known prostitutes, for detaining them if they were infected with venereal disease and for inflicting heavy punishments on the keepers of houses of ill-fame who knowingly harboured diseased women. A further Act gave even wider compulsory powers.

The passing of these Acts met with widespread disapproval in influential quarters. There was no doubt that this legalisation of prostitution (for that was what it amounted to) and the compulsory examination of the women was wholly repugnant to educated taste at the time. It was felt that the whole sordid business was humiliating and degrading to the nation as well as to the soldiers and the women themselves. A Royal Commission thought that the scheme was proving effective; but the public outcry was such that the Contagious Diseases Acts were repealed in their entirety in 1886.

Subsequently more and more knowledge about venereal diseases became available. The causative organism of gonorrhoea had been discovered by Albert Neisser in 1879 and the spirochaete of syphilis by Fritz Schaudinn in 1905. Moreover for syphilis the researches of Wassermann and Ehrlich had provided a new means of diagnosis and a valuable cure. The whole subject was coming more and more into the limelight and the far-reaching and revolting effects of venereal disease were becoming more fully and more generally recognized. Again it was on the continent of Europe that positive action was being taken. The legalization and control of prostitution continued in Denmark and Sweden well into the twentieth century and seemed to be having some effect; but in these countries the public outcry was just as loud as it had been in England fifty years before. In Sweden the doctors had been impressed by the success of the method; none the less, in face of public opinion, they reluctantly agreed—after years of wrangling—that the legal control of prostitution should be abandoned, *provided some other efficient scheme could be devised*. Denmark in 1906 and Sweden in 1918 brought in laws to provide for compulsory notification of venereal disease and for free treatment. Doctors were compelled to notify details of all cases of venereal disease, but they were not to divulge the names of the patients. The threat to disclose the names of the diseased was to be used as a lever to force them to submit to treatment. The patient's name remained a secret unless he failed to start or complete the prescribed course of treatment. Intensive contact examinations were to be undertaken both to find the source of the infection as well as to pick up any further cases that might have been infected by the original patient. Denmark went so far as to demand that a declaration or a medical certificate to the effect that a person was free from venereal disease should be produced before any marriage could take place.

There is little doubt that this scheme owed its success to the fact that it secured secrecy so long as the patient co-operated in undergoing thorough treatment. Similar legislation was enacted in other countries as a result.

In the United Kingdom it was found difficult or impossible to legislate until the public was more fully aware of the gravity of the situation. Accordingly a Royal Commission was appointed and it issued its final report in 1916. In this there was grave insistence not only on the evil effects of the diseases on the patient himself, but, more important still, on the disastrous results of congenital and hereditary syphilis on the next generation. Congenital syphilis was frequently a cause of antenatal death or of death in early infancy. The congenital syphilitic is of stunted growth and subnormal intelligence. Eyes, ears, skin, bones, joints, muscles, nervous system and brain may all be irretrievably damaged by this disease. The report stated that of 1,100 children in the London blind schools, 31·2 per cent were certainly and, in addition, 2·8 per cent probably due to syphilis . . . 'while as much as 25 per cent of all blindness had been attributed to gonorrhoeal ophthalmia'.

The social and economic effects were prodigious; loss of child-life and sterility often resulted, while blindness and idiocy added enormously to the expense of education and welfare. It was calculated that in the Navy and Army together, in 1912, nearly half a million working days were lost from venereal disease alone. The actual incidence among the population in general was difficult to assess, because the conditions were not notifiable so that there were no statistics. None the less information could be had from other sources. The Registrar-General could furnish the number of deaths certified as due to syphilis, but such a figure must certainly have been artificially diminished by the unwillingness of doctors to wound the susceptibilities of the relatives of the dead. Other more reliable information was obtained from the Navy, the Army, the Police, the Local Government Board's institutions and the Prison Commissioners, while the figures for general paralysis of the insane (a late manifestation of syphilis) could be obtained from the Lunacy Commissioners. The estimates of the Royal Commissioners were frightening. They affirmed their belief that not less than ten per cent of the whole population was infected with syphilis, while gonorrhoea was spread more widely still. It did not follow that these diseases were necessarily becoming more prevalent than before—indeed it was probable that there had been some decline—yet clearly it was time for action.

There were considerable difficulties to be faced. The facilities for diagnosis were very insufficient. Some voluntary hospitals, through the pious outlook of their benefactors (who did not believe that free treatment should be given to those who had acquired a disease through loose living), had regulations prohibiting them from treating venereal disease. The Commissioners expressed the hope that 'when the facts elicited from our inquiry are made public, the view that morality can be encouraged by denying medical treatment to those who by violating its laws have become a public danger will disappear'.

The advisability of making venereal disease notifiable was also considered. This had been done in some countries, but it had the very material disadvantage that it deterred patients from seeking medical advice and led to endless concealment and subterfuge. Furthermore, if the onus of notifying the disease is put upon the medical profession, the result is to drive the sufferers into the hands of unqualified practitioners. The Royal Commission called special attention to the calamitous effect of the treatment of venereal disease by such persons. This will hardly surprise anyone who has obtained an insight into the ignorance of the quacks by a perusal of the evidence given before the Commission. In spite of this the Government did not think it wise to prohibit any kind of treatment until some reliable alternative had been provided.

An important recommendation made by the Commission was that the Public Health Acts should be used to call into being a nation-wide scheme of treatment. This was done by the issue of the Public Health (Venereal Diseases) Regulations of 1916, which directed and empowered County and County Borough Councils to provide laboratory facilities for diagnosis and to prepare schemes for treatment and for the provision of salvarsan or other approved remedies. Treatment was to be free, the cost being borne by the councils, with a grant of three-quarters to be paid by the central authority. It was added that all information about patients was to be strictly confidential and to aid in ensuring secrecy it was advised that treatment should not be given at special centres but rather in departments of general hospitals. Local councils were also urged to provide information about venereal diseases, their dangers and their curability.

These schemes duly matured and did an immense amount of good. When a committee on the same subject reported in 1923 it was stated that no less than 179 approved centres were engaged in the diagnosis and treatment of such disease. There was good reason to suppose that there had been a decrease in the number of new cases.

In 1917, shortly after the new schemes for treatment began to work, it was decided to put a stop once and for all to the activities of quacks and mountebanks who were offering alleged cures for these diseases. The Venereal Disease Act prohibits the treatment of these complaints otherwise than by qualified practitioners, but only in areas where there is an approved scheme of treatment in operation. In such areas no one who is not a registered doctor may for direct or indirect reward treat or prescribe a remedy for, or give any advice directly or indirectly in connexion with the treatment of venereal disease. Advertisements are strictly forbidden, either of treatment or of any preparation intended for the prevention, cure or relief of such diseases. The point of forbidding the advertisement of preventives lies in the fact that there are none that are absolutely safe or fool-proof; consequently it is intended to prevent the spread of disease which might well occur if a false sense of security were engendered. There is no doubt, however, that careful self-disinfection and the issue of prophylactic packets have done much to lessen the incidence of disease in some branches of the Services.

Apart from treatment, the belief of the Commissioners was that prevention could best be achieved by educating young adults to lead clean and healthy lives, by insisting on the importance of early and thorough treatment and by warning the young against the enormous risks which sexual promiscuity entails. In 1917 the National Council for Combating Venereal Disease was set up. Later it changed its name to the British Social Hygiene Council. This is a voluntary body, but it is partially subsidized by the Government and local public health authorities. Its main activities are concerned with biological teaching and all kinds of educational propaganda concerned with sex and with healthy living.

In 1937 the Ministry of Health sent a Commission to Scandinavia to inquire into the working of the Danish and Swedish schemes outlined above. They found that these schemes were working well, but the Commission was not convinced that the results were materially different from the success achieved in countries where compulsory treatment was not in use.

Major wars are always accompanied by an increase in venereal disease and the Second World War was no exception. The actual increase does not seem to have been as large as was expected. There is no doubt that the advent of penicillin in the latter part of the war did much towards cleaning up the sources of infection. Unfortunately the early hope that penicillin would be able to control venereal disease at some low and tolerable level has not been fulfilled. None the less this drug and improved facilities for treatment have brought the venereal disease clinics in this country to a high pitch of efficiency.

It is now more than fifty years since these clinics were called into being by the Regulations of 1916. It will be noticed that this was more than thirty years before free treatment for all diseases was made available under the Welfare State. These fifty years have seen great advances in diagnosis and treatment. The clinics have increased in number from about 100 in 1917 to about 230 at the present time. There have been few changes in the actual organization of the services other than those brought about by the National Health Service. With the Welfare State the responsibility for the venereal disease clinics passed to the regional hospital boards, though the duties of looking after contacts and tracing defaulters remained with the local authorities. Whether the splitting-up of the venereal disease service in this way is an advance is open to doubt.

Recently there has been a considerable increase in the number of new patients. This in no way reflects on the efficiency of the venereal disease service, which in this country is probably as good as any in the world. Indeed it says much for our own service that the increase in disease has been small compared with that in most other developed countries; in spite of the fact that, with one exception, we have not resorted to compulsion. This exception was in the few years between 1942 and 1947 when, under a defence regulation (33B) brought in during the war, specialists were required to notify contacts and, through the magistrates, enforce treatment when necessary.

The recent increase in the number of new cases is undoubtedly the result of changing social patterns and the *prevention* of venereal disease (in the absence of any effective inoculations to produce immunity) must be considered as a social problem. The ultimate control almost certainly lies outside the sphere of pure medicine.

We have, then, to admit that treatment, as we have it today, has failed to control venereal disease. Publicity campaigns have also had no lasting impact on the epidemiological level. None the less, on the credit side, there have been outstanding achievements. The death-rate from syphilis began to go down almost as soon as effective treatment clinics became established. At that time over 1,000 infants died annually in England and Wales. Today the death of an infant from this cause is a rarity. The occurrence of congenital syphilis, apart from deaths, has also declined in a spectacular way. Blindness from syphilis used to be a terrible scourge. In 1930, for example, it accounted for about 12 per cent of all blindness; but now causes less than one half of one per cent. The death-rate from acquired syphilis has also fallen from about 140 to 10 per million in recent years. Blindness from gonococcal ophthalmia used to cause over one-quarter of all blindness in children. The Public Health (Ophthalmia Neonatorum) Regulations of 1914 ordered the notification of all cases, whether gonorrhoeal or not, of purulent discharge from the eyes of an infant starting within twenty-one days of birth. This ensured early diagnosis and prompt treatment; so that from being the commonest cause of blindness in children, gonorrhoeal opthalmia is now almost completely under control.

VIII. PURE AIR

This was one of the pressing problems which the industrial revolution brought with it. At first smoke was regarded merely as a nuisance, but later it became known that it was a serious menace to health, though the actual damage could be only roughly assessed. Firstly a smoky atmosphere caused a big loss of sunlight, particularly of the health-giving ultra-violet rays. This was worse in winter when the need for sunshine was greater. The loss of light must have contributed seriously to the incidence of rickets in children, though this was not known until the connexion between rickets, vitamin D and ultra-violet light had been worked out; though it had in fact been most strongly suspected as long ago as 1890 by an English missionary Theobald T. Palm,[1] who did his best to stress the value of 'sunshine as a means of health'. Secondly there was actual damage to the lungs from the inhalation of particles of soot, tar and sulphur products, contributing to chronic bronchitis and other respiratory troubles.

The extent of the problem may be dimly appreciated when it is realized that each individual inhales something like six tons of air every year and, during the same period, several million tons of solid matter, tar and sulphur dioxide are being emitted into the air from domestic and factory chimneys in the United Kingdom.

Fog occurs when there is what the meteorologists call an inverted temperature-gradient, that is to say when the coldest part of the air is that nearest to the ground, so that the water-droplets and the impurities they contain form dense clouds which hang about the streets of our cities and big towns. That fog can cause rapid death has been demonstrated only too clearly on various occasions and in many countries. Some 'London particular' fogs, in 1873 and 1880, for examples, caused conspicuous rises in the death-rate. There

[1] See above, p. 173, also Palm, T. A., 'The Geographical Distribution and Aetiology of Rickets', *Practitioner*, 1890, 40, p. 270.

was the so-called 'Belgian Death Fog' in December 1930. In the valley of the Meuse one single fog killed at least sixty-seven people. Inquiry showed that fog alone was the cause and that no special chemical fumes were connected with the deaths. The famous London fogs of 1952 are said to have caused upwards of four thousand deaths. It must be admitted that most of those who died in this way were previously in a low state of health, through old age or respiratory disease: but the fog itself was the precipitating cause of the disasters.

The worst polluters of the atmosphere were—and still are to a large extent—the numerous users of coal in the ordinary domestic fire. It was computed, about thirty-five years ago, that household fires were responsible for about 2·5 million tons out of a total of 3 million tons of solids belched into the air.

The Public Health Act of 1875, amended in 1926 by the Public Health (Smoke Abatement) Act, defined as a nuisance any fireplace which does not as far as practicable consume the smoke arising from the combustibles therein; and any chimney (not being the chimney of a private dwelling-house) sending forth smoke in such quantity as to be a nuisance. Smoke was held to include soot, ash and gritty particles. It was most unfortunate that the domestic hearth was held to be so sacred that the Act expressly excluded private chimneys from interference.

Some improvement did occur in the following thirty years, partly from the working of the 1926 Act. More probably it was the increasing use of smokeless fuels like anthracite, coke, oil and gas as well as the rapid expansion of the electrical industry that contributed to this end. The average annual deposit per square mile in London was as high as 392 tons in 1915–19, but had dropped to 289 tons by 1931.

The Clean Air Act of 1956 was a big step forward. This made it an offence for dark smoke to be emitted from chimneys in excess of a permitted period. This time domestic chimneys were included. Furthermore special smoke control areas were defined. Local authorities are required to draw up plans for such areas and can compel householders to adapt their fireplaces to burn smokeless fuels. These regulations have done much good, particularly in industrial areas; though a visit to these will convince anyone that much remains to be done. In the north the National Society for Clean Air attributes the slow progress in smoke control to over-generous allowances of free coal to the miners.[1]

There were other reasons than those of health which ought to have had considerable effect in urging the abolition of smoke. Buildings were rapidly being corroded by the chemical products of incomplete combustion of coal. Huge sums were being spent in extra illumination and laundry which could have been saved by cleaning the air. Moreover, since smoke was nothing else than the part of the fuel not burnt, millions of tons of coal could have been saved by ensuring complete oxidation of the coal. About three-quarters of the coal used in domestic fires is frankly wasted, whereas a properly conducted gas-works can use for heating pur-poses as much as 86 per cent of the energy value of the coal.

There is no doubt that, so far as coal is concerned, the situation is mending rapidly. Recently many of the outsides of the public buildings in big cities have been cleaned, the years of accumulated soot being removed at vast expense. It is the hopeful belief that, under the progressive modern conditions of smoke control, the blackening will not recur.

While the smoke menace is being overcome, we are still left with the pollution caused by the internal combustion engines of motor vehicles. The exhausts from these discharge large quantities of harmful chemicals into the air, especially carbon monoxide, hydro-carbons and acid fumes such as sulphur dioxide and nitrogen peroxide. Some control over this will have to be devised. It is widely believed that an appreciable proportion of lung cancer can be ascribed to atmospheric pollution. This problem will be dis-cussed in more detail in the epilogue.

IX. MENTAL ILL-HEALTH

The problem of mental ill-health is one which has been seriously attacked only in the last few decades and it is still far from having been solved. It was largely through ignorance or prejudice that doctors in the past failed to recognize the important part which stress played in causing ill-health of all kinds. Until quite recently

[1] *The Times*, 18th October 1967.

medical students were taught only about the grosser kinds of disorder of the mind, namely congenital deficiency, imbecility or
idiocy, and acquired insanity of several types, including those due
to such physical causes as arterial degeneration, syphilis (general
paralysis of the insane), alcohol and dangerous drugs. Today the
subject of psychology has also to include all the mental ill-health
acquired through the stresses and strains of modern life, leading to
breakdown of personality in many different ways.

A hundred years ago it was frank insanity—lunacy, as it was then
called—with which the law mainly concerned itself. Under
medieval law the insane had little or no protection. Their legal
acts were annulled and their property put under control; but there
was no kind of personal treatment whatever.

At the beginning of the nineteenth century the public attitude
towards the mentally deranged began to change. Attention was
called to the miserable condition of the insane, imprisoned without
inspection or treatment. At the same time the possibility that mad
people could be treated in a more humane and scientific way was
propounded and put into practice by physicians, such as Philippe
Pinel in France (at the Bicêtre and the Salpêtrière in Paris), W.
Tuke in England (at The Retreat in York) and B. Rush and I. Ray
in America. None the less with few exceptions the lot of the insane
was about as bad as it could be. J. E. D. Esquirol, a pupil of Pinel
wrote of them in 1817 'These unfortunate people are treated worse
than criminals, reduced to a condition worse than animals. I have
seen them naked, covered with rags and having only straw to protect them against the cold moisture and the hard stones they lie
upon; deprived of air, of water to quench thirst, and all the necessaries of life; given up to mere gaolers and left to their surveillance.
I have seen them in their narrow and filthy cells, without light and
air, fastened with chains in these dens, in which one would not
keep wild beasts. This I have seen in France and *the insane are
everywhere in Europe treated in the same way*.' Was not the King
of England himself confined in a strait-jacket at Windsor Castle?

In England the insane were for the most part incarcerated indiscriminately with criminals and paupers. There were a few
institutions—madhouses—where the insane were kept separately.
For example Bedlam (Bethlehem Royal Hospital) was rebuilt as an

asylum for the insane in 1676; but in 1815 a committee of the House of Commons, appointed to inquire into the 'provision to be made for the better regulation of madhouses', found this asylum in a disgraceful state. Patients were chained to the wall almost naked. Medical treatment, if it could be called such, was of a most inhumane kind, amounting to torture. The gradual progress towards separating the insane from the criminals and paupers and housing them in special institutions came about partly by voluntary efforts and subscriptions and partly by contributions from the rates. The reform of the madhouses in London was largely brought about by Lord Ashley (who later became Lord Shaftesbury) and his fellow members of a Metropolitan Commission set up by Act of Parliament in 1828. A number of Lunacy Acts were passed between 1829 and 1890, but they were mostly concerned with the registration and conduct of madhouses. The Act of 1845 set up a Permanent Board of Commissioners in Lunacy, which was to visit regularly all institutions, both public and private, where lunatics were held. Medical treatment for the mentally deranged was practically non-existent.

Later in the century better ideas about normal psychology were being propagated by many enlightened men. Henry Maudsley, the eminent alienist, advised a select committee in 1877 that, if insanity was to be cured, the importance of early treatment was paramount. But for the most part the tangle of legislation, culminating in the Lunacy Act of 1890, was concerned with procedure in certifying, admitting and caring for people who were demonstrably and (it was widely supposed) incurably mad. The 1890 Act was also designed to prevent improper certification and detention of people who were not mad at all; but this tightening up of the procedure for certification generally resulted in a 'lunatic' being far beyond any sort of cure by the time he had become sufficiently deranged to allow doctors to certify him without legal risk to themselves.

How late it was before modern psychiatric treatment became available may be seen from what Sir Clifford Allbutt, the Regius Professor of Physic at Cambridge, wrote in 1911; 'Sufferers from mental diseases are still regarded as troublesome persons to be hidden away in humane keeping, rather than as cases of manifold and obscure diseases, to be studied and treated by the undivided attention of physicians of the highest skill. The care of idiots . . . is making its way in England, and if as yet insufficient, is good of its kind.'

One of the difficulties about mental treatment was that there were almost no organizations for treating such illness, like the voluntary hospitals for the treatment of physical disease. Furthermore, as Allbutt pointed out, an enormous accumulation of lunatics of all sorts had pretty well paralysed public authorities which, in spite of huge expenditure on building institutions, massed them together more or less indiscriminately in barracks and expected that they could be adequately treated. He added; 'The life of the insane patient is as bright and the treatment as humane as a barrack life can be; but of science, whether in pathology or medicine, there can be little.'

A Royal Commission on Lunacy and Mental Disorder was appointed in 1926 and, among many recommendations, it advised that the treatment of mental disorder should be the business of local authorities; that they should try to treat mental illness just as thoroughly and universally as physical disease; and that early treatment should be available long before patients became certifiably mad. The Mental Health Act of 1930 put many of these recommendations on the Statute Book. Treatment for mental illness was to be available on a voluntary basis in hospitals or nursing homes. In this way early treatment was to be within reach of anyone needing it; and evidently the need was great, because within a few years a high proportion of those undergoing treatment were voluntary patients.

Before the Second World War other important improvements were brought in, in the first instance by voluntary bodies; the Child Guidance Council and the National Council for Mental Hygiene, which called into being respectively clinics for child guidance and arrangements for educating psychiatric social workers, who are now part of the accepted scheme of things.

Psychiatric social workers have a basic training in social science and also have a degree or other qualification in psychiatric social work and are attached either to hospitals or to local authorities' clinics. The child guidance organization brought new knowledge of family problems and it soon became clear that a child's psychological difficulties were inescapably tied up with those of his parents and that the whole family were really in need of treatment; not just the child himself. It was in this special field of 'family guidance' that the psychiatric social workers began to prove of great value in treating mentally sick people and their families.

In 1946 the National Health Service Act fused the prevention, treatment and after-care of mental illness and mental deficiency into the general health service, under the Ministry of Health. All mental institutions were put under the regional hospital boards and local authorities were required to undertake prevention and after-care of mental illness. In other words, for the first time mental illness was to be covered as completely as possible by the Welfare State on an equal footing with physical disease.

The Mental Health Act of 1959 was based on the findings of a further Royal Commission and brought the law concerning mental illness to the place it occupies today.

Treatment is now provided as part of the National Health Service, just as in any physical disease. The patient can consult his family doctor who can arrange for him to have specialist advice at an out-patient clinic at a hospital. Patients can be admitted for in-patient treatment in the normal way. When necessary, in the interests of society or of the patient himself, a mentally deranged person can be compulsorily detained; but the 1959 Act stressed that, wherever it was possible, mental illness should be treated like physical disease and that compulsion should be used only when absolutely necessary. In England and Wales only eight per cent of mental patients in hospital are there under compulsion. Indeed there are special safeguards to prevent a patient's being detained unnecessarily and he or his family can appeal to the mental health tribunal, of which there is one in each of the fifteen hospital regions of England and Wales. An important provision is that these tribunals are completely independent bodies, appointed by the Lord Chancellor, not the Minister of Health.

Local authorities must make provision for the prevention, care and after-care of people with mental disorder. They may provide suitable residential accommodation, like hostels, for those not ill enough to require hospital treatment or for those who are well enough to be discharged from hospital but have no home to go to. There is an increasing demand for such hostels, because of the growing recognition of the value of keeping such patients outside hospitals whenever possible. Local authorities can provide centres for occupational training for children or adults. Such training centres for children aim at improving their social behaviour and developing any skills they may possess in those below the mental level at which they could be expected to benefit from teaching in schools. The adult training centres are more in the nature of workshops where the patients can be trained in some occupation which they will be able to follow outside the centre once they have been trained. Those who are not well enough to reach this standard can be employed more or less permanently in the training centres. There is no doubt that these centres give a really valuable service to mentally sick people, because a man who finds himself at odds with society can be enormously helped by being encouraged to find satisfaction in some useful and productive work.

Finally a local authority must appoint one or more mental welfare officers, whose duty it is to get patients into hospital when their mental illness requires admission. Every area now has its own mental health service under the direction of a doctor trained to understand social and psychological problems. He is supported by a number of trained social workers who keep in touch with the mentally ill patients and their families as occasions arise.

It must be noted that the law in its present form stresses the importance of 'community care', as opposed to hospital treatment; for it is the growing belief that attention to the community and family aspect of mental illness will produce the best results in the prevention of mental disorder. The facilities for community care are available to patients leaving hospital or, better still, as an alternative to going into hospital. These facilities usually include out-patient clinics, attached as a rule to general hospitals, day hospitals, hostels, social clubs and occupational work centres. Community care for those leaving hospitals depends so vitally on the co-operation between the hospital and the various services provided by the local authority. The amount of co-operation that actually takes place varies enormously in different areas. What the future policy of the Ministry of Health will be must eventually depend on the results that all these various services can produce. It is really too early to venture a prediction of what the future may hold.

X. OLD AGE

Medicine in its widest sense has been directly responsible for producing one of the biggest problems of today, namely the care and cure of the aged. The need is a pressing one and it will almost certainly become greater in the foreseeable future. It has been calculated that by 1980 some eight millions of the population of this country will be over sixty-five. This has come about through a variety of causes, but all of them medical.

Firstly, in England and Wales the death-rate has been halved in the last 130 years. Secondly, the great loss of child-life has been checked. In early and mid-Victorian times all families, from the highest to the lowest, tended to have a large number of children (the Queen herself had nine) for two reasons: firstly the absence of effective birth-control measures and secondly there was the expectation that some of the children would die in infancy or childhood: as indeed they often did. In the early part of the nineteenth century about two-fifths of all deaths occurred among children under five years of age. This enormous death-rate is still operating in many under-developed and over-populated countries (though generally it does not occur on so large a scale as to prevent disastrous increases in the total population). In England and Wales the present infant mortality is of the order of 3 per cent of the total deaths.

By contrast, the death-rate among the elderly has soared, from 18 to nearly 70 per cent of the total deaths. The reason for this is that more and more people are living to sixty-five and beyond, because of improved social conditions. With the prevention of infant deaths by hygiene, immunizations, chemotherapy and antibiotics; with maternal mortality down; with major killing diseases, such as tuberculosis and diphtheria, virtually eliminated, and with the ravages of chronic diseases, like diabetes and pernicious anaemia controlled; the total result is that the average age of the population has been, and still is, increasing fast.

Medicine and the State

From Elizabethan times onwards responsibility for the care of old people was placed squarely on the shoulders of the younger members of the family. This was reaffirmed by the Poor Law Amendment Act of 1834. This law set up the Poor Law Commissioners with Edwin Chadwick as their secretary. Through its boards of guardians the commission gave relief to the poor in a way that was daunting enough to discourage as many people as possible from asking for it. Some relief was given to the aged under this Act; but it was made clear enough that poverty as such, especially in old age, was seen to be the result of negligence and therefore a disgrace. Outdoor relief, that is relief for the aged poor in their own homes, was given in some cases, but in general indoor relief was considered the ideal; that is to say relief given in infirmaries and institutions, which were generally run in such a way as to deter people from entering them. In Dickens's *Our Mutual Friend* we can read the opinion Mrs Betty Higden (the child-minder) held about the Poor House. 'Kill me sooner than take me there. . . . Do I never read how they are put off, put off, put off—how they are grudged, grudged, grudged the shelter, or the doctor, or the drop of physic or the bite of food? . . . Then I say I hope . . . I'll die without that disgrace.'

There were, on the other hand, some endowed charitable institutions, such as the Hospital of St Cross near Winchester, which offered pleasant asylum for the few aged poor that they were able to take in. This particular hospital dates back to the twelfth century, but there are more than forty other religious organizations still in existence that are four or five centuries old. In addition to these, some hundreds more endowed homes were founded in the nineteenth century and others still in the present century. In these early days the number of old people was comparatively small, although a very high proportion of them lived in extreme poverty, as was convincingly shown by Charles Booth in his ten volumes on *The Life and Labour of the People of London 1891–1897*. The urgent call for reform which arose about that time produced at length a Royal Commission on the Poor Law, which sat for four years without producing any improvement so far as the aged poor were concerned and they continued to depend on charitable institutions, or on poor-law relief as a last resort.

A beginning was made when Old Age Pensions were introduced in 1908. At first the pension was only 5 shillings a week, but in 1919 it was doubled. A means test was applied to all applicants. Later a scheme of contributory pensions was started. This was in effect a system of paying-in regular small sums during a man's working days to provide for a pension in old age.

In 1940 a big step forward was taken by the provision of extra pensions to be paid through the National Assistance Board. This *National* Assistance scheme must be distinguished from the hated *Public* Assistance. The former was to be administered by a central, as opposed to a local authority. In this way it was supposed that the disgrace attaching to *public* assistance would be avoided. This change in administration seemed to achieve its object, for the numbers of people receiving these extra pensions through the National Assistance scheme rose very rapidly in comparison with those who had been paid public assistance before.

Special houses for old people began to be built by local authorities shortly before the Second World War, but in small numbers only; and the programme, inadequate though it was in the first place, was totally interrupted by the war. After the war the project went ahead and an ever-increasing number of old people's houses and bungalows is being built.

A scheme for universal retirement pensions (a euphemism for old age pensions) was started under the National Insurance Act of 1946. This enabled men over sixty-five and women over sixty years of age to draw 26s. per week. This sum has been increased from time to time—accompanied, it may be said, by ever-mounting weekly payments exacted from the workers and their employers through the insurance stamps—and now[1] stands at 90s. There is no means test in this connexion, but the scheme works equitably, because substantial amounts of money are recovered by the State in the form of income tax and surtax from the richer among the pensioners.

The National Health Service Act of 1946, which set up the welfare state, also gave powers to local authorities to provide domestic help (usually called 'home help') where needed in cases of illness, confinement or where there are children who cannot be

[1] October 1967.

properly cared for and where there are old people at home unable to fend for themselves. This service can be charged for where the people are in a position to pay, but it can be provided free to those of very slender means. Domestic helps can do cooking for the elderly, clean their homes, do washing and mending and even shopping. They can also help with young children. This service is of necessity fairly costly, but it really pays its way because it is a preventive service, in that it helps to keep the old people from falling sick and having to be expensively treated in hospital.

At the same time home nurses began to be employed by local authorities. The Government provided a short course of training, lasting for three or four months, in preparing already trained hospital nurses for these special duties. This service has been much expanded recently, partly because patients are now often discharged from hospital before their treatment is complete and partly because of the ever-increasing numbers of elderly people. About half of all the home nurses' time is spent in nursing the aged or chronic sick. By 1964 there were over 10,000 such nurses in England and Wales.

Local authorities were permitted to give financial help to certain voluntary organizations which carried out home visits and provided home meals. Among such organizations we may mention particularly the Women's Royal Voluntary Service and the British Red Cross Society, which have done and are doing invaluable work.

Under the National Assistance Act local authorities were able to set up old people's homes which offered residential accommodation for the aged and infirm in need of care. There are now, in addition to many hundreds of old people's homes, numbers of voluntary institutions. Under the same Act these have to be registered with the local authority.

Apart from care, the question of treatment of the old had to be considered, both at home and in hospital. The general practitioner service and the home nurses provide for the first. Under the welfare state the institutional services which had been administered by the poor law were taken over by the regional hospital boards. All the old infirmaries—mostly hospitals attached to workhouses—were transferred and they were also renamed, in an attempt to remove any poor-law stigma which might be still attaching to them. The doctors in charge became properly paid instead of receiving mere pittances and specialists in the treatment of the aged were appointed to supervise these 'geriatric units' as they became known. The old infirmaries still exist, so far as the buildings are concerned, but the emphasis is now upon treatment and rehabilitation of the patients rather than merely the care of the aged.

A large fraction of the elderly suffer not only from physical ill-health, but also from mental illness and social distress. This makes it necessary that the health service for the old should be widespread in its scope. The hospital service by itself could not possibly cope with all the demands; so that the solution of the problem lies in well organized services designed to keep the old person in his own home whenever it is possible.

There is certainly a need for short-stay geriatric units where the patient's condition, mental as well as physical, can be thoroughly assessed and treatment begun. The units should be departments of general hospitals, so that all modern improvements in diagnosis and treatment can be brought to bear. To have such units attached to general or teaching hospitals is doubly important, in that they would be available to education for nurses and social workers as well as for students and doctors.

PART IV. EPILOGUE

Problems of today and the outlook for the future

EPILOGUE

THE OUTSTANDING PROBLEMS OF TODAY
AND THE OUTLOOK FOR THE FUTURE

W E have followed the course of many of the more important medical discoveries from the first half of the nineteenth century up to the present time. Any attempt to
predict the purely medical developments of the future would be
extremely rash: how rash, may be seen from the timid prophecies
put forward in the first edition of this book more than thirty years
ago. At that time no one foresaw the immense success of the new
chemotherapeutic agents, to be outdone in a few years by penicillin and other antibiotics. At the same time the clues were there,
had men been enlightened enough to follow them up. The first of
the sulphonamide drugs, prontosil, had already been launched in
1935 by Gerhard Domagk. Fleming's first demonstration of
penicillin at an international conference in 1936 had been largely
ignored. The electron microscope was born in 1931, so was still in
its infancy, though its future was assured.

Many of the other discoveries could hardly have been foretold
in detail. The astonishing success of insecticides (D.D.T. in
particular) in eliminating louse-borne diseases during the Second
World War, the advent of the new antituberculous drugs, the
immense development of hormones, both natural and synthetic,
the invention of effective anti-poliomyelitis vaccines, the use of
radioisotopes, the wonders of open chest and heart surgery—all
these were in the dim future and were nowhere clearly fore-
shadowed.

Infectious Diseases

The future of medicine must clearly lie in prevention. That at
least is the ideal. New cures will doubtless come from the extension

of existing methods—new chemotherapeutic drugs, antibiotics and so forth—; but in dealing with infectious disease it must be made clear from the outset that no *treatment* of a disease by itself has ever succeeded in eliminating infection altogether. It may be that in tuberculosis we could come close to this, but for the most part the future must concern itself with preventive medicine as opposed to treatment.

At present effective immunization is available against smallpox, yellow fever, diphtheria, whooping-cough, poliomyelitis, measles, tuberculosis and many forms of influenza. Two diseases for which active immunization is still sadly lacking are syphilis and gonorrhoea.

In spite of great improvements in health in many parts of the world, some communicable diseases remain unconquered and some others are actually becoming more widespread. The Report of the World Health Organization[1] states that since 1961 cholera has reappeared in countries which had been free of it for years. The El Tor variety appeared in the South Western Pacific regions and south-east Asia and began to spread to Africa and eastern Europe. In 1965 Iran was affected and Iraq in 1966. These outbreaks caused very considerable alarm in these countries and their neighbours. The old threat is a very real one, though modern treatment has greatly reduced the mortality.

Plague too has recently spread in South East Asia and South America. Insect-borne diseases are far from being under control despite energetic campaigns. This is particularly serious with the virus diseases carried by *Aëdes aegypti*, the mosquito responsible for the spread of yellow fever and dengue. The magnitude of the public health problems involved in keeping infectious disease under control is such that it seems almost beyond the capacity of the World Health or any other Organization. This is not surprising when it is realized that in Africa, in 1965, there were at least fourteen countries which had no medical school at all. The control of malaria, though theoretically quite possible, has failed in many parts of the world. That it is not under control is due not to lack of knowledge, but to deficiency of resources.

Leprosy is another communicable disease which is far from

[1] Geneva, 1965.

320

being under control. One of the difficulties in studying this complaint had been that no laboratory animal had been found susceptible. The recent discovery that mice can be infected, by special methods which overcome their natural immunity, has given fresh hope that progress will be made. With regard to the prevention of leprosy, the fact that leprosy and tubercle bacilli seem to be closely related prompted the use of B.C.G. as a protective measure. This is being tried in Uganda and, though it is too early to judge of the results, it seems likely that a substantial reduction in the incidence of leprosy will be secured.

The common cold has long demanded attention. From the 1920's onwards anti-catarrhal vaccines were tried. These usually contained a mixture of the pneumococcus, influenza bacillus, streptococcus, staphylococcus, micrococcus catarrhalis and Friedlander's bacillus. Unfortunately the results were disappointing. It gradually became clear that the actual cause was in the nature of a virus. In the last twenty years an immense amount of work has been done, particularly at the Medical Research Council's Common Cold Research Unit at Salisbury in Wiltshire. This unit began work in 1946 and most of its experiments have had to be done on human volunteers, because none of the common laboratory animals are susceptible. It appears that there are numerous distinct viruses—about ninety, according to a recent count—each of which may have several different strains; so that effective immunization against the common cold, though theoretically possible, may prove very difficult to achieve. One added difficulty is that cold viruses, unlike bacteria, do not invade the blood-stream, so that it is required to produce antibodies in high concentration actually in the secretions of the nose and throat. On the other hand there are grounds for encouragement. These different cold viruses tend to attack people one at a time, so that nasal material from a volunteer with a cold often contains one virus only. Furthermore there are reasons for believing that infection with one virus tends to suppress infection by another. Even so, the protection which one cold gives against a second is obviously not long-lasting: so that any effective immunizing substance would have to be given repeatedly.

In the last two years improved and simplified electron-microscopy techniques have produced finely differentiated photographs which show so much detail that it is possible to identify viruses from their photographs in a matter of five minutes. The electron microscope has now become a standard diagnostic tool.

In some diseases where active immunization is not available prevention can be achieved by chemical means. In particular malaria can be suppressed indefinitely by daily doses of suitable drugs, such as pyrimethamine or proguanil.

In the treatment of infectious diseases, the chemotherapeutic and antibiotic drugs, though enormously successful in most cases, have not fulfilled their early promise of wiping out epidemic diseases. The fact is that certain bacteria have contrived to outwit the doctor by producing strains that are resistant to the drugs. These resistant forms of organism are causing widespread concern in tuberculosis, malaria and venereal disease. Newer drugs and synthetic anti-biotics are of great help here: but it seems likely that the problems of resistance will continue to demand an unending supply of new drugs.

Effective chemotherapy against virus diseases is badly needed. Rapid progress is already being made in connexion with smallpox, cow-pox and herpes. It seems likely that in smallpox the new drugs will be used for prevention rather than treatment. For example, treatment with methisazone can be used to give temporary protection to unvaccinated people recently in contact with small-pox, until such time as they can be permanently protected by vac-cination. In this connexion it should be noted that a very high proportion of children and adults are not vaccinated today, so that if virulent smallpox breaks out anew in these islands (as well it may, with rapid modern travel), it will find many of us unarmed, and these will pay the penalty.

There are many other problems yet to be faced. Some of these are purely medical, others need legislation, while others still will require the close co-operation of medicine and the law.

The Main Causes of Sickness and Death

In spite of many successes, over which there is much cause for rejoicing, people continue to fall sick and to die. It is true that in this country death-rates are down, with some of the chief infectious diseases largely eliminated and many chronic conditions kept under control. It is true that the Welfare State has brought higher wages, fewer working hours, better houses and so-called social security, with free medical treatment for all. Nevertheless, in spite of all this, the doctors' waiting-rooms are crowded, the hospital waiting-lists grow longer and the drug bills mount ever higher. In short, the number of the sick is greater than ever. This is largely from the stresses and strains caused by the pace of modern life. It is probable that something like a quarter of all illnesses treated are the result of stress. This is not to say that they are all 'mental' cases. Indeed it is quite certain that stress can bring about many physical illnesses: in particular, high blood-pressure, duodenal ulcer, asthma, eczema, some forms of colitis and rheumatism. There is no doubt that the prevention of stress is one of the most pressing medico-social problems of the age.

As to deaths, in 1930 in England and Wales, out of a population of nearly forty millions, 455,427 died, giving a crude death-rate of 11·4 per thousand living. In 1966 the total population was over forty-eight millions and there were 563,624 deaths, with a crude death-rate of 11·7 per thousand. At first sight this would seem to show some deterioration, but when the figures are adjusted to show the Standard Mortality Ratio (a better guide) there has been a considerable improvement. The death-rate was nearly double a hundred years ago.

The main causes of death thirty years ago were, in order of numerical importance, arteriosclerotic and other heart disease, cancer, diseases of the respiratory system (including pneumonia) and tuberculosis. The same order of importance obtains today with the important exception of tuberculosis which has dropped out of the list of major killing diseases.

Heart Disease

Heart disease is due to a variety of causes and takes many forms; but there are certain diseases in which damage to the heart is especially likely to occur. Of these the most important are acute rheumatism (rheumatic fever) and chorea (popularly called St Vitus's dance), diseases quite apart from the conditions known as chronic rheumatism. Acute rheumatism for the most part attacks children of the relatively poorer classes: those of the well-to-do suffer proportionately much less. The earlier in life the disease occurs, the worse the heart is crippled. A very large proportion of all heart-disease is primarily rheumatic. The number of people dying of chronic rheumatic heart disease has not greatly changed in the last decade; but the deaths from rheumatic fever itself have been more than halved. This is almost certainly an indication of better social conditions in general and improved housing in particular.

Degeneration of the heart and arteries in middle and old age contributes to the high mortality. The increased pace of modern living may well be a contributory cause. The death-rate from arteriosclerosis and heart disease in the developed countries is highest in the United States: next comes the United Kingdom; whereas in France and in Japan the standardized death-rates from these causes are less than one-third as great.

Cancer

The second commonest cause of death is cancer. Deaths from all forms of malignant disease have been rising steadily ever since reliable figures have been available. In 1933 over sixty thousand people died in England and Wales from these causes. By 1965 the figure was 106,338 and in 1966 there were 108,158 deaths. More than one-third of the increase between 1965 and 1966 was due to lung cancer. The actual numbers of such deaths are much swollen by the alterations in the age distribution of the population; but, when due allowance has been made for this, the increase in cancer is very large indeed.

Years ago it was noted that mortality was highest in London and the County Boroughs and lowest in the rural districts, so that evidently the conditions of living must play some part in the causation. The actual cause of most types of cancer is not known, so that attempts at prevention cannot be scientifically planned. The causes must be environmental or endogenous, or a combination of both. A large proportion of cancer arises in the lungs, the digestive tract, the urinary tract and the uterus. All these organs have one thing in common, namely they have surfaces in contact with the outside world. As a result they are subject to repeated damage: so it seems very likely that the cause of such cancers will be found in external factors. Indeed in lung cancer this is almost certainly the precipitating cause in most cases.

In Great Britain the deaths from cancer of the respiratory system (trachea, bronchi and lungs) have been mounting year by year. In 1946 the deaths from this cause were 8,000, whereas in 1966 they numbered 27,025. The evidence that much of this is directly related to cigarette-smoking is largely statistical, but it is overwhelming. To quote but one example, many doctors in this country have stopped smoking altogether and it is very noteworthy that doctors form the only occupational group among which the incidence of lung cancer has declined in the last ten years. Here at least is one form of cancer which could be largely prevented. Unfortunately there are enormous vested interests in the sale of tobacco, the largest being held by the Treasury. The actual amounts of tobacco sold as cigarettes are quite staggering. In 1966 223·5 million pounds avoirdupoids were sold. This is less than in the years 1961–4, but is still much higher than it was in 1950.[1]

There is also good evidence that a proportion of lung cancer may be due to atmospheric pollution, apart from any question of cigarette-smoking. There is certainly a good case for reducing the pollution caused by industry as well as that coming from domestic chimneys.

Other forms of cancer can be prevented by careful attention to working conditions in factories. For example it was suspected some seventy years ago in Germany that workers in aniline dye factories were liable to develop cancer of the bladder, although this was not confirmed until forty years later. It was found that aniline itself was not the cancer-producing agent, but that other chemicals associated with the industry were responsible. Workers in this industry developed cancer of the bladder between ten and a hundred times more frequently than the general population of the country. With the co-operation of the industry the problem is now well under control.

[1] Ministry of Health, *On the State of the Public Health*, London, 1967, p. 84.

It is not impossible that stomach cancer may be caused by chemicals added to food to 'improve' its appearance, taste or keeping qualities. Certainly many foods have artificial colouring matters added to them, and there is always the possibility that some of these substances, eaten in quantity over very long periods, may cause cancer. The difficulty here is that experts are divided in their assessment of the danger. Moreover the actual effect of such damage may not become apparent for ten or twenty years and so it is difficult to pin down the true cause. Certain chemicals have been prohibited altogether, but there is not enough evidence to ban all colouring matters, though it is evidently a good working rule to advise that the less chemicals added to food the better.

As to the treatment of cancer, the most notable advance lies with early diagnosis. It is now generally agreed that the early diagnosis of cancer of the neck (cervix) of the uterus by microscopic examination of 'smears' taken from the cervix is a sound method. A nation-wide diagnostic service has been advocated, aiming in the first instance at 'screening' all women over thirty-five years of age at five-yearly intervals. The chief difficulty is the shortage of highly skilled pathologists. None the less good progress is being made and by the end of 1966 there were 306 such pathologists, fully trained in this specialized technique and 545 laboratory technicians. The number of specimens examined per month rose from 38,000 in 1964 to 109,000 by the end of 1966. It may be that lung cancer will also come to be diagnosed in its early stages by similar examination of the bronchial secretions: but this is not possible yet.

The actual treatment of cancer still lies in the hands of the surgeon, supplemented by radiotherapy with X-rays or gamma rays. In the latter connexion the use of radioisotopes has been rapidly developed. It is probable that certain cancers will be amenable to attack by administering specific radioisotopes having a particular affinity for cancer cells as opposed to normal tissues. When the new fundamental particles of matter began to be discovered by the physicists, it was hoped that some of them might be useful in treating deep-seated cancers: but of all these particles only the pi-meson, discovered in 1948, has shown any promise. The other particles are too few or too short-lived and therefore too ineffective.

Epilogue

Other methods of treating cancers have been by drugs. For example, success has been achieved with certain hormone preparations in controlling the spread of cancer of the prostate gland. So-called cyto-toxic drugs have been and are being tried. The idea is to find chemical substances more harmful to cancer cells than to normal tissues: but it must be admitted that success in this field has been limited. Some drugs have been used for treating childhood leukaemia (which has been classified as a cancer of the blood-forming organs). They have produced remissions and increased survival-rates, though they have not brought about any permanent cures.

Another line of attack has been the attempt to produce 'antibodies' to cancer cells, much as antibodies to bacteria and other foreign materials are engendered by the natural defence mechanism of the body. For example, tumours implanted in an animal may give rise to such antibodies. If these could be isolated by extracting the white blood-corpuscles of the animal, it should theoretically be possible to use the antibodies to treat cancer in human beings.

Many of these methods of treatment have succeeded in prolonging life: but it has been asked whether it is justifiable merely to extend the span of life when there is no hope of cure. This question has been expressly asked in connexion with childhood leukaemia. The answer is twofold. Firstly some of these children can be given a year or more of happy and healthy life in this way. Secondly it is quite justifiable to attempt to lengthen the child's life, simply in the hope that in a year or two a real cure may be found.

Mental Ill-health

When Macbeth asked his doctor 'Canst thou not minister to a mind diseased?' he presented a problem which looms large today. This has arisen mainly because of the failure of doctors to recognize its importance until comparatively recently. In the teaching hospitals thirty or forty years ago emphasis was placed on physical disease, almost to the exclusion of mental conditions. An average general text-book of medicine in the 1920's, containing about 1,000 pages in all, might devote as many as 16 to the 'psychoneuroses', and half of these would be taken up with hysteria.

Today the treatment and prevention of stress and anxiety have assumed gigantic proportions. Tens of millions of prescriptions are issued every year for states of anxiety and tension. Tranquillizers, sedatives and depressants are dispensed in huge quantities in private practice and in hundreds of general and mental hospitals and homes. It has been estimated that nearly half of Britain's hospital beds are occupied by people with mental trouble. At the same time only about one-tenth of the doctors employed in the hospital service are specialists in psychiatry. Evidently there is need for action to induce more medical students and young doctors to specialize in psychiatry if this unbalanced state of affairs is to be put right. Quite recently it was asserted by Sir Geoffrey Vickers to the Mental Health Research Fund that even today the time allotted to psychology and sociology in a medical student's pre-clinical studies varies from ninety hours to none.[1]

Rheumatism

Apart from the main causes of death, there are many ailments which produce much suffering and economic loss, but which many think are of secondary importance just because they do not kill. The most widespread and intractable of all is the condition generally called chronic rheumatism. This comprises a large group of diseases, which are probably quite distinct entities, but which have one thing in common, namely painful joints: though among 'rheumatic' conditions are also included painful conditions not directly associated with joints, such as sciatica and lumbago—often called fibrositis.

In the last thirty years tremendous efforts have been made to control rheumatism in all its forms. Research was greatly stimulated by the Empire Rheumatism Council, which was founded in 1935. The first specialized rheumatism department in a general hospital opened in 1938 at the West London Hospital, with four beds and some laboratory space.

The movement was hampered by the outbreak of war, but was resumed when peace returned. In 1961 the Empire Rheumatism Council changed its name to the Arthritis and Rheumatism

[1] *The Times*, November 8th, 1967.

Epilogue

Council and today it is the main support of rheumatic research. It is a voluntary body and not state-aided. In 1966 the Kennedy Institute of Rheumatology was opened in London, with five sets of laboratories and a clinical research division. Research has contributed much to our knowledge about this subject—mainly in biochemistry, immunity studies and biophysics—but none the less the cause remains unknown. There is no sure preventive or certain cure.

In the treatment of rheumatism precise diagnosis is of the utmost importance, because there are some fifty different diseases involved. There is no doubt that this precision in diagnosis has greatly advanced in recent years.

The commonest of all rheumatic conditions is rheumatoid arthritis, from which at least a million and a half persons are suffering in this country today. In treatment, rest and planned courses of exercise and physiotherapy are of great service. Numerous drugs have been tried, from aspirin onwards. Gold treatment was found to be of considerable value, but had corresponding disadvantages. The most powerful of all anti-rheumatic drugs are the cortico-steroids and, when first introduced, they were given in large doses and produced dramatic results: but unfortunately serious complications ensued, so that the new 'wonder drug' did not fulfil its early promise. Cortico-steroids are still used and are very helpful when given in small doses over long periods in severe cases of rheumatoid arthritis.

Much can be done to allay the worst pains of rheumatism and to restore the crippled joints in some degree: but how much remains to be done can be judged from the fact that, in this country, about thirty million working days are lost every year through this disease alone. It is clear that this unsolved problem is one of national importance.

Pure Air

Respiratory diseases play a large part in the sickness-rates in this country. Much is curable. Pneumonia and acute bronchitis yield to antibiotics: but we are left with thousands of chronic bronchitics, who have to be kept alive for years with intermittent treatment.

How much of this chronic respiratory disease is preventable? Much is due to the climate in which we have to live, but a big factor may be the quality of the air we are compelled to breathe.

In spite of much legislation and effort the problem of air pollution is still very much with us. While much improved so far as coal is concerned, the situation is getting worse in some other respects. None the less much pollution still comes from the burning of coal and oil, in industry, domestic fires and in petrol and diesel engines. Britain consumes about 200,000,000 tons of coal and 25,000,000 tons of oil per year and this pours into the atmosphere a million tons of dust and grit, two million tons of smoke and more than five million tons of sulphur dioxide.[1]

In some other parts of the world the situation is as bad, if not worse. New York suffers badly from a suffocating and sometimes a killing atmosphere. It has this extreme pollution in spite of its natural advantages, situated as it is on a wide river and open to the winds. The grass and the trees wilt under the atmospheric poisons and the human population suffers accordingly from respiratory affections. The city itself (to say nothing of the near-by industrial areas in New Jersey) spouts some 600,000 tons of sulphur (mostly as sulphur dioxide) each year into the air and, under conditions of an inverted temperature gradient, and because of the obstruction offered to the wind by the sky-scrapers, these poisons often linger in the city air. In 1966 New York had an air-pollution emergency lasting seven days, when, because of the high sulphur content of the air, it was found necessary to shut off municipal and private rubbish burners, to restrict the movement of cars and to order the local power stations to burn gas in place of coal or oil.

Another serious menace is carbon monoxide, which is present in considerable quantities in the exhaust gases of cars. The black smoke from imperfectly tuned diesel engines excites indignation, but it is quite likely that the invisible gases from car exhausts are a much greater danger. Carbon monoxide is fatal in high concentrations and in smaller doses it fixes some of the haemoglobin of the blood and so diminishes its oxygen-carrying capacity, leading to incoherent thought. How dangerous it can be in the proportions now present in town air is uncertain, but New York treats a con-

[1] Mellanby, K., *Pesticides and Pollution*, London, 1967, p. 33.

centration of 10 parts per million as an emergency. The situation is even worse in Tokyo where traffic congestion has caused a concentration of 50 parts per million. Los Angeles, with practically no industrial pollution, but with an enormous number of cars, has a special problem of its own. The bright sunshine acts chemically on the unburnt hydrocarbon from car fumes to produce a highly irritant chemical smog.

Many people seem to think that it is only necessary to fit a little black box to a car exhaust to make it safe, but the matter is not as simple as that. None the less in the United States stringent regulations are to come into force in 1968 limiting the discharge of carbon monoxide and unburnt hydrocarbons discharged from petrol engines. Even with these precautions there is still the danger from the lead compounds added to petrol as an anti-knock factor. This is certainly very widespread. Lead iodide, thought to be from these additions to petrol, has been found as far away from towns as the arctic regions.

In this country the Clean Air Act of 1956 has done much towards clearing the air of smoke, but the sulphur dioxide situation becomes worse. Where smokeless zones are enforced there is a switch to oil, which gives no smoke but plenty of sulphur which it is difficult to remove from the gases discharged into the air. In big power stations it can be done, but at a very high cost. The most practical way of limiting the concentration of sulphur dioxide is to have higher chimneys, so that the gas is well diluted before it descends on the towns. When this provision has been made in factories, there still remains the large quantity of sulphur dioxide produced by the increasing number of buildings burning oil for heating purposes.

There is no doubt that air pollution causes a great deal of respiratory disease, especially among the new-born and elderly. There is certainly a connexion between pollution and chronic bronchitis and probably lung cancer as well. As we have seen, the London fog of 1952 caused or at any rate hastened the deaths of 4,000 people. Following the indignation and interest aroused by this, the Medical Research Council founded its Air Pollution Unit in 1955 and a great number of measurements of pollution and physiological investigations have been carried out. Unfortunately, though there is no doubt that patients with chronic bronchitis are very seriously affected by dirty air, no direct proof is yet forthcoming that either smoke or sulphur in the concentrations that are found in London is the actual cause. It seems very likely: but, until it is proved, it seems hardly reasonable to spend millions of pounds in removing substances whose harmful effects are still in doubt.

Finally there is the grave problem of the pollution of the air from radioactive material and doubtless the medical officer of health of the future is going to find much of his time occupied with this.

Dental Caries

With the newer knowledge about nutrition, particularly about the part played by vitamin D in the formation of healthy teeth, it could have been hoped that dental caries would have diminished or even become a thing of the past. Far from this, dental decay in children is now commoner than it has ever been, and it has certainly increased since the end of the Second World War. The figures are most disheartening. Eighty-four per cent of the children entering school at five years have decayed teeth. It has been estimated that four tons of rotten teeth are removed every year from the children of England and Wales.

The development of the milk teeth depends on the diet of the mother during pregnancy and the child in early life. In this country these diets ought to be adequate in the light of modern knowledge, so that there must be some other cause for the children's bad teeth. There has been much controversy over the origins of dental caries. It is widely believed to be due to acids in the mouth, produced by the action of bacteria on carbohydrates. To cause decay the acids must act upon the teeth for an appreciable time. It therefore follows that there must be faulty eating habits and ill-cleaned teeth. Some classical experiments conducted at Vipeholm in Sweden clearly showed that the total amount of carbohydrate eaten bore no relation to the amount of dental caries that developed. What mattered was *when* the carbohydrate was eaten. The children who ate sugar between meals, particularly in the form of sticky sweets, had far more tooth decay than those who ate the same amount of sugar with their meals. Once again eating between meals has fallen into disrepute. These findings fit in well with the alarming increase in dental caries in this country when the war came to an end. Sweets, for so long severely rationed, became once more available to children in quantity and at all times of day.

There is no reasonable doubt that fluorides can prevent caries by producing resistant teeth. Any deficiency of fluoride in the diet could be made good universally by the addition to fluoride to water supplies. This is the official policy of the Ministry of Health, the British Medical Association and the British Dental Association. Yet at the present time only a small minority of local authorities have undertaken to put fluoride in their water. By the end of 1966 only 112 authorities had voted in favour of this measure. There has been a great deal of well-meant opposition to fluoridation, based largely on muddled-thinking about interference with the liberty of the subject and the undesirability of what has been stigmatized as 'mass medication'. If the subject is considered dispassionately it will be found that fluoridation is not a new and untried experiment, because in many parts of the world water containing fluorides has been drunk for centuries. Moreover in the United States some 58 million people are drinking water containing fluoride with nothing but good results. All the available information about fluoridation goes to show that probably no other single act in the whole of preventive medicine could achieve so effective a result with complete safety. Yet with all that is known about the appalling condition of the children's teeth, we still await any widespread action to put this remedy into effect.

Congenital Disease

There are many thousands of persons alive in this country today who have suffered all their lives from ailments varying from slight physical or mental disability to complete crippling blindness or idiocy. Many of these are cases of preventable congenital disease.

The number of registered blind persons in this country rose from 25,840 in 1919 to 62,458 by 1932. Much of this blindness dated from birth or the first year of life. One of the main causes used to be *ophthalmia neontorum*, generally due to gonorrhoea. This used to account for one quarter of all blindness in children, but it is now almost completely under control in the developed countries. Similarly, in 1930, congenital syphilis was the cause of 12 per cent of blindness, but now the figure is less than 0·5 per cent. These facts are a great tribute to the efficiency of the venereal disease service, but with the recent increases in the incidence of such diseases there is no room for complacency and the supreme importance of treatment for pregnant women cannot be over-emphasized.

With these forms of blindness under control there are still others that can be prevented by appropriate action. In 1941 Norman Gregg discovered that German measles (rubella) in a pregnant woman could lead to physical deformity in her child. He reported on seventy-eight babies blind as a result of cataract (and many of them had serious congenital heart defects as well). All the mothers had suffered from German measles—an otherwise quite harmless disease—in the early months of pregnancy. This discovery led to the development of an anti-rubella serum for expectant mothers who come into contact with German measles.

When all these forms of blindness have been prevented, there will still be the cases of congenital defects due to heredity. People who are blind from this cause ought on no account to procreate children, for there is no doubt that certain gross defects of the eye are purely hereditary. The mischief done by the marriage of one blind person may be immense. One pedigree[1] of a man with aniridia (absence of the iris, or coloured part of the eye) showed that in three generations he was directly responsible for no less than 113 blind persons out of a total of 118 descendants. This, of course, is an exceptional case, but the danger of hereditary blindness is very real.

There are many other hereditary malformations, not only of the body, but also of the mind. The only sound method of prevention is by segregating individuals who are mentally defective. The numbers are huge and the cost of following this policy in its entirety would be prohibitive. Consequently many of the higher grades of mental defectives are perfectly free to procreate indefi-

[1] Risley pedigree (1915): but the authenticity of this has been called in question.

nitely. Birth control, compulsory sterilization of defectives and *proved* carriers of mental defect, legalized abortion in some cases—prohibition of marriage and so forth—have all been suggested as means of prevention. It should be added, however, that many mentally defective children are engendered by seemingly normal parents, so that the restrictive measures mentioned would probably have little effect in reducing the numbers.

Iatrogenic Disease

Iatrogenic is a word which has been coined to describe disease produced by the physician. It derives from two Greek roots, *iātrós* physician and *gennân* to produce (via the French gène). Unfortunately there seem to be a growing number of these illnesses brought about by treatment.

By far the commonest of the iatrogenic diseases is cow-pox, a comparatively harmless condition which may follow vaccination. In England and Wales between 1951 and 1960 there were some 5 million cases, but they were for the most part mild and without complications. In the past other diseases have been transmitted by such procedures as blood transfusion and vaccination. Blood donors have to be strictly 'screened' to guard against the possibility of passing on diseases—syphilis or malaria for example—to the recipient.

There are a large number of diseases which have been caused by modern powerful chemotherapeutic substances, and some reports about the damage that is being done are quite frightening. In one American University hospital the recovery of one patient out of five is said to have been complicated by untoward effects produced by the treatment.[1] Most of these troubles are due to the frankly toxic action of the drugs—euphemistically described by the makers as 'side-effects'. These are often damaging and sometimes disastrous. For example, fatal anaemia has followed the over-prolonged administration of the antibiotic chloramphenicol.

Perhaps the most lamentable occurrence of all was the thalidomide disaster which took place within the last decade. A large number of children were born with gross multiple deformities,

[1] Weatherall, M., *British Medical Journal*, 1965, I, p. 1174.

amounting in many cases to absent or incompletely developed arms and legs. The cause was traced to this drug, thalidomide, which had been thought to be a safe and reliable soporific and which had been given to the mothers during pregnancy. This horrible event made it plain that new drugs were being put on the market without adequate testing of their effect in every possible circumstance in which they might come to be used.

The Ageing Population

One of the most serious difficulties that this country has to face is that of the ageing population. If the present trend continues, in about ten years' time about 8,000,000 of our total population will be over sixty-five years of age. Are we prepared for this? The answer is certainly 'No'. On the other hand we have to admit that prophecies about future statistics have frequently been belied by events. Thus in 1934 Sir Josiah Stamp wrote, 'We are now on the eve of the greatest event in the population history of this country, for we reach our maximum population in two or three years, and thereafter a gradual decline is anticipated, with some far-reaching changes in age distribution'. Figures for the expected decrease in the population were based on the number of women of child bearing age and the current fertility-rates. The changes in the age distribution have undoubtedly come about: but, so far from declining, the total population of the United Kingdom and Republic of Ireland has shown an increase in every year (except 1941) since 1934. In that year it was 48·7 millions and in 1965 54·4 millions. At present, though the births still exceed the deaths, this excess is getting smaller. It is probable that the downward trend of the birth-rate, which began in 1965, is due to the use of oral contraceptives.

The net result of the saving of life by the elimination of disease, together with the falling birth-rate, must be that the average age of the population will continue to increase. How far this process will be allowed to continue must be for the rising generation to decide. It is only too plain that if the present progress over the control of disease goes on, the developed countries will gradually become nations composed largely of old men and women in their dotage, being kept alive by large numbers of doctors, nurses, technicians and machines, all of which could be better employed in attending to the needs of the younger and healthier members of the community. This, the logical conclusion of the successful pursuit of medicine, is the doctors' dilemma of the immediate future. Is the object of medicine to keep people alive as long as possible? If not, at what point do we deliberately decide to let them die?

Conclusion

The last hundred years have seen many successes. First and foremost they have brought us a workable system of preventive medicine. Secondly they have given us new methods of diagnosis and cures for many individual diseases and have shown us the paths along which we may hope to come to further victories. Thirdly they have brought a vast increase in knowledge based upon sound experimental work. Progress in the future must make use of many of these accumulated facts.

With all this to our credit, we should be rash to be over-jubilant. A note of warning must be struck. At the present time there is a grave disproportion between the amount of available knowledge and the relatively few methods of applying it. Medicine is in danger of being overwhelmed by unco-ordinated facts. There are many thousands of scientific periodicals of varying worth, many of them directly or indirectly medical, which are piling up an unwieldy mass of data. The pace of progress is so great that no busy doctor can hope to catch up with many branches of his subject. Daily medicine is becoming more complicated. It has been said that a science which is truly progressing tends to become more simple, not in the sense that it may be more easily understood by the non-technical inquirer, but in that it brings more and more facts under one comprehensive scheme. The latter kind of simplicity we cannot claim for medicine.

Wherein lies the remedy that shall save us from a traffic chaos when all the streets of thought are choked with facts? This is the chief question for the future to answer. None the less it is evident from the viewpoint of today that medicine is going to rely more and more upon machines. Automation in medicine is at hand.

The use of machines in medicine could be one answer to the world-wide shortage of doctors. Already automatic laboratories exist for carrying out biochemical and other investigations at a pace far beyond anything that trained men could achieve. For example there is a machine for grouping blood samples, which can label them at the rate of two specimens per minute. Another machine can do twelve different major chemical analyses of body-fluids at the rate of sixty samples an hour.

There is little doubt that computers will soon become part of the normal equipment of hospitals. They would be used to store and analyse accumulated data and to make diagnoses. Lord Cohen of Birkenhead, President of the General Medical Council, opening a symposium on automation in medicine, pointed out that when the blood-pressure machine—now a standard tool for every doctor—was introduced in 1880, the *British Medical Journal* remarked that 'by such methods we pauperize our senses and weaken our clinical acuity'. It was to be regretted that today automation often provoked a similar reaction among many clinicians. 'Medicine,' said Lord Cohen, 'must learn to accept these techniques, to use them and to master them.'[1]

As the horizon of knowledge spreads slowly in every direction from the centre, one individual can hope to master only an increasingly narrow sector of the whole. Specialism becomes inevitable and unity in medicine can therefore be achieved only by increasingly large teams of workers, backed by machines. Can we hope for some intellect, mechanical or human, which may integrate the scores of separate branches into a whole living tree? Hopefully let us make medicine speak the words which Robert Browning put into the mouth of the dying Paracelsus:

> '. . . . . If I stoop
> Into a dark tremendous sea of cloud,
> It is but for a time; I press God's lamp
> Close to my breast; its splendour, soon or late
> Will pierce the gloom: I shall emerge one day.
> You understand me? I have said enough?'

[1] *The Times*, November 14th, 1967.

BIBLIOGRAPHY

THE works contained in this list are mainly non-technical, the bibliography being intended for the use of non-medical readers who may wish for further information.

ABRAHAM, J. A., *Lettsom; His Life, Times, Friends and Descendants*, London, 1933.

AITKIN, D. M., *Hugh Owen Thomas—His Principles and Practice*, London, 1935.

BAAS, J. H., *Grundriss der Geschichte der Medizin und des Heilenden Stundes*, Stuttgart, 1876.

—— The same. *Outlines of the History of Medicine and the Medical Profession*. Translated by H. E. Handerson, New York, 1889.

BALDRY, P. E., *The Battle Against Bacteria*, Cambridge, 1965.

BALL, J. M., *The Sack-'em-up Men. An Account of the Rise and Fall of the Modern Resurrectionists*, Edinburgh and London, 1928.

BANTING, F. G., *The History of Insulin, Edinburgh M. J.*, 1929. 36: 1–18.

BARON, J., *The Life of Edward Jenner, M.D.*, London, 1827.

BATEMAN, T., *Reports on the Diseases of London*, London, 1819.

BECLERE, A., *The Work of Madame Curie*, Quarterly Review, 1935, CCLXIV, 22.

BELL, E. M., *Octavia Hill*, London, 1942.

BEST, C. H., Obituary of F. G. Banting, *Canada. M. A. J.*, 1941, 44: 327–8.

BIGELOW, H. J., *A History of the Discovery of Modern Anaesthesia (In A Century of American Medicine, 1776–1876)*, Philadelphia, 1876.

BOOTH, C., *Life and Labour of the People in London*, London, 1895–7. 10 volumes.

BRIDGES, R., *An Account of the Casualty Department, St Bartholomew's Hospital Reports*, 14: 167–82, 1878.

BRITISH MEDICAL ASSOCIATION, *Secret Remedies*, London, 1909.

—— *More Secret Remedies*, London, 1912.

BROCKINGTON, C. F., *The Health of the Community*, London, 1965.

—— *A Short History of Public Health*, London, 1965.

BROWN, L., *The Story of Clinical Pulmonary Tuberculosis*, Baltimore, 1941.

BROWN, P., *American Martyrs to Science through the Roentgen Rays*, Springfield, Illinois, 1936.

BROWNLEE, J., *An Investigation into the Epidemiology of Tuberculosis in Great Britain and Ireland*, London, 1918.

BUER, M. C., *Health, Wealth and Population in the Early Days of the Industrial Revolution*, London, 1926.

BULLOCH, W., *The History of Bacteriology*, Oxford, 1938.

BURTON, E. F. and KOHL, W. H., *The Electron Microscope*, New York, 1942.

BURTON, W., *An Account of the Life and Writings of Hermann Boerhaave*, London, 1743.

CARR-SAUNDERS, A. M. and WILSON, P. A., *The Professions,* Oxford, 1933.

CASTIGLIONI, A., *History of Tuberculosis*, New York, 1933.

CHEYNE, W. W., *Lister and His Achievements*, London, 1925.

CHRISTIAN, H. A., Tribute to Professor Folin, *Science*, 1935, 81: 37–8.

CLAY, R. M., *The Mediaeval Hospitals of England*, London, 1909.

COOK, E., *The Life of Florence Nightingale*, 2 vols., London, 1913 and 1914.

COOPER, B. B., *The Life of Sir Astley Cooper, Bart.*, 2 vols., London, 1843.

CREIGHTON, C., *A History of Epidemics in Britain from A.D. 664 to the Extinction of the Plague*, Cambridge, 1891.

CREIGHTON, C., *A History of Epidemics in Britain from the Extinction of the Plague to the Present Time,* Cambridge, 1894.

CURIE, E., *Madame Curie*, Paris, 1938.

CURIE, M., *Pierre Curie*, Paris, 1923.

DICKENS, C., *American Notes*, London, 1842.

DRUMMOND, J. C. and WILBRAHAM, A., *The Englishman's Food*, London, 1939.

ECKSTEIN, G., *Noguchi*, New York and London, 1931.

ERICHSEN, J. E., *On Hospitalism and the Causes of Death after Operation*, London, 1874.

ESDAILE, J., *Mesmerism in India*, London, 1846.

——*The Introduction of Mesmerism (with the Sanction of the Government) into the Public Hospitals of India*. Second Edition, London, 1856.

FARR, W., *Report on the Cholera Epidemic of 1866 in England*, London, 1868. Section on vital statistics in J. R. McCullough's *A Statistical Account of the British Empire*, London, 1837.

FINER, S. E., *Life and Times of Sir Edwin Chadwick*, London, 1952.

Bibliography

FISHBEIN, M., *The Medical Follies*, New York, 1925.

FLEXNER, S. and FLEXNER, J. T., *William Henry Welch and the Heroic Age of American Medicine*, New York, 1941.

FOSTER, M., *Claude Bernard*, London, 1899.

FOSTER, W. D., *A History of Parasitology*, Edinburgh and London, 1865.

GARRISON, F. H., *An Introduction to the History of Medicine*, Fourth Edition, Philadelphia and London, 1929.

—— *History of Pediatrics (Abt's Pediatrics,* Philadelphia, 1923, Vol. 1, pp. 290–322*).*

GLASSER, O., *Wilhelm Conrad Röntgen and the Early History of Roentgen Rays*, London, 1933.

GODLEE, R. J., *Lord Lister*, London, 1917.

GORDON, H. L., *Sir James Young Simpson and Chloroform*, London, 1897.

GORGAS, M. D. and HENDRIK, B. J., *William Crawford Gorgas, His Life and Work*, Philadelphia and New York, 1924.

GRAVES, R. J., *Studies in Physiology and Medicine*, London, 1863 (containing *The Life and Labours of Graves*).

GREENWOOD, M., *Epidemics and Crowd Diseases*, London, 1935.

GRISCOM, J. H., *The Sanitary Condition of the Labouring Population of New York*, New York, 1845.

GUY'S HOSPITAL REPORTS; Memoir of *Adrian Stokes*, London, 1928, lxxviii, 1–17.

HABERLING, W., *Johannes Müller, das Leben des rheinischen Naturforschers*, Leipsig, 1924.

HAEHL, R., *Samuel Hahnemann, His Life and Work*, 2 vols. Translated by M. L. Wheeler and W. H. R. Grundy, London, 1923.

HAMMOND, J. L. and B., *The Age of the Chartists*, London, 1930.

—— *Lord Shaftesbury*, London, 1923.

HEALTH OF TOWNS COMMISSION, *Report*, London, 1844.

—— *Second Report*, London, 1845.

HIRSCH, A., *Handbook of Geographical and Historical Pathology*. Translated by C. Creighton, 3 vols. London, 1883.

HOLMES, O. W., *Medical Essays, 1842–1882*, London, 1891.

HOWARD, J., *The State of the Prisons in England and Wales*, Warrington, 1777.

—— *An Account of the Principal Lazarettos in Europe*, Warrington, 1779.

IRVINE, K. N., *B.C.G. Vaccination in Theory and Practice*, Oxford, 1949.

KEITH, A., *Menders of the Maimed*, London, 1919.

KELLY, H. A., *Walter Reed and Yellow Fever*, New York, 1906.

KOREN, J., *The History of Statistics*, New York, 1918.

LAENNEC, R.-T.-H., *Traité de l'Auscultation Mediate et des Maladies des Poumons e du Coeur*, Paris, 1828 (containing *Notice sur la Vie et les Travaux de Laennec,* by A. L. J. Bayle).

LAMBERT, R., *Sir John Simon and English Social Administration,* London, 1963.

LAZARUS, A., *Paul Ehrlich*, Vienna, 1922.

LEWIS, R. A., *Edwin Chadwick and the Public Health Movement,* London, 1952.

LEWIS, T., *Willem Einthoven* (memoir), *British Medical Journal*, 1927, II, 664.

LITTLE, E. M. (compiled by), *History of the British Medical Association,* 1832–1932, London, 1932.

LONG, E. R., *A History of Pathology*, Baltimore, 1928.

McCULLUM, W. G., *William Stewart Halsted*, Baltimore, 1930.

MANSON-BAHR, P. H. and ALCOCK, A., *The Life and Work of Sir Patrick Manson,* London, 1927.

MEAD, R., *A Short Discourse Concerning Pestilential Contagion and the Methods to be used to Prevent it.* Fourth Edition, London, 1720.

MEADE, R. H., *A History of Thoracic Surgery*, Springfield, Illinois, 1961.

MEGROZ, R. L., *Ronald Ross, Discoverer and Creator*, London, 1931.

MELLANBY, K., *Pesticides and Pollution*, London, 1967.

MITCHELL, R. J. and LEYS, M. D. R., *A History of London Life*, London, 1958.

MUNK, W., *The Gold Headed Cane*, London, 1884 (Drs Radcliffe, Mead, Askew, Pitcairne, Baillie and others).

MYER, J. S., *The Life and Letters of Dr William Beaumont, including hitherto unpublished data concerning the case of Alexis St Martin*, St Louis, 1912.

NEUBERGER, M., *Essays in Medical History* (translated), New York, 1932.

—— *History of Medicine* (translated by E. Playfair), Vol. I, 1910; Vol. II, Part I, 1925, London and Oxford.

NEWMAN, G., *Health and Social Evolution* (Halley Stewart Lecture, 1930), London 1931.

—— *Interpreters of Nature. Essays*, London, 1927. (Contains chapters on Sydenham, Boerhaave, John Hunter, Keats, Pasteur and Osler.)

—— *The Rise of Preventive Medicine*, Oxford, 1932.

NEWSHOLME, A., *Medicine and the State*, London, 1932.

OSLER, W., *Oliver Wendell Holmes*, Bull. Johns Hopkins Hospital, 5; 85–8, Baltimore, 1894.

—— *The Evolution of Modern Medicine*, New Haven, 1921.

Bibliography

PACKARD, F. R., *History of Medicine in the United States,* 2 vols., New York, 1931.

PAGET, S., *Sir Victor Horsley,* London, 1919.

PAGET, S., *John Hunter, Man of Science and Surgeon (1728–1793),* London, 1897.

PALM, T. A., *The Geographical Distribution and Aetiology of Rickets. Practitioner,* 40: pp. 270–321, London, 1890.

PARISH, H. J., *A History of Immunization,* Edinburgh and London, 1965.

POOL, E. H., and McGOWAN, F. J., *Surgery at the New York Hospital One Hundred Years Ago,* New York, 1930.

POOR LAW COMMISSIONERS, *Sanitary Condition of the Labouring Population of Great Britain,* London, 1842.

POSNER C., *Rudolf Virchow,* Vienna, 1921.

POWER, D'A., *Eponyms—Spencer Wells Forceps. Brit. J. Surg.,* 14. 385–7, 1927.

PUTNAM, J. L., *Isotopes,* London, 1960.

RICHARDSON, B. W., *The Health of Nations. A Review of the Works of Edwin Chadwick,* 2 vols., London, 1887.

RIESMAN, D., *American Contributions to Nosography* (Shattuck Lecture) *New England J. Med.,* 1938, 219: 591–611.

ROLLESTON, H. D., *The Right Honorable Sir Thomas Clifford Allbutt, K.C.B.,* London, 1929.

ROWNTREE, B. S., *Poverty, A Study of Town Life,* London, 1901. *Poverty and Progress,* London, 1941.

SIGERIST, H. E., *Great Doctors. A Biographical History of Medicine.* Translated by Eden and Cedar Paul, London, 1933.

SIMON, J., *English Sanitary Institutions,* London, 1890.

SIMPSON, J. Y., *Anaesthesia, Hospitalism etc.,* Edinburgh, 1871. (Works of Sir James Y. Simpson, Vol. II.)

SINCLAIR, W. J., *Semmelweiss; His Life and Doctrine. A Chapter in the History of Medicine,* Manchester, 1909.

SINGER, C., *A Short History of Medicine,* Oxford, 1928.

SNOW, J., *On the Mode of Communication of the Cholera.* Second Edition, London, 1855.

SPENCER, H. R., *The History of British Midwifery,* London, 1927.

STRACHEY, L., *Eminent Victorians,* London, 1918 (contains an essay on Florence Nightingale).

TAYLOR, F. L., *Crawford W. Long and the Discovery of Ether Anesthesia,* New York, 1928.

TENON, M., *Mémoires sur les Hôpitaux de Paris,* Paris, 1788.

THACKRAH, C. T., *The Effects of the Principal Arts, Trades and Professions . . . . . ,* London, 1831.

A Hundred Years of Medicine

TOPLEY, W. W. and WILSON, G. S., *The Principles of Bacteriology*. Second Edition, Baltimore, 1936.

TILANUS, C. B., *Surgery a Hundred Years Ago*, London, 1925.

TILDEN, W. A., *Famous Chemists, the Men and their Work*, London, 1921.

TRUDEAU, E. L., *An Autobiography*, New York, 1916.

VALLERY-RADOT, R., *La Vie de Pasteur*, Paris, 1900.

WAKSMAN, S. A., *The Conquest of Tuberculosis*, London, 1965.

WALKER, M. E. M., *Pioneers of Public Health*, Edinburgh, 1930.

WATSON, F., *The Life of Sir Robert Jones*, London, 1934.

WALSH, J. J., *Makers of Modern Medicine*, New York, 1907 (contains essays on Morgagni, Auenbrugger, Jenner, Laennec, Müller, Schwann, Claude Bernard, Pasteur, Virchow and others).

WEBB, S. and WEBB, B., *English Prisons under Local Government*, London, 1922.

—— *English Poor Law History*, Part II, *The Last Hundred Years*, 2 vols., London, 1929.

WEBSTER, N., *A Brief History of Epidemics and Pestilential Diseases*, 2 vols., Hartford, Conn., 1799.

WILLIAMS, J. H., *A Century of Public Health in Britain, 1832-1929*, London, 1932.

WILSON, R. H., *The Beloved Physician, Sir James Mackenzie*, London, 1926.

WOODHAM-SMITH, C., *Florence Nightingale*, London, 1950.

WUNDERLICH, C. A., *On the Temperature in Disease*. Translated by W. B. Woodman, London, 1871.

ZIMMERMAN, L. M. and HOWELL, K. M., *History of Blood Transfusion*, Ann. Med. Hist. 4: 155, 1932.

INDEX

Index

Index

Index

Rheumatism, acute, 324
  chronic, 328–9
Rickets, 172–3, 304
Ricketts, H. T., 101, 114
Rickettsiae, 101, 114
Rocha Lima, H. da, 114
Röntgen, W. C., 156 *et seq.*
Ross, Ronald, 108
Round worms, 143
Roux, Pierre, 120
Rowntree, B. S., 260
Rowntree, Leonard, 261
Royal Army Medical Corps, 241
Royal College of Physicians, 53
  Surgeons, 53
Rubella, 334
Rubner, Max, 82
Ruge, Carl, 195
Rush, B., 307
Ruskin, John, 259
Russell, 'sea-water', 33, 136
Rutherford, E., 166

Sabin, Albert, B., 130
Saenger, Max, 202
St. Vitus's Dance, *see under* Chorea
Salk, Jonas, E., 129
Salvarsan, 131
Sanatorium, 289
Sanitary Commission, Royal, 257
Sanitary Inspectors, 268
Santorio, Santorio, 66
Sayre, L. A., 209
Scarlet fever, 51, 97
Schäfer, E. S., 149, 220
Schaudinn, Fritz, 131, 298
Schick test, 122
Schiff, Moritz, 147
Schimmelbusch, Carl, 178
Schindler, Rudolf, 197
Schistostomes, 141
Schleiden, M. J., 61
Schönlein, J. L., 28, 95
School meals, 277
School Medical Service, 276 *et seq.*,
  291
Schwann, Theodor, 61–62
Scurvy, 171–2
Scutari, 238 *et seq.*
Secretin, 149
Sellors, Sir Thomas Holmes, 233
Semmelweiss, Ignaz, 92–93, 201
Serum, immune, 120 *et seq.*
Shaftesbury, Anthony Ashley Cooper,
  7th Earl of, 250, 308
Shenstone, Norman, 229

Shakespeare, William, his father's
  insanitary behaviour, 247
Shiga, Kigoshi, 106
Shock, surgical, 180, 224
Silicosis, 287
Simon, Gustav, 206
Simon, Sir John, 252 *et seq.*
Simpson, Sir J. Y., 34, 72 *et seq.*, 200
Sims, Marion, 190
Skłowdowska, Marie, *see* Curie, Marie
Skoda, Josef, 28
Sleeping-sickness, 97, 111 *et seq.*
Smallpox, 45, 100, 117–18
Smellie, William, 55
Smith, Andrew, 239
Smoke nuisance, 304 *et seq.*
Snow, John, 104–5
Souttar, H., 231
Spiegel, E. A., 225
Spirochaete of relapsing fever, 114
  of Syphilis, 131
Stadfeldt, A. S., 201
Stahl, G. E., 21
Stamp, Sir Josiah, 336
Stanley, W. M., 99
Starling, E. H., 148
Steenbock, H., 170, 172
Stegomyia fasciata, 110, *see also under*
  Aëdes aegypti
Stilboestrol, 154
Stokes, Adrian, 110
Stokes, William, 27
Streptomycin, 134–5, 139, 176, 211
Sulphonamide drugs, 131–2
Suprarenal capsules, 146
Sydenham, Thomas, 19
Syme, James, 34
Syphilis, 97, 131, 297 *et seq.*
  congenital, 299
Szent-Györgyi, A., 172

Takaki, K., 169
Takamine, Jokichi, 149
Tape-worms, 142–3
Tarnier, Etienne, 202
Testosterone, 153
Tetanus, 122
Tetany, 153
Tetracycline, drugs, 135
Thackrah, C. T., 282
Thalidomide, 335–6
Thiamin, 171
Thiersch, Carl, 194
Thomas, H. O., 212
Thomson, Sir William, *see* Kelvin,
  Lord
Thoracic surgery, 226 *et seq.*

Thoracoplasty, 138
Thucydides, 117
Thudicum, J. L. W., 143, 189
Thyroid gland, 146 *et seq.* 192 *et seq.*
Thyroxine, 148, 192
Toison, J., 223
Travers, Benjamin, 180
Trench fever, 113, 115
Treves, Sir Frederick, 189
Tristan da Cunha, 173 *et seq.*
Trudeau, E. L., 136
Trypanosomes, 110
Tsetse-fly, 111–12
Tuberculosis, 105, 126 *et seq.*, 135 *et seq.*, 207, 230, 276, 289 *et seq.*
Tuke, W., 307
Typhoid fever, 124
Typhus, 45, 48, 114, *see also under* Gaol fever

Uranium, 163
Urine, chemical tests in, 69

Vaccination, *see under* Jenner, Edward
Acts 1840 and 1841, 248
Vaccines, 124 *et seq.*
Vasopressin, 150
Venereal disease, 275, 296 *et seq.*
Disease Act 1917, 301
Veronal, 76
Vesalius, Andreas, 18
Villemin, Jean, 137
Virchow, Rudolf, 62 *et seq.*
Virus, filterable, 98–99, 322
Vitamins, 169 *et seq.*, 304

Voit, Karl von, 82
Volkmann Richard von, 194

Waksman, Selman, 134
Waldeyer, Wilhelm, 194
Wassermann test, 125, 298
Water-supply, infection from, 104–5
Weese, H., 75
Weill-Hallé, B., 127
Welch, Thomas, 196
Wells, Horace, 71
Wells, Spencer, 179, 203
Wertheim, Ernest, 203
Whipple, George, 175
White Phosphorus Prohibition Act 1908, 286
Whooping-cough, 97
Wickham, L., 165
Williams, F. H., 137
Wöhler, Friedrich, 79
Women's Royal Voluntary Service, 315
Wood, Alexander, 182
Wren, Sir Christopher, 181
Wright, Sir Almroth, 124, 132
Wucheria bancroftii, 144
Wunderlich, K. A., 66
Wycis, H. T., 225

X-rays, 137, 156 *et seq.*, 184, 195, 212 *et seq.*, 326

Yellow fever, 100, 109–10, 129
Yersin, Alexandre 113, 120
Young, Hugh, 178